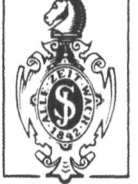

# Treatment in Clinical Medicine
Series Editor: John L. Reid

*Titles in the series already published:*

**Gastrointestinal Disease**
Edited by C.J.C. Roberts

**Rheumatic Disease**
Hilary A. Capell, T.J. Daymond and W. Carson Dick

**The Elderly**
W.J. MacLennan, A.N. Shepherd and I.H. Stevenson

**Cardiovascular Disease**
A. Ross Lorimer and W. Stewart Hillis

**Neurological Disorders**
David Parkes, Peter Jenner, David Rushton and David Marsden

*Forthcoming titles in the series:*

**Endocrine and Metabolic Disease**
Colin M. Feek and Christopher R.W. Edwards

**Hypertension**
B.N.C. Prichard and C.W.I. Owens

Anne E. Tattersfield · Martin W. McNicol

# Respiratory Disease

With 29 Figures

Springer-Verlag
London Berlin Heidelberg New York
Paris Tokyo

Anne E. Tattersfield, MD, FRCP
Professor of Respiratory Medicine, Respiratory Medicine Unit,
City Hospital, Hucknall Road, Nottingham NG5 1PB, England

Martin W. McNicol, MB, ChB, FRCP
Consultant Physician, Cardiothoracic Department, Central
Middlesex Hospital, Acton Lane, Park Royal, London NW10 7NS,
England

ISBN-13: 978-3-540-16209-4     e-ISBN-13:978-1-4471-3132-8
DOI: 10.1007/978-1-4471-3132-8

British Library Cataloguing in Publication Data
Tattersfield, A.E.
Respiratory disease. – (Treatment in clinical medicine).
1. Respiratory organs – Diseases
I. Title  II. McNicol, Martin W.  III. Series
616.2  RC731
ISBN-13:978-3-540-16209-4

Library of Congress Cataloging-in-Publication Data
Tattersfield, Anne E. (Anne Elizabeth), 1940–
Respiratory disease
(Treatment in clinical medicine)
Includes bibliographies and index.
1. Respiratory organs – Diseases. 2. Respiratory organs – Diseases – Chemotherapy.
3. Respiratory agents. I. McNicol, M.W. II. Title. III. Series. [DNLM: 1. Respiratory
Tract Diseases.  WF 140 T221r]  RC731.T38  1987  616.2  87–9570

© Springer-Verlag Berlin Heidelberg 1987
Softcover reprint of the hardcover 1st edition 1987

Filmset by Tradeset Photosetting, Welwyn Garden City, Hertfordshire.

2128/3916-543210

# Series Editor's Foreword

*Respiratory Disease* is the sixth in a series of monographs on "Treatment in Clinical Medicine".

Drs. Tattersfield and McNicol are well qualified to tackle the volume on respiratory disease. Anne Tattersfield is Professor of Respiratory Medicine at Nottingham University Medical School and Martin McNicol is a Consultant Physician to the Cardiothoracic Unit at the Central Middlesex Hospital in London. They both have extensive practical clinical experience in chest medicine as well as being active contributors to research in the field. They are particularly suited to address the interface between respiratory medicine and clinical pharmacology and therapeutics as they have for many years been involved in studies of drug action in man and optimizing therapy for pulmonary disease.

As with previous volumes in this series, the book is divided into two parts. Firstly, pathophysiology, clinical features and general management of the important areas of respiratory medicine are reviewed. In the second part the clinical pharmacology and use of specific drugs and drug groups are considered in depth. This part includes not only drugs used exclusively in respiratory diseases but also groups like the corticosteroids which have wider applications. A chapter is devoted to oxygen therapy, and the roles of respiratory stimulants and cough suppressants are also covered. At the end of each chapter a list of suggested reading is provided as an introduction to the literature for the reader who wishes to explore a topic in more depth.

This book should be useful to a wide range of doctors, medical students and other health personnel. It does not deal exclusively with rare specialist diseases but reviews all the common problems encountered in chest medicine in clinical practice, including respiratory tract infections and lung tumours. Where appropriate, as in the case of tuberculosis, attention is drawn to differences in clinical features and management between Western Europe and Third World countries.

Bethesda, Maryland, U.S.A.                                    John L. Reid
April 1987

# Preface

Respiratory disease is a major health problem worldwide. The pattern of disease varies enormously in different parts of the world and continues to change rapidly. In the Third World respiratory infection accounts for some 15 million deaths a year in children under the age of five, and tuberculosis continues to kill over one million people a year. In industrialised countries the dramatic decline in mortality from respiratory infection has been replaced by an epidemic increase in mortality from diseases due to smoking and atmospheric pollution such as lung cancer and chronic bronchitis. Respiratory disease now accounts for one-fifth of all deaths in the United Kingdom, and much disability in addition — one-third of all absences from work and one-quarter of all general practitioner consultations.

In the developed countries the approach to respiratory disease has undergone radical change. With new investigative procedures such as fibreoptic bronchoscopy, computer-assisted tomography and improved microbiological techniques it is very unusual not to be able to make a definitive diagnosis. The approach to functional assessment has been transformed by the increasingly wide availability and application of physiological measurement techniques.

This book is concerned with the application of this new knowledge and better understanding of the pharmacological action of drugs to the management and treatment of patients. Relatively few respiratory disorders other than infection can be cured, but patients with chronic respiratory disease, the major group in industrialised societies, can be helped. Optimum management requires a good working knowledge of the drugs available and an understanding of their place in treatment.

*Respiratory Disease*, a monograph in the series on *Treatment in Clinical Medicine*, approaches the problems in two ways. In the first half the background to each of the main respiratory diseases is reviewed — aetiology, physiological consequences, clinical features, diagnosis and prevention — with a particular emphasis on management and treatment. The second half of the book discusses the main drugs used in respiratory practice in more detail and combines a pharmacological appraisal with a more personal assessment of their role and value in treatment. Practical aspects of management are emphasised. Where there is uncertainty we have described our own practice. We believe that *Respiratory Disease* will fill a gap between textbooks of respiratory medicine where management and treatment are usually not covered in detail, and textbooks of pharmacology which describe drug actions but are not normally concerned with practical management problems. This book has been written for the doctor beginning to specialise in respiratory medicine. We believe that it may also be useful for the respiratory physician, and that it provides a 'state of the art' view of the treatment of respiratory diseases which may be of value to the research fellow considering studies on the therapeutic aspects of respiratory disease. We hope that the senior medical student of an enquiring turn of mind will find it helpful.

## Acknowledgements

Several colleagues have answered queries as they arose or reviewed chapters at different stages of gestation. We would particularly like to thank Mark Woodhead, Fiona Moss and Martin Church for useful comments and advice. We have received the greatest possible secretarial help and support from Jane Galletti, Alicia Etherington and Margaret Dowling, for which we are extremely grateful.

Nottingham and London                    Anne E. Tattersfield
1987                                      Martin W. McNicol

# Contents

# Abbreviations

| | |
|---|---|
| A-aDO$_2$ | alveolar–arterial oxygen tension difference |
| BAL | bronchoalveolar lavage |
| COMT | catechol-$O$-methyl transferase |
| cyclic 3′,5′-AMP | cyclic 3′,5′-adenosine monophosphate |
| FEV$_1$ | forced expiratory volume in one second |
| IPPB | intermittent positive pressure breathing |
| KCO | TLCO corrected for lung volume |
| MAO | monoamine oxidase |
| PaCO$_2$ | carbon dioxide tension in arterial blood |
| PaO$_2$ | oxygen tension in arterial blood |
| PDI | phosphodiesterase inhibition |
| PEEP | positive end expiratory pressure |
| TLC | total lung capacity |
| TLCO | transfer factor for carbon monoxide |
| sGaw | airway conductance (Gaw) corrected for lung volume |
| VC | vital capacity |

# 1 Assessment of Patients with Respiratory Disease

Generalisations about disease patterns inevitably oversimplify. However, it is true to say that patients with respiratory disease fall primarily into one of two categories: those with an *anatomical* illness such as a respiratory infection or lung cancer, and those with a *physiological* disease where problems of lung function predominate, such as asthma or chronic bronchitis. Although the incidence of anatomical disease is probably greater, the physiological diseases are chronic and often incurable, and they cause considerable disability. Their management dominates the work of most respiratory physicians.

The diagnostic approach to these two types of problem is very different. For the anatomical illness a conventional approach to history, examination and investigation with a view to making a specific diagnosis is clearly appropriate. The resources for this type of investigation, while not as complex as, for example, cardiac catheterisation, are becoming increasingly sophisticated. The chest X-ray remains the essential starting point however, supplemented by other imaging techniques such as tomography, computed tomography (CT) scanning, isotope scanning and ultrasound as appropriate. Fibreoptic bronchoscopy has transformed anatomical diagnosis in the last few years and its full potential has not yet been realised. It permits visual inspection of the bronchial tree, sampling of bronchial and alveolar secretions and tissue biopsy. The examination is easily carried out and can be repeated readily even in the ill patient. Complications are uncommon but include pneumothorax, haemoptysis and fever. Discrete shadows not accessible to the bronchoscope are usually approached by percutaneous needle biopsy using needle aspiration, or cutting needle biopsy under imaging control, and again the complication rate is low in experienced hands. Other biopsy techniques such as mediastinoscopy and limited open thoracotomy are improving and increasing in importance. By selecting appropriate investigational techniques, it is now very unusual not to be able to make an "anatomical" diagnosis when needed. Table 1.1 provides a commentary on the available investigations.

The approach to physiological diagnosis is different. Diagnosis of the main functional disorder is usually not difficult. The essential starting point here is simple spirometry. The majority of patients are suffering from chronic airways obstruction, and a good history usually makes the underlying diagnosis clear. The emphasis in these patients is on the assessment of severity, progression and

**Table 1.1.** Anatomical investigations

| Investigation | Comments |
| --- | --- |
| *Sputum* | |
| Appearance | Very helpful |
| Microscopy | Valuable for ill patients and when TB possible |
| Culture | Can be misleading, essential for TB |
| Cytology | Value depends on local service |
| *Radiology* | |
| Chest X-ray | Essential for anatomical diagnosis |
| PA +/− lateral | Lateral useful for localisation |
| +/− other views | |
| Tomography | For "difficult" lesions |
| CT scan | Still being evaluated, used mainly for assessment of mediastinal masses and nodes, more sensitive for metastatic tumours |
| Ultrasound | Occasionally for pleural disease |
| *Blood tests* | |
| Neutrophils | For infection |
| Eosinophils | Sometimes useful in supporting the diagnosis of asthma, pulmonary eosinophilia |
| Blood culture | Useful for bacteriological diagnosis in pneumonia |
| Precipitating antibodies, autoantibodies, serum, angiotensin-converting enzyme, $\alpha_1$-antitrypsin | Additional tests helpful in specific conditions |
| *Pleural aspiration* | |
| Protein, cells, culture and cytology | Essential if cause of effusion not known |
| Biopsy | Helpful mainly in TB, should be routine if cause of effusion uncertain |
| *Fibreoptic bronchoscopy* | |
| Bronchial | |
| Secretions ⎱ | Bacteriology of infection, especially |
| Washings ⎰ | opportunistic infection |
| Brushing | Cytological diagnosis of carcinoma |
| Biopsy | Histology of superficial lesions, sarcoid |
| Alveolar lavage | Assessment of cell numbers and type in sarcoid and alveolitis |
| Transbronchial biopsy | Useful in opportunistic infection, sarcoid; less helpful in interstitial disease because sample may be unrepresentative |
| *Rigid bronchoscopy* ⎫ | Methods of obtaining tissue for bacteriology, |
| *Percutaneous biopsy* ⎪ | cytology and histology |
| *Mediastinoscopy* ⎬ | |
| *Thoracoscopy* ⎪ | |
| *Thoracotomy* ⎭ | |
| *Mediastinotomy/scalene node biopsy* | Useful in diagnosis of sarcoid, diagnosis and assessment of carcinoma |
| *Lung biopsy* | |
| Needle: aspiration | Under X-ray control — good for nodules — |
| biopsy | cytology or histology |
| Trephine | Done blind — more risk of pneumothorax but better sample; used mainly for diffuse lung disease |
| Thoracoscope | Useful for diagnosis of obscure pleural disease |
| Open | Requires operation, but safe and gives good sample |

disability. Experience and knowledge of the natural history of the disease are required to advise patients sensibly and predict the likely course of the disease. Although the problems of these patients are chronic and not "curable", they can be helped to a varying extent by treatment, and the assessment of response to treatment is a fundamental part of management. Measurement of lung function in these physiologically disabled people is as essential as knowing the creatinine level in renal failure or the blood pressure in hypertension. In a smaller group of patients, mainly those with alveolitis, there is a need for both functional assessment and anatomical diagnosis.

The range and complexity of methods of testing lung function have increased greatly though appropriate use of a few simple tests is all that is needed for the majority of patients. Measurement of peak expiratory flow rate (PEF) from a peak flow meter and forced expiratory volume in 1 second ($FEV_1$), and vital capacity (VC) from a spirometer is easily carried out and highly reproducible. Repeated measurements in the home or working environment are especially useful. These tests are not particularly sensitive to the very early airway changes of chronic bronchitis and emphysema but they detect change long before symptoms occur. Efforts to detect very early changes of airways obstruction are irrelevant to clinical practice.

Blood gas analysis is essential for management of acute problems. Sensible interpretation is important, however, since errors occur more often than is generally realised, for a variety of reasons related both to blood sampling and calibration techniques. For severely disabled patients simple exercise tests such as the 6-min or 100-m walk test are probably the most appropriate method of assessing the effect of drugs or oxygen therapy since exercise limitation by breathlessness is the patient's major symptom. Placebo effects are important however, so that ideally a matched study with appropriate placebo should be carried out. This makes the tests in these disabled patients rather time consuming and for this reason many laboratories only use them to assess drugs such as oxygen where the implications of long-term prescribing are greater.

Other measurements of pulmonary function are in general more sophisticated than spirometry and more sensitive to small changes, but they are almost invariably less repeatable both within and between laboratories. They are useful for a minority of patients for whom the diagnosis is not straightforward and for some relatively unusual conditions. Understanding the tests and their limitations is important since blind application of the most sophisticated battery of lung function tests is most unlikely to provide a clear-cut diagnosis. Using particular tests to answer specific questions is a much more fruitful approach. Measurement of lung volumes and carbon monoxide transfer may be helpful in the initial diagnosis and assessment of patients, but their overall contribution to diagnosis and management compared to spirometry is relatively small. More detailed tests of airflow obstruction, such as airway resistance or indices derived from flow volume loops, require more complex equipment and again give less repeatable results. They are important research tools, but, with the occasional exception of some patients with upper airways obstruction, have little place in diagnosis or day-to-day management. Exercise testing with monitoring of tidal volume and end-tidal $PCO_2$ is useful in patients where disability appears to be greater than would be expected from the results of other lung function tests.

In patients with chronic disease, symptoms and perception of disability are greatly modified by attitudes, fears and expectations. This is well recognised in disease for which little treatment is available, but it can be just as important when there is good specific therapy. Patient compliance is crucial in diseases like asthma and in slowly resolving infections like tuberculosis since neither antituberculous drugs nor the most potent bronchodilators will benefit the non-compliant patient. In assessing response to treatment, a combination of the patient's symptoms and the results of more objective tests (lung function tests, chest X-ray) should normally be used. An apparently poor response to treatment may be due to failure of the treatment to improve the underlying condition, to change in the patient's response to his symptoms, or to non-compliance. Finally, when disease is incurable, an essential part of treatment is to help patients to come to terms with disability so that they can be as active as possible despite it.

## The Breathless Patient

In any book on respiratory medicine a statement of the general approach to the breathless patient is almost obligatory. Ours is as follows. Breathlessness is usually due to cardiac or respiratory disease; other causes are relatively rare. On the basis of the history, particularly the symptoms associated with shortness of breath, it is usually possible to separate cardiac from respiratory problems. In cardiac dyspnoea there is often a background history of cardiac disease, hypertension, chest pain or oedema, while in respiratory disease a history of cough or sputum, or of seasonal or other influences is more striking. Features of the breathlessness itself are often unhelpful; nocturnal shortness of breath is experienced more often by patients with respiratory disease than by patients with cardiac failure with whom it is traditionally associated.

If the history does not discriminate between cardiac and respiratory causes of dyspnoea, physical examination and a few investigations will usually do so without difficulty. If there are no clinical signs of cardiac failure, the heart is not enlarged and the blood pressure, chest X-ray and ECG are normal, cardiac causes of dyspnoea are extremely unlikely.

Respiratory causes of dyspnoea are commonly associated with airways obstruction. Spirometry establishes the presence and severity of airways obstruction, but the underlying cause is usually found from the history, which is also the primary indicator of severity. In dealing with patients with obstructive respiratory disease, identification of asthma is most important since treatment has much more to offer the asthmatic than the bronchitic or emphysematous patient. The diagnosis should not be difficult. In practice it is usually made after considerable delay, largely because of failure to measure $FEV_1$ or PEF at the time of symptoms. Failure to diagnose asthma can have major adverse consequences, particularly in a child. The main challenge in chronic obstructive lung disease is to detect airways obstruction early enough for preventative measures to be effective. The severity of the airways disease is often not appreciated until the patient presents with symptoms, when the $FEV_1$ is often reduced by more than 50%. Physical examination of the breathless patient with obstructive respiratory disease rarely does more than confirm a diagnosis based on the history and exclude other causes of shortness of breath.

In interstitial lung disease, dyspnoea and cough usually precede hypersecretion and the adventitious sounds heard on chest auscultation are helpful diagnostically. Diffuse shadowing on the chest X-ray and a restrictive spirometric pattern are characteristic.

## The History

In the history, careful detailing of the variability of symptoms, attacks of breathlessness and the assessment of severity of symptoms are particularly helpful.

*Variability.* All breathless patients experience some variability in their symptoms but this needs to be quantified by comparing good and bad days. The young asthmatic may play football one day and be unable to go to school the next. The patient with severe emphysema may have to stop more often on the stairs on a bad day, but will probably stop once or twice on a good day.

*Attacks of breathlessness.* These represent the extreme of variability and should be documented carefully. Breathlessness occurring over seconds rather than minutes suggests pulmonary embolism or inappropriate hyperventilation. Asthma and pulmonary oedema are usually more gradual in onset. When attacks are a conspicuous feature, precipitating factors should be identified — commonly exercise in the young asthmatic, but also respiratory infection, allergic or other factors including occupational exposure.

*Severity.* The patient's expectations greatly influence their assessment of severity. The variable airflow obstruction of asthma is more likely to cause symptoms. An apparently short history of dyspnoea in patients with chronic obstructive lung disease usually relates to an expectation of declining performance with advancing years rather than being a true estimate of the duration of disease.

Patients often have difficulty in describing the nature of their breathlessness and the descriptions are rarely useful. Patients with asthma may find greatest difficulty in either inspiration or expiration, and although patients with restrictive disorder sometimes describe a feeling of inability to expand the chest, the symptom is also often associated with functional dyspnoea. "Air hunger" tends to be associated with metabolic acidosis, pulmonary oedema or pulmonary emboli, but the description is not particularly helpful in practice. A recent change in the pattern of dyspnoea should be regarded as a symptom requiring investigation, for it often signals a new development or a complication of the primary disease.

Symptoms at night may be prominent. Patients with asthma often present with cough and breathlessness during the night and these are often the last symptoms to be relieved by treatment. Breathlessness on waking is characteristic both of patients with asthma and chronic bronchitis. Patients with either condition will usually reach for an inhaler on waking but the response of the bronchitic is usually slower — an hour or two of coughing and clearing secretions may be required before the day begins properly.

## Other Causes of Dyspnoea

The possibility of pulmonary embolism should always be considered since this is a treatable condition. If routine assessment fails to show a good cause for shortness of breath, anaemia and acidosis as in chronic renal failure should be excluded.

Inappropriate hyperventilation is not uncommon though it presents with symptoms such as dizziness or tinnitus more often than with breathlessness. When dyspnoea does occur it is usually unrelated to exertion. The patient may associate it with stress or anxiety but not necessarily so.

## Investigation of the Dyspnoeic Patient

A chest X-ray should usually be taken on first assessment, except in uncomplicated asthma in children where it is probably not justified.

Pulmonary function tests are not normally indicated in patients in whom breathlessness can clearly be accounted for by cardiac causes or other problems such as renal failure. They are indicated for patients in whom breathlessness appears to be due to respiratory causes, in whom the cause is unknown, and where breathlessness appears to be greater than would be expected from a known problem such as mild heart failure.

Investigation of respiratory function in the breathless patient has four objectives:

1. To demonstrate whether respiratory function is normal or abnormal
2. To identify the type of abnormality
3. To provide a measure of severity and response to treatment
4. To demonstrate a link with provocative factors

The $FEV_1$ and FVC measured before and after an inhaled $\beta_2$ agonist provides a great deal of information. It separates patients into those with normal spirometry, those with a restrictive disorder and those with airways obstruction. It assesses the severity of the restrictive or obstructive disorder, and it assesses the degree of reversibility in patients with airways obstruction. For the majority of patients with airways obstruction, no further investigations are required to establish the diagnosis. Regular peak flow readings at home or work are useful for patients with a history suggesting asthma who have normal function when seen in the clinic. They are also helpful in assessing the variability of airflow obstruction in asthmatic patients, particularly at night, and to help to identify provocative factors. The response to other drugs (ipratropium, steroids, oxygen) may be measured using spirometry or a simple exercise test such as the 6-min walk test.

**Table 1.2.** Physiological assessment

| | In diagnosis | In follow-up |
|---|---|---|
| Peak flow rate | Only useful in airway obstruction; part of examination like BP | Follow-up of asthma, regular charting at home and work, for nocturnal breathlessness and to assess variability and response to treatment, diagnosis of occupational asthma, etc.: *underused* |
| Spirometry | Better hospital assessment — more information | Essential for follow-up |
| | Classifies obstructive and restrictive, and assesses | $FEV_1$ for obstructive disorders |
| | severity and response to treatment | VC for restrictive disorders |
| Exercise test | Assess exercise tolerance | Assess response to oxygen or other |
| e.g. 6-min walk | Determine limiting factors | therapy — must use placebo |
| 100 m walk | Diagnose exercise-induced asthma | |
| Bicycle or treadmill | | |
| Arterial blood gases | Assessment of hypoxaemia and $CO_2$ retention | To assess $CO_2$ retention and adequacy of oxygen therapy |
| Lung volumes | May help to sort out mixed problem, e.g. asbestosis + chronic bronchitis | Probably no more useful than VC |
| KCO | May help in Goodpasture's syndrome and restrictive disorder; can help to separate emphysema and bronchitis, ?necessary, probably overused | Value in follow-up not certain except perhaps in Goodpasture's syndrome |
| Flow-volume curve | May diagnose upper airways obstruction, but not entirely reliable | $FEV_1$ is better for follow-up for tracheal stenosis or after tracheal surgery, when diagnosis known |
| Airway resistance | Not a routine test | No place in follow-up |
| Isotope scans of ventilation and perfusion | Diagnosis of pulmonary embolism and vascular disease; not very specific in patients with lung disease | No place in routine follow-up |
| Clearance | Investigation of abnormal | Research only |
| lung | ciliary function, mainly in | |
| nose | specialised centres | |
| Sleep studies | For symptoms consistent with sleep apnoea syndrome, obscure underventilation and polycythaemia | Occasionally to monitor therapy |
| Tests of muscle function | Acutely in myasthenia gravis or polyneuritis; lying vs. standing VC for diaphragmatic function; VC most useful clinically | Serial VC useful to monitor change |
| Non-specific bronchial reactivity | Possibly additional test to support diagnosis of asthma if spirometry normal in clinic | Mainly research technique |
| Bronchial challenge for sensitising agents | Confirmation of sensitisation if occupational asthma suspected and unable to confirm by PEF readings at work | None |

Other physiological methods of assessment are listed in Table 1.2, and are discussed in more detail in relation to specific diseases in subsequent chapters.

# Useful References

Gibson GJ (1984) Clinical tests of respiratory function. Macmillan, London
Howell JBL, Tattersfield AE (1981) Methods in clinical pharmacology — Respiratory system. Macmillan Press, London
Lane DJ (1985) Tissue biopsy of the lung: clinical applications. J R Coll Phys Lond 19: 184–188
Macfarlane J (1985) Lung biopsy. Br Med J 290: 97–98

# 2 Autonomic Control of Airway Function

The sympathetic and parasympathetic limbs of the autonomic nervous system modulate many aspects of lung function: airway and vascular smooth muscle tone, mucus secretion, surfactant production, ion transport, and release of mediators from resident cells such as mast cells.

Understanding of β-adrenergic and parasympathetic control of airway function has advanced rapidly over the last 4 decades as a result of the identification of highly specific agonists and antagonists. The role of the α-adrenergic limb is less clear because the respective receptor agonists and antagonists are much less specific. There are still considerable gaps in our understanding of autonomic control of airway calibre, including the role of β-adrenoceptors which are present in large numbers on bronchial smooth muscle but are curiously remote from sympathetic nerve endings. In normal subjects they appear to play little part in control of airway calibre, despite their importance in the treatment of airways obstruction. The role of other possible neural controls such as local axon reflexes and the non-adrenergic, non-cholinergic nerves (NANC) is uncertain.

## Receptors (Table 2.1)

The activity of the parasympathetic nervous system is mediated through cholinergic receptors: nicotinic receptors in autonomic ganglia and muscarinic receptors on bronchial smooth muscle, mast cells, epithelial cells and mucus-secreting cells.

Sympathetic control is mediated through both β- (inhibitory) and α-adrenoceptors (mainly excitatory). Both are widely distributed in the lungs — on cholinergic ganglia, bronchial smooth muscle, pulmonary blood vessels, mast cells, submucosal cells and, in the case of β-adrenoceptors, on epithelial and alveolar cells. β-Adrenoceptors on bronchial smooth muscle, cholinergic ganglia and epithelium are $\beta_2$-adrenoceptors, those on alveoli a mixture of $\beta_1$- and $\beta_2$-adrenoceptors. Postsynaptic $\alpha_1$-adrenoceptors are found on bronchial smooth muscle and $\alpha_2$-adrenoceptors on cholinergic ganglia.

**Table 2.1.** Autonomic control of airway calibre

| | Preganglionic Parasympathetic and sympathetic | Postganglionic Parasympathetic | |
|---|---|---|---|
| Nerve endings | Ganglia | Bronchial smooth muscle Submucosal glands | |
| Action | Neurotransmission | Bronchoconstriction | ?Bron |
| Neurotransmitter | Acetylcholine | Acetylcholine | Norac |
| Receptors | Nicotinic | Muscarinic | $\alpha$ |
| Site of receptors | Ganglia | Bronchial smooth muscle | Small |
| | | Submucosal cells | Bronc |
| | | Epithelial cells | Choli |
| | | Mainly large airways | Subm |
| | | | Blood |
| Antagonist | Hexamethonium | Atropine | $\alpha_1$-Pra |
| | | Ipratropium | Inc |
| | | | Ph |
| | | | $\alpha_2$-Yc |

Autoradiographic receptor mapping in man is at an early stage. In animals β-adrenoceptors are distributed fairly evenly throughout the airways, with the highest concentration in bronchioles. α-Adrenoceptors are more numerous in small airways and muscarinic receptors in larger bronchi.

# Nerves

### Parasympathetic Nerves

Preganglionic vagal fibres terminate in a mesh of ganglia close to the airway, from which short postganglionic fibres pass to bronchial smooth muscle and mucus-secreting cells (Fig. 2.1). Innervation is maximal in the trachea and large airways, with a gradual reduction to little or none in small airways. Acetylcholine, the neurotransmitter released from vagal efferent fibres, is formed by the acetylation of choline by acetyl coenzyme A (Fig. 2.2). It is stored in intracellular vesicles and released in response to calcium-dependent depolarisation of the nerve terminal. Acetylcholine is rapidly removed by acetylcholinesterase, thus ensuring that the rapid response characteristics of the neuroeffector junction are maintained.

The action of acetylcholine is prolonged by acetylcholinesterase inhibitors such

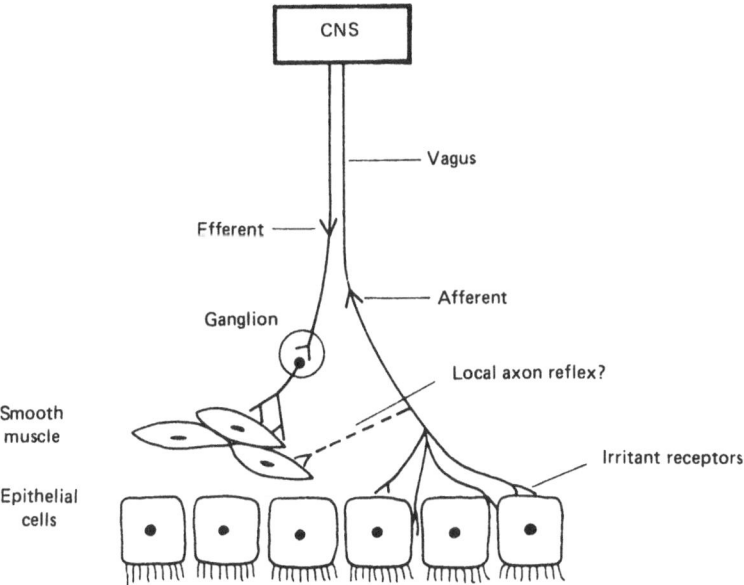

**Fig. 2.1.** Afferent and efferent cholinergic pathways in the vagus. Acetylcholine is released from both pre- and postganglionic nerve terminals to stimulate nicotinic and muscarinic receptors respectively.

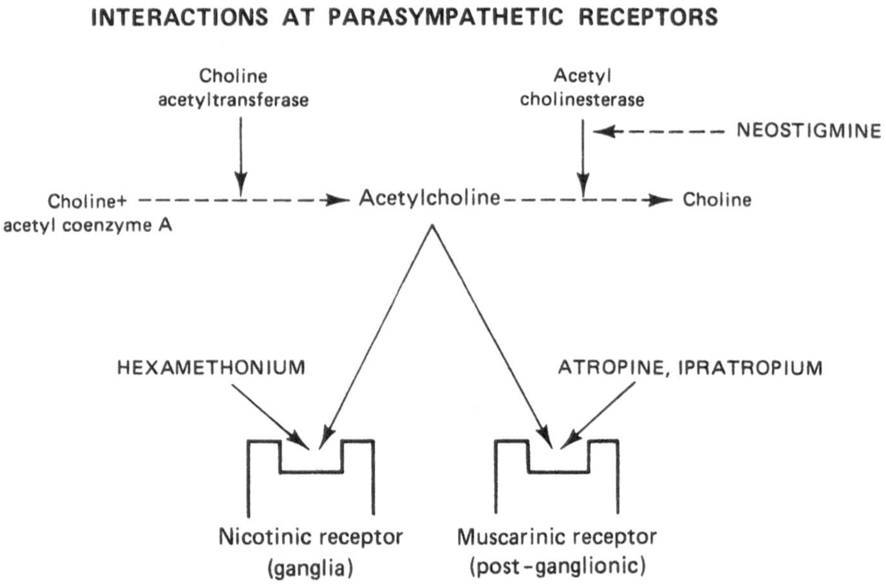

## INTERACTIONS AT PARASYMPATHETIC RECEPTORS

**Fig. 2.2.** Acetylcholine production and breakdown; interaction with other drugs.

as edrophonium or neostigmine. Its effect on muscarinic receptors is blocked by competitive receptor antagonists such as atropine and ipratropium.

### Sympathetic Nerves

Adrenoceptors can potentially be stimulated by sympathetic nerves or by circulating catecholamines, predominantly adrenaline. The neurotransmitter noradrenaline is synthesised from tyrosine in sympathetic nerve terminals and stored in granules to be released following sympathetic nerve stimulation. Noradrenaline stimulates both postsynaptic receptors and presynaptic $\alpha_2$-receptors which then inhibit further noradrenaline release. It is rapidly removed from the synaptic cleft, partly by diffusion and metabolic degradation, but mainly by two active catecholamine uptake mechanisms, uptake 1 into sympathetic nerve terminals where the majority is returned to storage granules and uptake 2 into non-neuronal tissue such as smooth muscle, to be degraded by catechol-O-methyltransferase and monoamine oxidase. The half-life of noradrenaline is fairly short — about 2 min — so that under normal circumstances it is not considered to be a circulating catecholamine.

The paradox in the lung is that despite the presence of numerous adrenoceptors on bronchial smooth muscle, sympathetic nerve endings are rarely found in close proximity to bronchial smooth muscle, in contrast to pulmonary blood vessels, submucosal glands and parasympathetic ganglia, where they are easily identified (Fig. 2.3). This suggests that stimulation of bronchial smooth muscle adrenocep-

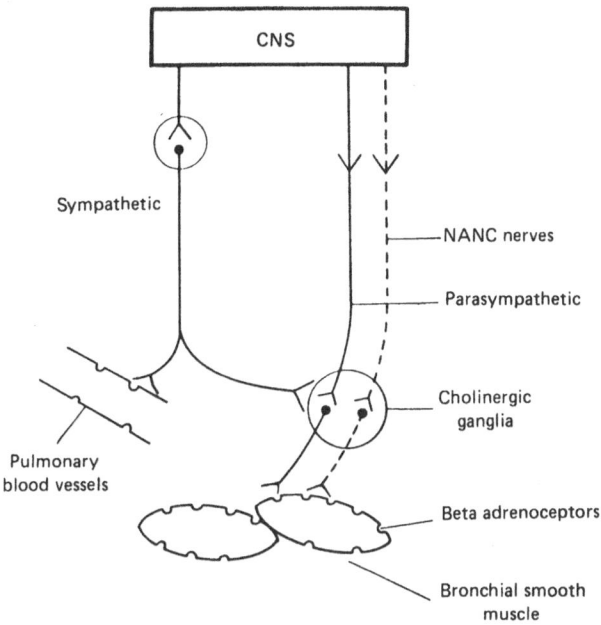

**Fig. 2.3.** Scheme outlining how sympathetic nerves may influence airway calibre.

tors in vivo is more likely to be due to circulating catecholamines, though there is no direct proof of this (see below).

## Non-adrenergic, Non-cholinergic (NANC) Inhibitory Nerves

The NANC nerves travel in the vagus nerve, synapse in parasympathetic ganglia and pass to bronchial smooth muscle, mucus-secreting cells, epithelium and pulmonary blood vessels. Electrical field stimulation of human bronchial smooth muscle demonstrates neurally mediated relaxation which is not inhibited by β-adrenoceptor antagonists. It was originally thought that the NANC postganglionic transmitter might be a purine such as adenosine triphosphate and hence the nerves were originally described as purinergic. Current evidence suggests that this transmitter is more likely to be a peptide, possibly vasoactive intestinal polypeptide (VIP). The role of NANC in normal airways and in disease is speculative at present.

## Local Axon Reflex

In guinea-pig trachea, part of the bronchoconstriction following electrical field stimulation is inhibited by a substance P antagonist and not by atropine. This has led to the suggestion that a local axon reflex might release substance P but there is as yet no direct evidence for this in man.

# Autonomic Control of Airway Calibre

## Normal Subjects

Normal subjects have some bronchomotor tone at rest due to vagal parasympathetic activity. This is deduced from the fact that atropine and ipratropium cause bronchodilatation with a 30%–100% increase in specific airway conductance (sGaw) in most subjects. The purpose of this resting bronchoconstrictor tone is not certain but it may provide some stability to airways and allow fine local adjustments of airway calibre to help to match ventilation with perfusion. There is no evidence of any corresponding sympathetic tone to normal airways. Neither α- nor β-adrenoceptor antagonists have caused any change in airway calibre in the majority of studies of normal subjects, even when sensitive measures of airway calibre, such as sGaw, are used.

β-Agonists cause a similar degree of bronchodilatation as antimuscarinic drugs in normal subjects, an effect attributed to functional antagonism of resting vagal tone on bronchial smooth muscle. α-Adrenoceptor agonists do not alter airway calibre in normal subjects.

Both infused adrenaline and inhaled noradrenaline cause bronchodilatation in normal subjects. Since both have a more potent action on α- than on β-adrenoceptors, the preponderance of the β-adrenoceptor-mediated bronchodilatation emphasises the overwhelming importance of β-adrenoceptors in the airways.

## Asthmatic Patients

Asthmatic patients, like normal subjects, bronchodilate with antimuscarinic drugs, confirming that they also have resting parasympathetic tone. It is often suggested that vagal tone might be increased in patients with asthma, as a result of increased afferent traffic from airway irritant receptors (see Fig. 2.1). This is difficult to test directly. Asthmatic subjects are hyperreactive to the parasympathetic neurotransmitter acetylcholine so the response to an antimuscarinic drug such as ipratropium would be expected to be larger in patients with asthma even if vagal tone were normal. At present there is insufficient evidence to determine whether vagal activity is increased in asthma or not. The fact that patients with asthma usually respond better to a β-agonist than to an antimuscarinic drug (in contrast to patients with chronic bronchitis) argues against increased vagal activity being of primary importance in asthma.

The main difference between asthmatic and normal subjects is that the former have resting sympathetic bronchodilator tone, as evidenced by the bronchoconstriction which occurs when β-adrenoceptor antagonists are given. The source of this increase in sympathetic tone is not known. Possible mechanisms include increased stimulation from sympathetic nerves, increased levels of circulating catecholamines or increased responsiveness to normal levels of sympathetic stimulation. The main arguments are as follows.

1. *Sympathetic nerves.* The lack of nerve terminals close to bronchial smooth muscle makes it unlikely that increased sympathetic nerve activity is stimulating bronchial smooth muscle directly in asthma. Stimulation could, however, be due to sympathetic inhibition of presynaptic vagal activity at cholinergic ganglia or to overspill of noradrenaline from pulmonary blood vessels. Tyramine, which releases noradrenaline from sympathetic nerve terminals, does not cause bronchodilatation in asthmatic subjects, arguing against increased sympathetic nerve discharge at any site.

2. *Circulating catecholamines.* Resting levels of both adrenaline and noradrenaline are similar in normal subjects and patients with mild asthma. Patients with acute severe asthma show rather smaller changes than might be expected from the degree of stress, with no increase in adrenaline levels and only a two- to threefold increase in circulating noradrenaline levels. Initially, studies suggested that the rise in catecholamines during exercise was less in asthmatic patients than in normal subjects, but recent work in which the severity of exercise has been carefully matched has shown similar changes in both groups.

3. *End-organ responsiveness to sympathetic stimulation.* This is difficult to study in man. Our own recent studies suggest that airways of patients with mild asthma may be slightly more responsive to adrenergic agonists than those of normal subjects. Small differences in airway responsiveness between normal and asthmatic subjects, even subjects with mild asthma, must be interpreted cautiously because differences in baseline airway calibre will influence the quantitative response.

Thus although increased sympathetic drive is clearly present in patients with asthma its source has still to be clarified.

It has been suggested that asthma might be due to impaired β-adrenoceptor function or partial β-blockade. This idea generated considerable interest despite the fact that it was inherently unlikely; first, because asthmatic subjects are very responsive to small doses of β-agonists and second, because normal subjects given very high doses of β-adrenoceptor antagonists do not develop asthma. The subsequent claim that α-adrenoceptor activity might be increased in asthma, or that asthma might be due to an imbalance in α- and β-adrenoceptor function, is more difficult to refute because of the lack of specificity of the drugs used to probe α-adrenergic function. However, recent evidence from studies of the airway response to a range of adrenoceptor agonists in normal and asthmatic subjects argues strongly against any such α/β-adrenoceptor imbalance.

# Useful References

Barnes PJ (1984) The third nervous system in the lung: physiology and clinical perspectives. Thorax 39: 561–567

Barnes PJ (1986) Neural control of human airways in health and disease. Am Rev Resp Dis 134: 1289–1314

Carstairs JR, Nimmo AJ, Barnes PJ (1985) Autoradiographic visualization of beta-adrenoceptor subtypes in human lung. Am Rev Resp Dis 132: 541–547

Ind PW, Causon RC, Brown MJ, Barnes PJ (1985) Circulating catecholamines in acute asthma. Br Med J 290: 267–270

Laitinan A (1985) Autonomic innervation of the human respiratory tract as revealed by histochemical and ultrastructural methods. Eur J Respir Dis (Suppl 140) 66: 140: 42P

Richardson JB (1979) Nerve supply to the lungs. Am Rev Resp Dis 119: 785–802

Tattersfield AE, Leaver DG, Pride NB (1973) Effects of β-adrenergic blockade and stimulation on normal human airways. J Appl Physiol 35: 613–619

Tattersfield AE (1987) The site of the defect in asthma — neurohumoral, mediator or smooth muscle. Chest, in press

# 3 Lung Defence Mechanisms

Airways are constantly exposed to atmospheric pollutants, inhaled organisms and nasal secretions. They are also less commonly exposed to foreign bodies, food, drink and gastric contents. Thus airways are, of necessity, provided with a fairly elaborate defence mechanism designed to remove foreign material from the airways, protect the epithelium from sudden change in the local environment, and prevent the lung from becoming infected.

The upper respiratory tract, with its convoluted and somewhat obstructed courses, serves to warm and humidify the inspired air and also to screen out the majority of large particles. The larynx prevents gross soiling of the lower respiratory tract and the geometry of the tracheobronchial tree ensures that any remaining large particles impact on the mucous layer lining the larger bronchi, to be removed by coughing. Smaller particles trapped in the mucous layer are removed by mucociliary clearance. Tracheobronchial mucus also has considerable antimicrobial activity against both viruses and bacteria through the actions of proteins such as immunoglobulins and other constituents. Tight junctions between epithelial and mucus-secreting cells prevent excessive transudation of fluid or movement of large molecules. Alveolar stability is maintained by surfactant. Alveolar secretions contain macrophages with an important phagocytic role.

These different host defence mechanisms combine to filter out virtually all particles larger than 2 $\mu$ from inspired air before they reach the terminal bronchiole, and also to ensure that inhaled organisms are expelled or killed. Considering that at least 10 000 litres of air are inhaled every day, the defence mechanisms are extremely efficient. They can, however, be overwhelmed by a massive insult or be damaged by chronic irritants. Mucociliary transport is impaired to a greater or lesser extent in virtually all patients with respiratory disorders, occasionally as a primary problem, but much more often as a secondary effect of the disease or the factors causing disease such as cigarette smoke.

## Cough

The cough reflex is an extremely important protective mechanism for clearing sputum, ridding the respiratory tract of foreign bodies and protecting the lung against large changes in pH or ionic composition. It consists of a sensory vagal component originating in irritant receptors in the upper airways, a cough centre in the medulla and a motor output which passes to the diaphragm, intercostal and abdominal muscles. Recent work suggests that the afferent limb of the cough reflex is stimulated by change in ionic composition of the fluid lining the airways, and when the tight epithelial junctions are opened to allow intraepithelial receptors closer contact with airway lining fluid. Irritant receptors in the nose and airways may protect the lung by stimulating mucus secretion and bronchoconstriction via other nervous reflexes.

Cough can be suppressed at any point of this reflex, e.g. the afferent limb by local anaesthesia, central connections by sedatives and opiates, and the efferent limb by neuromuscular problems causing muscle weakness. Drugs designed to suppress cough usually act centrally, though unfortunately none of the drugs available acts specifically on the cough centre so central nervous system depression is a frequent side-effect.

# Mucus

Mucociliary clearance depends on both the quantity and quality of mucus produced and its interaction with ciliary function. In the airways mucus consists of a liquid sol phase about 5 μm deep, adjacent to the epithelium and covering the cilia, with a gel phase of similar thickness lying above it. The gel layer is propelled forward by cilia beating in the sol phase.

Mucus is a complex material with several important functions.

1. To provide a mucous blanket to facilitate ciliary action and remove unwanted particles.
2. To provide a pool of antimicrobial proteins, e.g. secretory IgA, lysozyme, interferon, complement.
3. To protect the epithelium from irritants, pH change and enzymatic degradation, e.g. $\alpha_1$-antitrypsin.
4. To humidify inspired air.

It is difficult to measure normal mucus production in man or to obtain uncontaminated mucus from the bronchial tree. Normal adults probably secrete around 100 ml a day, some from epithelial goblet cells, but most from submucosal mucous and serous cells. The constitution of mucus varies down the bronchial tree, but in normal airways is thought to consist of:

| | |
|---|---|
| water | 95% |
| salts and small molecules | 1% |
| mucus glycoprotein | 2%–3% |
| other proteins, including immunoglobulins, transferrin, $\alpha_1$-antitrypsin | 0.1%–0.5% |
| lipids | 0.3%–0.5% |

The main macromolecule in mucus, mucus glycoprotein, contains a polypeptide core with branched sugar chains along its length which help to protect it from proteolytic degradation. However, some naked peptide regions remain and are vulnerable to enzymatic degradation. Disulphide double bonds crosslink smaller glycopeptide subunits within the glycoprotein molecule and provide crosslinks between molecules. The sol phase of mucus contains protein and some small glycoproteins, whereas the more viscous gel phase contains macromolecular glycoprotein, proteins and lipids. Gel formation appears to be due mainly to disulphide crosslinking between glycopeptide subunits within and between molecules. The complex viscoelastic properties of mucus allow it to behave more like a liquid when a strong force is applied and more like a solid when weak forces are applied.

Some of the constituents of mucus, such as IgG, IgM and $\alpha_1$-antitrypsin, derive from plasma by transudation, whereas others, such as lysozyme, transferrin, IgE and secretory IgA, are produced locally by mucus, mast, serous and plasma cells. Some are bacteriocidal (lysozyme, transferrin and interferon), some enhance bacterial adherence to phagocytic cells (complement, opsonins), whereas others protect the airways from proteolytic enzymes ($\alpha_1$-antitrypsin).

Mucus secretion is increased by $\beta_2$-agonists, parasympathomimetic drugs and some of the putative mediators of asthma such as leukotrienes and prostaglandins. It is reduced to some extent by atropine. The patient's general hydration is probably important in ensuring normal mucus production.

# Cilia

Cilia extend throughout the respiratory tract down to the respiratory bronchioles. Their spontaneous co-ordinated rhythmic action at 6–20 Hz is independent of nervous control or mechanical stimulation, but it is altered by change in pH, chemical factors, temperature and radiation. Cilia are 5 μm in length and beat mainly within the mucous sol layer, their tips just engaging the gel layer to propel it forward on the sol layer. Ciliary beat frequency can be measured relatively non-invasively from nasal mucosa removed from the inferior turbinate by cytology brush.

Primary abnormalities of ciliary function are rare — about 1 in 20 000 of the population. In the autosomal recessive disorder primary ciliary dyskinesia (immotile cilia syndrome), there is partial or complete absence of ATPase-containing dynein arms in cilia in several sites including airways, nose, middle ear, fallopian tubes and spermatozoan tails. Subjects usually develop bronchiectasis and recurrent sinusitis in early childhood and about 50% have situs inversus (Kartagener's syndrome). Despite poorly functioning cilia, patients usually have only mild to moderate disability from chest infections and often have a normal life span. This is in marked contrast to patients with cystic fibrosis where the primary abnormality is in mucus, emphasising the major importance of mucus.

Secondary impairment of ciliary function is far more common. It occurs with smoking, cold, alcohol, infection and inhaled irritants and is present in most patients with airway disease. Squamous metaplasia disrupts the normal clearance mechanism in cigarette smokers. Recent studies suggest that ciliary activity in man is inhibited by factors released from certain bacteria such as *Pseudomonas aeruginosa* and *Haemophilus influenzae* and also by elastases released from neutrophils; both may be important in patients with chronic bronchial sepsis. Whether cholinergic and $\beta$-adrenoceptor agonists increase ciliary activity is disputed, but at most their effect is likely to be small.

## Mucociliary Function in Disease

The production of sputum is abnormal and indicates mucus hypersecretion. When in excess of 100 ml a day, it is described as bronchorrhoea. Increased mucus secretion is a normal protective mechanism against inhaled irritants and infection, but prolonged stimulation of mucus secretion leads to hyperplasia and hypertrophy of mucus-secreting glands and what was initially a protective mechanism then becomes part of the disease. Airway mucus from patients with mucus hypersecretion contains more mucus glycoprotein and more tissue fluid transudate including serum-derived immunoglobulins and lipids. The difference in mucus composition between subjects with the same disease, however, is large.

Impairment of mucociliary clearance is clearly of great importance in predisposing the lung to infection, and recently attempts have been made to measure integrated mucociliary function in man. Clearance in the lungs has been measured by marker techniques using fluoroscopy or bronchoscopy, or by the rate of clearance of inhaled radiolabelled aerosols using gamma cameras or scintillation counters. The rate of clearance of an inhaled aerosol is influenced by the initial deposition of the marker, by coughing and by alveolar deposition. Allowances are made for these factors in calculating mucociliary clearance but these are based on certain assumptions so the techniques are relatively crude and at present are more useful for comparing patient groups or the effect of drugs than for assessing individual patients. Patients with mucociliary problems in the airways may have similar problems in the nose, and the nasal mucosa is rather more accessible for study. Nasal clearance can be measured by coloured tracers, radio-opaque or radioactive particles or by placing saccharin in the inferior nasal turbinate and observing the time taken for a sweet taste to appear. These techniques are designed to give a global assessment of mucociliary clearance; when clearance is impaired they do not shed light on the underlying cause.

There is some reduction in mucociliary clearance measured by radiolabelled aerosols in cigarette smokers, in normal subjects at night, in patients with $\alpha_1$-antitrypsin deficiency and in asymptomatic asthma. It is most impaired, however, in patients with chronic bronchitis, cystic fibrosis and bronchiectasis. It is normal in subjects with autonomic dysfunction. It has usually increased with $\beta$-agonists and been unaffected by ipratropium.

# Epithelial Integrity

The epithelial lining of the respiratory tract provides an important barrier, restricting passage of fluid and molecules in both directions. Animal studies suggest that damage to epithelium opens up the tight junctions between cells. This could be an advantage in man if it allowed greater transudation of plasma antimicrobial constituents such as immunoglobulins, but it could be detrimental if it allowed exogenous molecules such as antigens greater access to mast cells. Epithelial permeability has recently been assessed in man by measuring clearance of low molecular weight solutes such as technetium-labelled diethylene-triamine penta-acetic acid — $^{99m}$Tc-DTPA (mol. wt. 492 daltons).

Epithelial permeability to $^{99m}$Tc-DTPA is increased in cigarette smokers but normal in patients with asthma. Measurement of epithelial permeability may have a role in detecting early disease but further studies are needed.

# The Response of the Lung to Inhaled Organisms

The lower respiratory tract is normally sterile despite being exposed to large volumes of air containing potential pathogens. Organisms which reach the alveolus either sediment or exit with the next exhalation. The organisms which remain are normally phagocytosed and killed by macrophages in the fluid layer lining the alveoli with the help of other antibacterial factors such as IgG and complement. Experimental work in animals suggests that a large number of organisms have to be inhaled to produce infection in a normal lung. In the presence of infection, macrophages liberate chemotactic and activating factors which attract other cells to enhance the lung defences. Macrophages move by migration either towards the airways and the mucociliary lining or into the interstitium and lymphatics.

Respiratory infection occurs when the defence mechanisms are overwhelmed or, more commonly, when they fail to function normally. This is often due to a virus infection of the upper respiratory tract which causes the tight junctions between epithelial cells to become more permeable. Once the lower respiratory tract is involved, mucociliary clearance is disrupted and removal of secretions impaired. The main factors contributing to the development of infection are as follows.

1. *Increased contamination of the lower respiratory tract with infected secretions.* Some aspiration of upper respiratory tract secretions is not uncommon during normal sleep. Aspiration of infected secretions from an upper respiratory tract infection is increased when normal laryngeal reflexes are lost or cough is depressed. Contamination is more likely when the upper airways are bypassed, as with tracheal intubation.

2. *Impaired removal of secretions.* This is of major importance and may be due to several factors, including loss of the cough reflex, respiratory muscle weakness,

impaired mucociliary clearance and airways obstruction. Endotracheal intubation impairs secretion removal; pain and postoperative sedation depress cough. Prolonged bed rest and associated respiratory muscle weakness with poor cough and low lung volumes predispose to secretion retention and atelectasis. In chronic bronchitis and bronchiectasis, mucus hypersecretion, impaired mucociliary clearance and stagnant secretions provide a nidus for infection while local airways obstruction predisposes to atelectasis of the distal lung which may then become infected.

Significant anatomical abnormalities disrupt normal secretion clearance mechanisms and predispose to infection. The importance of anatomical factors varies greatly. In generalised bronchiectasis and cystic fibrosis, the combination of abnormal mucociliary function and gross disruption of airway anatomy is clearly important, as are the lesser abnormalities in localised bronchiectasis. Patients with bronchial carcinoma often develop persistent or recurrent infection of the distal lung as a consequence of partial obstruction. Infection may also occur in any grossly damaged part of the lung, as in pulmonary infarction. However in most primary community acquired pneumonias, lower repiratory tract infection occurs in the presence of both normal anatomy and apparently normal defence mechanisms prior to infection.

3. *Impaired immunity*. A poor immune response allows relatively non-pathogenic organisms to become invasive and pathogenic. Colonisation either by normal upper respiratory tract flora or by normally relatively non-pathogenic organisms often resistant to antibiotics is common, and may be encouraged by overgenerous antibiotic use. Colonisation shades off into invasion in the more severely ill patients.

# Useful References

Bienenstock J (1984) Immunology of the lung and upper respiratory tract. McGraw Hill, New York

Greenstone M, Cole PJ (1985) Ciliary function in health and disease. Br J Dis Chest 79: 9–26

Higenbottam T (1984) Cough induced by changes of ionic composition of airway surface liquid. Clin Resp Physiol 20: 553–562

Lopez-Vidriero MT (1984) Lung secretions. In: Clarke SW, Pavia D (eds) Aerosols and the lung. Butterworths, London, pp 19–48

Wilson R, Roberts D, Cole P (1985) Effect of bacterial products on human ciliary function in vitro. Thorax 40: 125–131

# 4 Asthma

The gratifying decrease in morbidity in patients with asthma over the last 30 years is the result of improved understanding of the disease, improved management and the introduction of several new drugs. All the drugs used currently, other than theophylline, have been introduced in the last 40 years, and even with theophylline the formulation has changed. This progress has unfortunately not been associated with any reduction in deaths from asthma.

## Definition

Like many easily recognised diseases, asthma is difficult to define. A widely accepted definition describes it as "a disease characterised by wide variations in resistance to flow in intrapulmonary airways over short periods of time", but this begs the question of how wide the variations should be. The American Thoracic Society definition includes "an increased responsiveness of the trachea and bronchi to various stimuli . . .", emphasising the change in bronchial reactivity. Others would argue that until the relationship of bronchial hyperreactivity to the clinical syndrome of asthma is defined more clearly, it is premature to include it in a definition.

Problems in defining asthma are unimportant to clinicians. They are crucial, however, for epidemiological studies and these have been severely hampered by the lack of a widely accepted working definition. As a consequence it is impossible to say, for example, whether the prevalence of asthma in Britain has changed over the last 40 years. Serious efforts are now being made to develop a definition of asthma which will at least allow a measure of change in prevalence to be made over time and allow comparisons between countries.

## Prevalence

The reported prevalence of asthma has varied considerably within countries and to a greater extent between countries. Some of this variation is due to different criteria and methods used to define asthma. Studies which merely ask people whether they have asthma have, not surprisingly, found much lower prevalence rates than studies which have looked at the symptom of wheeze (between 3% and 30% to take the extremes recorded in Britain). There do, however, appear to be real differences in prevalence between countries. Most studies from Australasia have reported relatively high prevalence rates (5%–19%) compared to those from Scandinavia (0.7%–4.2%), with Britain in between (3%–12%). Very high prevalence rates have been found in certain isolated communities such as Tristan da Cunha and the Western Caroline Islands (45% and 75%), while in others such as the New Guinea highlands a prevalence of only 0.3% was found in 1974. Prevalence rates in general are higher in more westernised communities than in the Third World, and in urban rather than rural areas in Third World countries. The majority of migrant studies have shown that immigrants develop the prevalence rate of the community they join within one generation.

Asthma is roughly twice as common amongst boys than girls, whereas hay fever is equally common. In adults the sex ratio is closer to unity, though there is a suggestion that older women are more likely to be labelled as asthmatic whereas men presenting with the same symptoms would be labelled as bronchitic.

# Pathology

Pathological information has been obtained from patients who have died from asthma and from patients with asthma dying from other causes. Biopsy material from living patients has been available relatively infrequently because bronchoscopy carries a small risk of increasing bronchoconstriction in asthmatic patients. Patients dying from acute episodes of asthma have bulky over-distended lungs which fail to deflate when the chest is opened. The airways are thickened and plugged with sticky opaque secretions. Microscopically, the main features are marked thickening of the basement membrane, bronchial smooth muscle hypertrophy and damaged epithelium, much of which is shed. The bronchial wall contains inflammatory cells, the most frequent and characteristic being the eosinophil. The number of neutrophils, lymphocytes and plasma cells is more variable. Mast cells appear to be normal in number but they contain fewer granules, implying that degranulation has occurred. The mucus within the airways contains eosinophils and eosinophil granule major basic protein, epithelial cells, Charcot–Leyden crystals and Curshmann's spirals of glycoprotein. Mucus is often impacted in small airways in severe asthma and is occasionally seen in alveoli, having presumably moved in a retrograde direction.

In a few patients dying from a very acute episode of asthma there have been few pathological changes in the airways, a finding compatible with death being due to overwhelming bronchial muscle constriction. More commonly, however, patients with an apparently short attack of asthma have widespread inflammatory changes, suggesting that moderately severe asthma had been present for some time. Patients with incidental asthma dying from other causes usually have similar though less marked airway changes, even when asthma was asymptomatic prior to death.

Bronchoalveolar lavage has been carried out recently in a few patients with asthma. Mast cell numbers have not been particularly high, though there is some evidence that they release more histamine when incubated with antigen or IgE.

# Aetiology

Aetiology can be considered in terms of the factors which cause or predispose to the initial development of asthma, and factors which provoke attacks of asthma in predisposed individuals. The latter are considered on page 31.

The factors which determine why asthma occurs in a particular individual are still far from clear. Genetic factors play a role since asthma occurs more commonly amongst relatives of both atopic and non-atopic patients. There is evidence that bronchial hyperreactivity and atopy are inherited independently, and that asthma is more likely to occur when both are present. The concordance rate for asthma amongst monozygotic twins, although higher than that amongst dizygotic twins, is still only 19%, suggesting that environmental factors are more important than genetic factors. Migrant studies support this since immigrants rapidly develop the prevalence of their adopted community. It appears, therefore, that although genetic factors are important, an environmental factor is necessary for full expression of the disease.

The environmental factor or factors responsible are unknown. Respiratory infection and exposure to antigen early in life have been considered as possible causes of asthma but there is little supporting evidence. The preventative value of breast-feeding for the first few months of life is still disputed, so any effect, if it does exist, must be small. Certain occupational factors can cause asthma "de novo".

## Pathophysiology

The precise sequence of immunological, biochemical and pathophysiological events which cause the clinical syndrome of asthma is still not clear despite intensive investigation in the last few years. Any mechanism put forward to explain asthma must account for the following features.

1.  *Clinical.*
    a)  The majority of patients have bronchial hyperreactivity.
    b)  The majority of patients are atopic.
2.  *Pathological.*
    a)  Smooth muscle contraction.
    b)  Increased secretions.
    c)  Mucosal oedema.
    d)  Inflammatory cells in the airways.

## Non-specific Bronchial Hyperreactivity

One of the hallmarks of asthma is increased bronchial reactivity to non-specific stimuli such as histamine, methacholine, cold air and exercise. There is a good correlation on the whole between the response to different stimuli within subjects. Bronchial hyperreactivity is present in the great majority of subjects with asthma though there is some overlap with normal and atopic non-asthmatic subjects. It is also present in many patients with airway problems other than asthma, particularly those with chronic bronchitis where it may, in part at least, be secondary to airway narrowing. In asthma, however, hyperreactivity is thought to be due mainly to increased "twitchiness" of bronchial smooth muscle.

Exercise-induced asthma has been shown to be related to respiratory heat loss during exercise, though whether it is respiratory heat loss as such or the osmotic effects of respiratory water loss is not clear as yet. Isocapnic hyperventilation with dry air or cold dry air will also produce bronchoconstriction in proportion to respiratory heat loss. The mechanisms underlying the two may not, however, be identical since there is evidence of mediator release with exercise, but not with cold air.

## Atopy

The majority of patients with asthma are atopic, with immediate positive skin test responses to several different antigens. The antigen producing the greatest response varies in different geographical locations, with house dust mite and cat fur being the commonest antigens identified in Britain. Subjects with a positive skin test will usually have a bronchoconstrictor response to the same antigen if inhaled. This suggests that local antigens may be relevant to "everyday" asthma by providing one of the triggers which maintain bronchoconstriction from day to day.

When an asthmatic patient inhales an antigen to which he or she is allergic in the laboratory there is usually an early bronchoconstrictor response. This is maximal 10–15 min after inhalation and recovers over 1–2 h. In many patients it is followed by a late bronchoconstrictor response 4–12 h later. The late response occasionally occurs without an early response. The early response is attenuated by prior inhalation of a β-agonist, sodium cromoglycate and by regular treatment with inhaled steroids for several days prior to challenge. The late reaction is reduced by sodium cromoglycate or steroids prior to challenge but, once established, is more refractory to treatment, though it will respond to high doses of β-agonist. The late response is associated with the development of increased non-specific reactivity for the next few days and sometimes longer, and often with an increase in symptoms, particularly at night. For this reason it has been suggested that the late response may be a good model of "everyday" asthma, though the concentration of antigen inhaled in a challenge test is very much greater than that inhaled in daily life. The magnitude of the bronchoconstrictor response to antigen challenge has been shown to depend on two factors — the patients' non-specific reactivity and their allergic status as judged by the response to skin prick tests.

In view of the widespread epithelial damage in asthma, it was thought that airway permeability might be increased, allowing antigen greater access to cells below the mucosal surface and encouraging more rapid diffusion of mediators. Studies in smokers and in animals following induced inflammation showed increased lung permeability to low molecular weight agents such as diethylene-triamine penta-acetic acid (DTPA, mol. wt. 492 daltons) due to widening of intra-epithelial cell tight junctions. Surprisingly, however, measurements of airway permeability have been normal in asthmatic patients; and there is no correlation between permeability and bronchial reactivity in smokers.

## Mechanism of Bronchoconstriction

Although mucosal oedema and increased secretions are prominent pathological features of asthma, most work in vivo has concentrated on bronchial smooth muscle contraction, partly because it is easier to study and partly because discovering the cause of the increased bronchial smooth muscle "twitchiness" appears to be fundamental to unravelling underlying mechanisms in asthma. Increased smooth muscle contraction could *a priori* be due to:

1. impaired neurohumoral control,
2. increased release of mediators making the muscle "twitchy", or
3. an inherently twitchy muscle.

From the evidence, reviewed here briefly, increased release of mediators appears to be most probable.

### *Abnormalities of Neurohumoral Control*

1. *Increased vagal tone*. The shedding of epithelium in asthma is likely to expose airway irritant receptors to inhaled stimuli and this could cause reflex bronchoconstriction through the vagus. There are as yet no direct measurements of vagal efferent tone in patients with asthma and no definite evidence that it is increased in man (see Chap. 2). The fact that atropine and ipratropium usually produce a greater clinical response in patients with chronic bronchitis than in patients with asthma argues against a primary role for the vagus in the aetiology of asthma.

2. *Partial β-blockade*. There is little evidence to support the theory that asthma is due to partial β-blockade. Normal patients taking β-adrenoceptor antagonists do not get asthma, whereas asthmatic patients respond to very small doses of β-agonists which they would not do if β-adrenoceptors were partially blocked.

3. *Non-adrenergic inhibitory system and local axon reflexes*. Non-adrenergic non-cholinergic nerves or local axon reflexes may be important in asthma, but without specific antagonists it is impossible to say.

4. *Humoral control and circadian rhythms*. Patients with asthma deteriorate if they develop Addison's disease or receive β-adrenoceptor antagonists, showing that endogenous secretion of cortisol and adrenaline is important in maintaining

airway calibre. They are not of aetiological importance, however, since levels of circulating endogenous cortisol and catecholamines have usually been normal in asthmatic patients at rest and show normal circadian rhythms. Circadian changes in these hormones, even if normal, may contribute in a permissive sense to nocturnal asthma.

A diurnal swing in airway calibre is seen in normal subjects and this is greatly enhanced in patients with asthma. Nocturnal asthma occurs when a large diurnal swing is superimposed on poor overall control. It occurs despite sleep deprivation. In workers changing shift, the diurnal swing changes over 2–3 days as their endogenous diurnal rhythms change. It is currently attributed to the coincidence of several adverse effects at night: colder temperature, increased concentration of antigen, low adrenaline and cortisol levels, and reduction in treatment.

Many studies have found some evidence of abnormal autonomic function in patients with asthma, but the changes have usually been small and it seems unlikely that neurohumoral dysfunction is of primary aetiological importance. Increased vagal activity or local axon reflexes may contribute but direct evidence is lacking.

## Increased Local Concentrations of Mediators Making the Muscle "Twitchy"

On present evidence, abnormal or excessive release of mediators is the most likely mechanism underlying bronchoconstriction. Several putative mediators are capable of constricting bronchial smooth muscle, attracting inflammatory cells, increasing mucosal oedema and altering the production and constitution of mucus. Which mediators are important and which cells are releasing these mediators is under intense investigation at present. Histamine and neutrophil chemotactic factor can be measured in venous blood and are used as markers of mediator release rather than as evidence that either is itself necessarily important. Both are increased following antigen- and exercise-induced bronchoconstriction but not by isocapnic hyperventilation or methacholine challenge. The inhibition of antigen- and exercise-induced bronchoconstriction by sodium cromoglycate (SCG) suggested that mast cells are involved, but interpretation is complicated since SCG may have other actions (see Chap. 19). Mediators are almost certainly being released from other cells and there has been increasing interest in eosinophils, epithelial cells, neutrophils, platelets, basophils and lymphocytes and in possible interactions between cells.

It has been suggested that all putative mediators for asthma should be assessed by the following criteria, based on "Koch's postulates".

1. The mediator should reproduce the pathophysiological features of asthma when administered to man.
2. The mediator should be identified in body fluids during an episode of clinical asthma.
3. Pharmacological antagonism of the putative mediator should ameliorate or modify the disease process.

Although many of the vast number of new putative mediators (probably over 50) fulfil the first of these postulates, none as yet fulfils all three. The development of specific antagonists to mediators such as the leukotrienes will help to clarify the role of individual mediators. If, as appears to be more likely at present, several mediators are interacting to cause bronchoconstriction, the problem could take some time to unravel.

### An Inherently "Twitchy" Muscle

An abnormally reactive muscle would respond excessively to normal stimulation by nerves and mediators. This, on present evidence, appears to be unlikely. On the few occasions when bronchial smooth muscle from asthmatic patients has been studied in vitro it has behaved normally, and a primary abnormality in smooth muscle would not account for changes in mucus and mucosal oedema, nor for the accumulation of inflammatory cells.

Thus on balance it is likely that asthma is due to the excessive release of mediators from one or more cells and that these mediators make the bronchial smooth muscle twitchy, cause oedema and increase mucus production. The interaction of cells and mediators is likely to become clearer in the next few years but it needs to be emphasised that the "cell–mediator" approach is orientated to explain *how* bronchoconstriction occurs. It will not necessarily answer the crucial question of *why* mediators are released in excessive amounts in asthmatic patients.

# Pattern of Disease

Asthma usually presents in early childhood or in middle age (Table 4.1). Asthma starting in childhood is usually associated with skin atopy and atopic disorders (hay fever, allergic rhinitis and eczema), when it is described as extrinsic. Patients with extrinsic asthma develop IgE antibodies after exposure to common environmental antigens and usually have immediate positive skin prick tests to several common antigens, including house dust mite in Britain. Attacks of asthma may be provoked by allergen but are also provoked by various non-allergic factors such as infection, exercise, drugs and cold. There is often a marked diurnal fluctuation, with most severe airways obstruction around 6 a.m. to 8 a.m., the "morning dip". Marked variation in airflow obstruction on different days is common and the $FEV_1$ or peak flow rate can vary from normal or near normal to extremely low or unrecordable values during severe episodes. Approximately 75% of children will have normal pulmonary function between episodes. Asthma usually improves and may disappear during adolescence.

Patients with late onset asthma usually develop their first symptoms in middle age and are more likely to have intrinsic asthma with no evidence of atopy. When first seen, these patients usually show a moderate amount of airways obstruction which can be reversed to some extent by bronchodilators. Diurnal variation and day-to-day fluctuations in airways obstruction are usually present but less marked

**Table 4.1.** Main clinical features of asthma related to age of onset

| | Asthma starting in childhood | Late onset asthma |
|---|---|---|
| Age of onset | Usually starts age 2–5 years | Any time after adolescence, peak onset 20–50 years |
| Pattern | 75% have acute episodes and are well in between, 25% have some chronic disability with acute attacks superimposed; worse in June and September; morning dipping very common | Variability less with increasing age; a proportion develop progressively increasing airways obstruction despite treatment |
| Features of allergy | Usually atopic; skin test positive in 80%–90%; mild eosinophilia common | Usually non-atopic; eosinophilia common |
| Response to treatment | After 2 years of age usually respond well to $\beta_2$-agonists; inhaled steroids and sodium cromoglycate useful for prophylaxis if needed | Moderate response to $\beta_2$-agonist and inhaled steroids initially; tends to get less responsive with time; more likely to need oral steroids |

than in the younger extrinsic asthmatics, and a proportion are consequently diagnosed incorrectly as having chronic bronchitis. The disease is more likely to progress with the development of more chronic airflow obstruction, with less variability and reversibility. β-Agonists are effective initially but additional treatment is often needed, including inhaled steroids and ipratropium. Oral steroids are needed for exacerbations initially but some patients are not controlled on maximum doses of inhaled steroids and need regular oral steroids to maintain an acceptable $FEV_1$, exercise tolerance and lifestyle.

## Associations

Patients with allergic aspergillosis have extrinsic asthma, complicated by episodes of fever, pleuritic pain and breathlessness due to eosinophilic pneumonia. This can lead to airway damage and proximal bronchiectasis. They have a positive immediate skin test response to *Aspergillus fumigatus*. Polyarteritis and carcinoid syndrome are extremely rare causes of asthma.

## Complications

Asthma is a common disease and significant complications are rare. They include the following.

1. Chest cage deformities, particularly "pigeon chest" and Harrison's sulcus in children with severe asthma.
2. Growth retardation in young patients with severe asthma.

3. Collapse or consolidation of a lobe or even a whole lung following impaction of a large mucous plug. Patients may cough up plugs or casts of the bronchial tree, consisting largely of mucus and eosinophils. This occurs more often in allergic aspergillosis.

4. Right ventricular hypertrophy and cor pulmonale in patients with chronic severe asthma.

5. Pneumothorax, mediastinal and surgical emphysema on rare occasions. Surgical emphysema occurs when overdistended alveoli rupture into the lung interstitium, allowing air to track back via the hila to the mediastinum.

## Factors Provoking Asthma

Attacks of asthma are often precipitated by different factors in the same patient. The relative importance of each varies between patients.

1. *Infection.* Patients often give a history of an upper respiratory tract infection before an attack of asthma. These symptoms are assumed to be due to viral infections but there have been few studies. There is some evidence that rhinovirus infections are more likely to provoke asthma.

2. *Allergy.* Eighty per cent of young patients with asthma have positive skin tests to common allergens such as house dust mite, compared to 20%–30% of the general population. Exposure to specific antigens will often precipitate attacks of asthma, particularly in young people. How much allergens contribute to airflow obstruction in patients with more chronic asthma is less clear.

The importance of food intolerance is difficult to assess. The yellow food-colouring agent tartrazine causes bronchoconstriction in a small number of patients, often those who are sensitive to non-steroidal anti-inflammatory drugs such as aspirin. Eggs, milk, nuts and wheat are the foods most often implicated as causing asthma, but few studies have looked at this carefully. Alcohol will cause bronchodilatation in some patients but it can also make asthma worse, either the alcohol itelf or, more commonly, its congeners.

3. *Exercise.* Vigorous exercise, particularly on a cold dry day, will cause asthma to deteriorate in more than 80% of children and young adults with asthma.

4. *Atmosphere.* Asthma is usually worse on cold dry mornings, when there is a strong wind, in a stuffy smoky atmosphere and in the presence of cigarette smoke.

5. *Psychological factors.* Asthma has often been labelled as a psychosomatic disorder, and some doctors and many lay people think that psychological factors are important. There is little evidence to support this. Patients with psychological problems and asthma undoubtedly can use their asthma, like any other illness, to manipulate their environment. There is no evidence, however, that patients with asthma have more psychological problems than the general population, after allowing for the psychological sequelae of any severe illness. Studies in which asthma was attributed to the effect of suggestion in patients inhaling normal saline are widely quoted, but more recent studies have shown that bronchoconstriction

was due to the cooling effect of the inhalation and quite independent of suggestion. Hyperventilation with airway cooling may explain why exacerbations may follow laughter or excitement in children.

6. *Drugs.* The main drugs known to cause asthma are shown in Table 4.2. Drugs can cause bronchoconstriction through pharmacological actions which could be anticipated (e.g. β-adrenoceptor antagonists) or by an unexpected or idiosyncratic effect. Very occasionally, patients bronchoconstrict after taking medication prescribed for asthma.

7. *Occupational factors.* Occupational asthma is "asthma caused by a specific agent in the work place" and over 200 such agents have been reported. The prevalence of occupational asthma is unknown but has been estimated to be at least 5% of patients with adult asthma. Prevalence will have been underestimated in some surveys since patients with respiratory problems often leave the industry and many cases are undoubtedly missed. Some of the main agents causing occupational asthma are shown in Table 4.3. They can be divided into 4 main groups.

a) High molecular weight compounds which cause IgE antibody production. This group includes laboratory animal products, wheat and biological enzymes. The prevalence of asthma is often high amongst workers involved with these substances (20%–40%) and most patients are atopic, with high IgE levels and positive skin tests both to common allergens and to the causal agent.

b) Low molecular weight compounds. Many smaller compounds such as isocyanates, acid anhydrides and plicatic acid from western red cedar cause

**Table 4.2.** Drug-induced asthma

*A    Predictable pharmacological effects*
1.  β-*blocking drugs.* Approximately 50% of patients with mild asthma bronchoconstrict if given a β-adrenoceptor antagonist. Deterioration can be sudden, severe and fatal; patients have died from timolol eye-drops. Problems are less common with cardioselective drugs, but still occur. There is no way of identifying patients at risk so *all* β-blocking drugs must be avoided in *all* patients with asthma.
2.  *Anticholinesterase drugs.* Drugs such as neostigmine and edrophonium used for myasthenia gravis cause bronchoconstriction in asthmatic patients. Pilocarpine eye-drops have done so rarely.
3.  $PGF_{2\alpha}$ used to induce abortion — causes bronchoconstriction in asthmatic patients.

*B    Less predictable/idiosyncratic effects*
1.  *Non-steroidal anti-inflammatory drugs.* Up to 5% of asthmatic patients bronchoconstrict following aspirin and other cyclo-oxygenase inhibitors; a few patients (<1%) bronchodilate with the same drugs. Bronchoconstriction can be dramatic. Patients are more likely to be middle aged with nasal polyps, but this is by no means invariable. Some patients sensitive to cyclo-oxygenase inhibitors bronchoconstrict to intravenous steroids and 10%–40% are also sensitive to tartrazine.
2.  *Drugs for asthma.* Rare but documented with inhaled ipratropium bromide, β-agonists and sodium cromoglycate and with inhaled and parenteral corticosteroids. In many it appears to be due to the propellant.
3.  *Other drugs.* Bronchoconstriction occasionally complicates the use of opiates, thiopentone and certain muscle relaxants and has been attributed to histamine release. Anaphylactic reactions to any drugs, e.g. iron dextran, can cause severe bronchoconstriction.

Table 4.3. Some causes of occupational asthma

| | | Associated work |
|---|---|---|
| Metal salts | * Platinum, chrome, nickel | Metal workers |
| Chemicals | * Isocyanates such as TDI | Polyurethane manufacturers |
| | * Epoxy resin curing agents Phthalic acid anhydride Trimellitic anhydride | Paints, plastics workers |
| | * Colophony and solders | Electronic workers |
| | Reactive dyes and diazonium salts | Dyers and photocopiers |
| | Persulphates, henna | Hairdressers |
| | Ethylenediamine and paraphenylenediamine Formaldehyde | Lacquer and rubber workers |
| | * Azodicarbonamide | Blowing foam plastics |
| Pharmaceutical agents | * Antibiotics, penicillins, cephalosporins sulphonamides, spyramycin | |
| | Piperazine *cimetidine *Ipecacuanha, *ispaghula powder | Pharmaceutical workers |
| *Enzymes | *Bacillis subtilis* | |
| | Pancreatic enzymes | Biological detergent makers |
| *Animals, birds and fish | Sera and secretions | Laboratory staff |
| Vegetable dusts | Wood dust, vegetable gums | Sawmill workers, cabinet makers, printers |
| | * Grain dust and flour, *castor bean, coffee bean, cotton dust | Coffee workers, farmers |

*Prescribed causes of occupational asthma in the United Kingdom.

asthma. They may act as haptens, combining with body proteins to form antigens. Subjects are usually non-atopic and skin tests are rarely helpful. The prevalence in the exposed population is usually low ($< 5\%$).

c) Gases and fumes. Irritant gases and fumes such as smoke and ammonia will occasionally lead to persisting symptoms and increased bronchial reactivity.

d) Pharmacological agents. In byssinosis, for example, asthma appears to be due to a histamine-releasing agent, possibly endotoxin, in cotton bract.

Occupational asthma should not be considered as a homogeneous entity since the natural history varies considerably. The prevalence can be as low as 5% for people working with isocyanates and up to 50% for workers exposed to platinum or proteolytic enzymes. The latent period between first exposure and the development of symptoms varies both between patients and between agents, averaging 3 months for platinum to 4 years for colophony. The time between subsequent exposure and the development of symptoms depends on frequency of exposure and the type of response. Patients may develop an immediate response within 1 h of exposure, a late response several hours after exposure, or both. Symptoms are sometimes worse at the beginning of the week (cotton, humidifiers) but more often deteriorate throughout the week. Recovery may occur rapidly after removal from the occupational hazard but it is more likely to be protracted and incomplete.

## Physiological Changes in Asthma

### Airways Obstruction

The first and most obvious functional consequence of asthma is an increase in airway resistance and reduction in air flow. The airway changes result in changes in lung volumes, gas exchange, exercise tolerance and work of breathing. Airflow obstruction is most conveniently measured as the $FEV_1$ or peak flow rate (PEF). It can be documented in greater detail by measurements such as specific airway conductance or flow at different lung volumes from a flow–volume curve, but these are unnecessary for routine use. Most patients with asthma appear to develop fairly generalised narrowing of intrathoracic airways, although some patients show a predominantly large airway response.

As asthma increases in severity, the maximum expiratory flow rate which can be achieved at any lung volume falls progressively and eventually reaches the flow rates necessary for tidal breathing. Minute ventilation can then only be maintained by increasing inspiratory flow (and so reducing inspiratory time), or by increasing the lung volume at which the patient breathes to allow greater expiratory flow rates (Fig. 4.1).

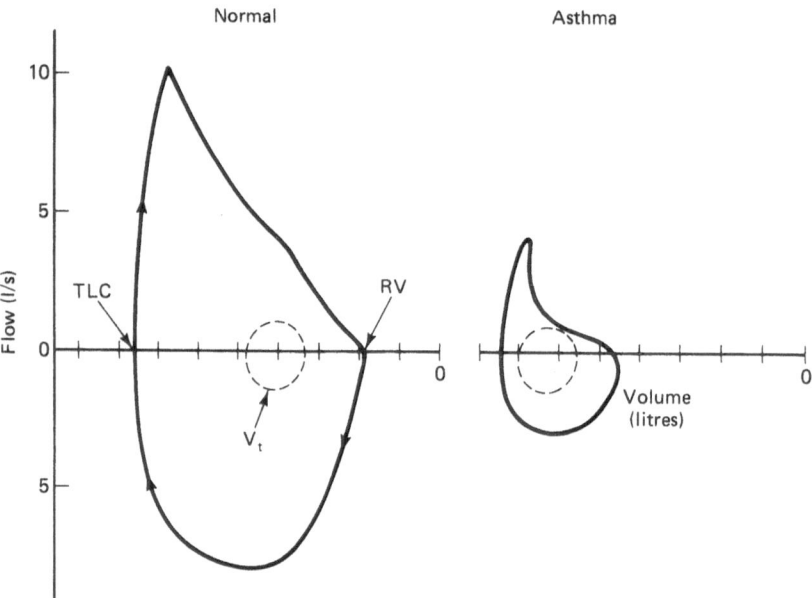

**Fig. 4.1.** Maximum flow volume curves from a normal subject and an asthmatic patient with tidal ventilation ($V_t$) superimposed. The patient breathes out with maximal effort from total lung capacity (TLC) to residual volume (RV) and then breathes in with maximal effort to TLC; for the asthmatic patient maximum flow rates are decreased at all lung volumes, and the expiratory flow rate during tidal expiration is the maximum possible. Any increase in tidal volume can only be achieved by increasing inspiratory flow rate to allow more time for expiration or by increasing lung volume so that maximum flow rates are greater.

Reversibility of airflow obstruction by drugs such as β-agonists is one of the hallmarks of asthma, but the subject is confused when it comes to pinning down exactly what is meant by reversibility. Reversibility shows a bell-shaped relationship to lung function, being greatest in patients with moderate bronchoconstriction. It is reduced when the $FEV_1$ is high because the capacity for response is reduced, and it is reduced when the $FEV_1$ is very low because oedema and mucus are making a greater contribution to airway narrowing. Patients with mild to moderately severe asthma will usually show an increase in $FEV_1$ or PEF of 15% or more in response to a bronchodilator. In patients with a low $FEV_1$, a 15% increase is within the variability of repeat measurements, and within the range of responses seen in patients with chronic bronchitis. However, a response of 15% is a reasonable compromise for epidemiological purposes and therapeutic trials, but it is arbitrary, and this criterion alone will exclude some patients with asthma and may include some without.

## Lung Volumes and Elasticity

Asthma is associated with an increase in residual volume, a reduction in vital capacity and, in some patients, an increase in total lung capacity (TLC) (Fig. 4.2). A substantial increase in TLC of more than 2 l was first noted in patients with acute severe asthma in whom residual volume on admission to hospital was sometimes higher than total lung capacity after recovery. Similar increases in TLC have since been documented during attacks of asthma induced acutely by exercise and inhalation challenge. There is now some doubt about the magnitude of the changes in TLC since recent work has shown that at least some of the increase

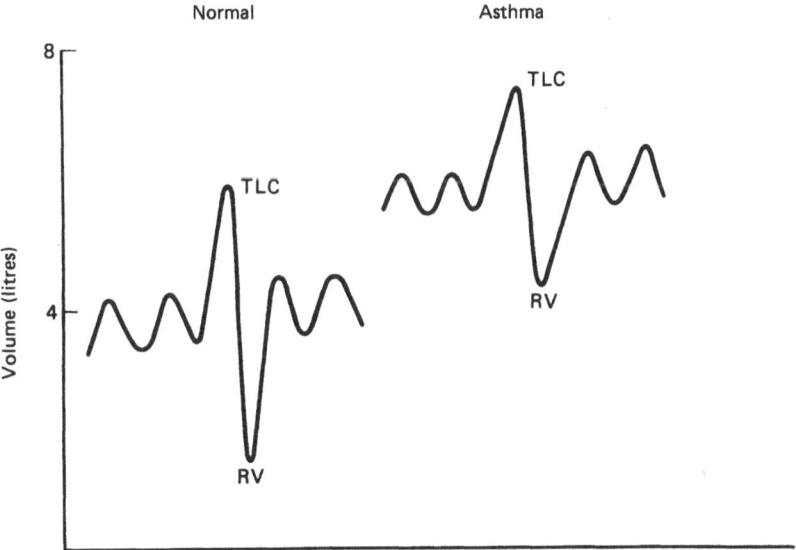

**Fig. 4.2.** Change in lung volumes during an attack of asthma.

measured in the body plethysmograph is artefactual, due to underestimation of alveolar pressure by pressure measured at the mouth in patients with severe airways obstruction. The increase in residual volume is a much more consistent finding, with values of two or three times normal being common in severe asthma. Lung recoil pressure in patients with asthma tends to be lower at all lung volumes, so that the static pressure–volume curve shows parallel displacement.

The increase in functional residual capacity (FRC) during attacks of asthma means that patients are breathing at a higher lung volume, where both lung recoil pressure and airway calibre are increased. The increased work of breathing needed to overcome the increased elastic load plus the need to increase inspiratory flow rates may explain why patients often find inspiration more difficult than expiration during attacks of asthma.

### Gas Exchange

Ventilation–perfusion ($\dot{V}/\dot{Q}$) lung scans show marked regional inhomogeneities in the distribution of both ventilation and perfusion in asthma. Inter- and intraregional $\dot{V}/\dot{Q}$ mismatching accounts for the characteristic abnormalities in arterial blood gas tensions — low values for both oxygen ($PaO_2$) and carbon dioxide ($PaCO_2$). Areas with a high $\dot{V}/\dot{Q}$ ratio will compensate for areas with a low $\dot{V}/\dot{Q}$ ratio for $CO_2$ delivery but not for $O_2$ uptake, because of the different shapes of the dissociation curves. The low $PaCO_2$ is attributed to increased respiratory drive from receptors in the lung. As airflow obstruction increases, $PaO_2$ and $PaCO_2$ fall progressively until the point is reached where the ventilation needed to maintain the low $PaCO_2$ cannot be sustained and ventilatory failure supervenes (Fig. 4.3). This occurs late in the natural history of deteriorating asthma. A normal $PaCO_2$ in the presence of a low $FEV_1$, PEF and $PaO_2$ denotes a serious situation. The patients should be monitored closely and consideration given to intubation and intermittent positive pressure ventilation if the situation cannot be reversed rapidly.

The transfer factor for carbon monoxide is relatively well preserved in asthma and this helps to distinguish asthma from emphysema in patients with hyperinflation and large lung volumes.

## Diagnosis

The diagnosis of asthma should not be difficult. Nevertheless many surveys have shown that clinically significant disease is being missed, particularly in children. Nocturnal cough and breathlessness is a common but insufficiently recognised initial presentation. Recurrent episodes of wheezing or cough in children are often treated inappropriately with antibiotics and not bronchodilators. There is sometimes a reluctance to use the word asthma for young children in case this causes parental anxiety. However, the diagnosis of wheezy bronchitis can be more frightening and when parents have been asked, the majority felt happier with the

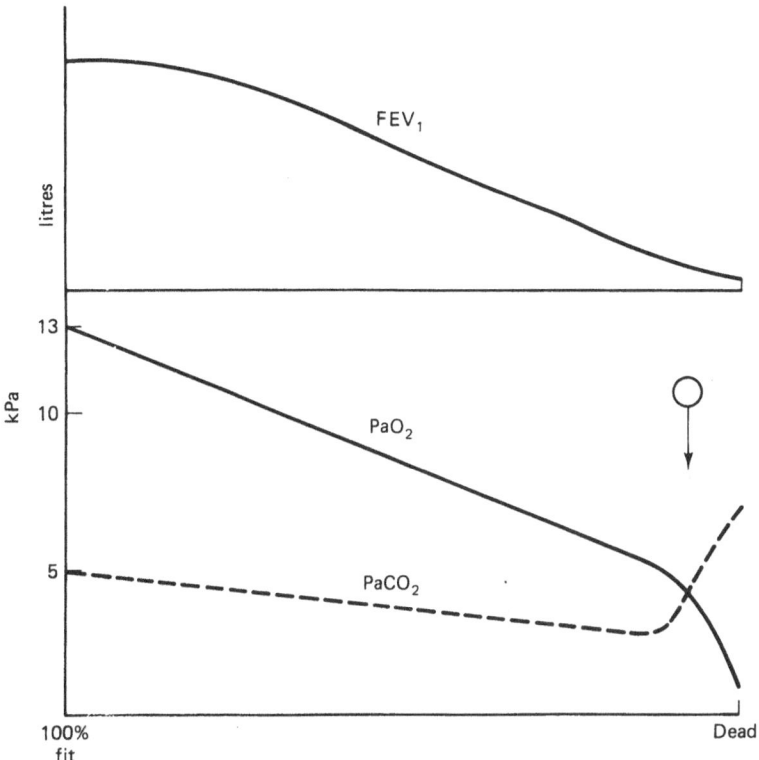

**Fig. 4.3.** Change of $FEV_1$, $PaO_2$ and $PaCO_2$ during progressive deterioration with asthma. The *arrow* shows the danger point when $PaCO_2$ is normal, but rising, and when mechanical ventilation is usually needed urgently.

diagnosis of asthma, as long as it was followed by an explanation and appropriate treatment. In older children and adults, failure to make the diagnosis is most commonly due to failure to make appropriate measurements of airway function in patients with breathlessness, wheeze or cough.

The diagnosis of asthma is confirmed by demonstrating airflow obstruction which fluctuates with time, with bronchodilators or, if necessary, with a bronchoconstrictor challenge. The best way to confirm the diagnosis in patients with mild or intermittent symptoms is to measure $FEV_1$ or PEF at a time when symptoms are present. This is achieved most easily by giving the patient a peak flow meter to make regular recordings through the day with additional recordings when wheezy. Patients unable to make reliable peak flow measurements should be asked to visit the laboratory when symptomatic. An alternative approach is to provoke bronchoconstriction by an exercise or cold air provocation test, or by an inhalation challenge of histamine or methacholine. Bronchial hyperreactivity is present in most patients with asthma, but the results overlap with those of cigarette smokers and patients with chronic bronchitis and need to be interpreted in context. These tests are safe in patients with mild asthma when carried out carefully by experienced personnel but they are more time consuming and less pleasant for the patient than PEF monitoring or bronchodilator tests and are not usually necessary. Challenge with specific antigens or sensitising agents is needed very occasionally for patients with suspected occupational asthma.

Sputum and blood eosinophil counts are often increased in patients with asthma, and skin prick tests to common allergens are often positive. These can be useful corroborative evidence when the diagnosis is not straightforward, but the tests lack specificity and are not necessary for most patients. Serum levels of allergen-specific IgE correlate well with skin prick tests and provide no useful additional clinical information.

### Differential Diagnosis

1. The differentiation of chronic bronchitis and emphysema from late onset asthma can be difficult and indeed some patients have features of both diseases. In clinical practice it is unnecessary to classify these patients precisely; the important thing to determine is whether they respond to bronchodilators and steroids. A steroid trial should be carried out in all patients with severe airways obstruction to exclude the possibility of asthma (see Chap. 18).

2. Upper airways obstruction due to tumour or lymphadenopathy will occasionally be mistaken for asthma. It usually presents with rapidly progressive airways obstruction and inspiratory stridor when the obstruction is severe. The spirometer trace of volume against time may show a straight-line response, and flow–volume curves often show a characteristic pattern. Tracheal tomograms or bronchoscopy will usually confirm the diagnosis.

3. Acute left ventricular failure may cause wheezing and rhonchi on auscultation, particularly in patients with pre-existing airways obstruction. A careful history, detection of other clinical signs of heart failure and a chest X-ray should clarify the diagnosis.

## Assessment

Once the diagnosis of asthma has been made, the next step is to ascertain which provocative factors are important, the severity of the disease, and the patient's knowledge of and attitude to asthma.

1. *Provocative factors.* A good history should establish the important provoking factors. It is important to ask about both nocturnal and exercise-induced asthma since these may require specific management. Particular care should be paid to the patient's occupation and to any suggestion that the patient's asthma may be worse at work and better at the weekend or when on holiday. Two-hourly

PEF measurements throughout the day can help to identify industrial causes or other precipitating factors. Provocation tests in the laboratory are occasionally necessary, particularly when the patient is exposed to several possible agents at work.

2. *Severity*. It is important to be able to relate the patients' perception of the severity of their asthma obtained from the history, with the severity of airflow obstruction assessed by PEF or $FEV_1$ on different occasions. A patient with a small reduction in peak flow from 500 l/min to 400 l/min may be more distressed than a patient with a peak flow rate of 100 l/min. Patients with poor perception of their asthma are at greater risk of undertreatment, while patients with high perception may need more reassurance. There is some evidence to suggest that perception of breathlessness is less in patients with a low $FEV_1$ and in those with greater bronchial reactivity, possibly because these patients have experienced greater fluctuations in airway calibre in the past.

3. *Patients' knowledge of and beliefs about their symptoms and asthma*. Outdated or erroneous views about asthma are common. Many patients believe that psychological factors are important in causation and are often very relieved to hear that this is rarely the case. A patient may have been misinformed about treatment, and may be unnecessarily worried about inhalers or steroids.


# Management

The aim of management is to ensure that as many patients as possible are able to lead a normal active life, including exercise and sport if desired.


### The Patient's Role

Patients with asthma should be encouraged and taught to manage the disease themselves as far as possible. They need to understand the nature and natural history of asthma and the different ways in which treatment may help. Many patients do not understand how drugs should be used. It is not uncommon for a prophylactic drug to be taken during an acute attack rather than a bronchodilator. Careful explanation takes time, perhaps 30 min initially with reinforcement later, but it will save time and improve management in the long run.

Home peak flow monitoring is particularly useful for patients with marked variability, for those who tend to underestimate the severity of their asthma, and for patients requiring repeated admission to hospital. It seems reasonable now to aim for the majority of patients with asthma to own a peak flow gauge. These cost under £10, a small price to pay for the increased ability to manage their own asthma and the increased confidence this brings. Most patients will only need to make occasional measurements until they realise that their asthma is deteriorating, but for patients who underestimate the severity of their asthma more regular measurements will be required. Patients need to know the acceptable range of PEF values for them and when to increase treatment.

## General Health Measures

Smoking by the patient or any relatives with whom he is in close contact must be strongly discouraged. Dusty occupations or those associated with occupational asthma should be avoided. Patients developing occupational asthma should be removed from any contact with the sensitising agent. Those who within the last 10 years have been involved with one of the categories of sensitising agents recognised as causing occupational asthma in the United Kingdom (see Table 4.3) can claim disablement benefit. General safety measures to reduce exposure of workers to sensitising agents such as proteolytic enzymes are important. Dust masks and respirators are often recommended but in practice the masks are often ineffective and, because of the discomfort, compliance is usually low.

### Self-help Groups

Many patients and parents of children with asthma wish to know more about asthma and to meet and discuss matters with patients and parents in a similar position. The Asthma Society and Friends of the Asthma Research Council* was established in 1980 and now has over 100 branches throughout Britain. It has produced several pamphlets and books for asthmatic patients and produces a newspaper, *Asthma News*. Local branches arrange meetings and several run swimming groups for asthmatic children.

### Alternative Medicine

Studies of hypnosis, acupuncture and ionisation have shown minimal or no benefit when subjected to control trials. Yoga was of some benefit in one study.

## Preventative Measures

### Allergen Avoidance

Allergen avoidance is usually possible for patients who get clearly defined attacks of asthma after contact with specific allergens. Some animal and occupational contacts can be avoided or at least minimised. Other allergens, such as house dust, are ubiquitous and impossible to avoid. It is important not to recommend major and expensive changes in lifestyle unless there is good evidence that such a change will be helpful. Simple measures such as not using feather pillows, vacuuming frequently and enclosing the mattress in a polythene cover can be tried for patients with significant nocturnal symptoms, but the benefit is unlikely to be substantial.

*Address: 300, Upper Street, London N1 2XX.

The house dust mite thrives in a warm humid environment, so a reduction in humidity may be useful. Attempts to reduce the house dust mite population by chemical means have been disappointing.

### Hyposensitisation

Hyposensitisation to allergens would be most likely to benefit patients whose asthma is made worse by animals, grass pollen or house dust. However, trials of different allergens to date, including house dust mite, have shown little or no benefit as far as asthma is concerned. Any marginal benefit has to be weighed against the occasional severe adverse reaction which in asthmatic patients can be fatal — estimated at 1 death per 750 000 injections. If desensitising vaccines are used facilities for full cardio-respiratory resuscitation must be immediately available. The development of a more specific antigen may improve response in the future but at present we believe that the largely negative response does not justify the risk involved for patients with asthma.

# Drug Treatment

The introduction of new drugs and reformulation of old drugs have completely changed the management of asthma over the last 30 years. The aims of drug treatment in asthma are as follows.

1. To allow patients to lead as normal a life as possible and to participate in as much sport and exercise as they wish.
2. To reduce the frequency and severity of episodic attacks and nocturnal asthma by improving round-the-clock control.
3. To achieve good control of asthma with minimal side effects and minimal long-term risk from medication.
4. To encourage independence and allow patients to manage their asthma themselves as far as possible.

The drugs are potent and skill is needed to achieve the best balance between benefit to the patient and side effects. The choice of drug, route of administration and dose are all important. The inhaled route is preferred for β-agonists and corticosteroids whenever possible since this achieves the same benefit with fewer side effects than both the oral and intravenous routes.

The response to drugs varies considerably between patients so the response to any new treatment must be assessed after a few days or weeks to ensure that there is a useful response. Assessing the response to treatment should take account of change in PEF or $FEV_1$ in conjunction with the patient's symptoms and exercise tolerance. Drugs should not normally be continued unless there is some objective evidence of improvement. Assessing the adequacy of treatment overall needs to be realistic. Many patients do not achieve 100% normal pulmonary function. For some this is because their asthma is very severe, and for others because some of their airflow obstruction is irreversible. For many, however, it is because they have few symptoms and prefer to have slightly impaired function and take less treatment. This approach is reasonable in adults as long as they are not having significant nocturnal symptoms or severe intermittent attacks. A rather different approach is needed for children since they are less able to ask for, or take, treatment as necessary. There is evidence that many children are losing time from school and not participating in sport because of inadequate treatment. Poor control in children may cause more permanent long-term deleterious effects on lung function, though this is unproved.

Patients frequently suffer from being prescribed appropriate drugs but receiving inadequate information on how the drug should be taken. Booklets and a comic are available and helpful, but in no way replace the obligation on the doctor to explain the reason for each treatment, how and when it should be taken and potential side-effects as appropriate.

## Specific Drugs

The only drugs of proven efficacy in asthma are:

$\beta_2$-Agonists
Corticosteroids
Sodium cromoglycate
Antimuscarinic drugs
Methylxanthines.

Drugs such as $\alpha$-adrenoceptor antagonists, calcium antagonists and antihistamines inhibit non-specific bronchial reactivity to some extent but are of no help to patients with asthma.

It is impossible to give absolute guidelines as to how patients with asthma should be treated since decisions about which drugs and what dose are based on several factors. Broad guidelines for the use of drugs in different presentations of asthma are given below.

1. *Mild episodic asthma.* Drugs should be given by inhalation whenever possible. A metered dose aerosol of a $\beta_2$-selective agonist will effectively deal with the majority of episodes of acute asthma with minimal side-effects. If asthma is mild and attacks infrequent, it should be taken "as necessary"; with more frequent attacks, the patient should be advised to take the inhaled $\beta_2$-agonist regularly every 4–6 h. Patients unable to use a pressurised aerosol should try alternative inhalers, such as the dry powder inhaler or a spacing device (see Chap. 14). An oral preparation is a less satisfactory alternative.

2. *Mild to moderate symptomatic asthma.* Patients with more persistent symptoms should again start with a $\beta_2$-agonist inhaler. This will need to be taken

at regular intervals ranging from 3 to 6 h, depending on severity. If symptoms and airways obstruction persist despite 6 to 8 inhalations of a β-agonist a day, inhalation technique should be rechecked. If this is correct, additional treatment is needed. A prophylactic drug should be added, either an inhaled steroid or sodium cromoglycate. In young atopic patients a trial of sodium cromoglycate for 1 month may be tried. An inhaled steroid is usually preferred since nearly all patients show some response and side-effects are rare and mild. If symptoms persist, a higher dose of inhaled steroid should be given. The incidence of oral candidiasis may be reduced by giving the inhaled steroid through a spacing device, and by the patient taking a drink after using the inhaler. These patients may require short courses of oral steroids for temporary episodes of deterioration.

3. *Exercise-induced asthma.* Exercise-induced asthma may be a sign of inadequate control generally, so the patient's regular treatment should be assessed, and $\beta_2$-agonists or inhaled steroids added or increased as necessary. Inhalation of a $\beta_2$-agonist or sodium cromoglycate prior to exercise will usually prevent exercise-induced asthma. Both are allowed by the Olympic Committee!

4. *Nocturnal asthma.* Patients who complain of cough or wheezing at night usually have inadequate daytime control of their asthma. This should be looked at carefully and additional treatment given to improve overall control. If symptoms persist, the late night dose of inhaled $\beta_2$-agonist and steroid should be doubled and both given through a large (750 ml) spacing device (see Chap. 14). If symptoms still occur, an oral slow release preparation of either theophylline or a $\beta_2$-agonist should be added.

5. *More severe chronic asthma.* A small proportion of patients are inadequately controlled on maximum doses of inhaled steroid and maximum recommended doses of $\beta_2$-agonist, with or without sodium cromoglycate. Additional treatment is then needed — an additional bronchodilator (ipratropium bromide or a theophylline), oral steroids, or higher doses of $\beta_2$-agonist by nebuliser (Table 4.4). Inhaled ipratropium bromide will usually have a small additional bronchodilator effect. It is often not very useful clinically but it is very safe and is worth trying particularly in older patients and those who have smoked and where asthma may be complicated by bronchitis. The relatively high incidence of side-effects with theophylline and the need for repeat blood tests for adequate control limit its value severely. It can be tried at this stage if the patient is sensible but should only be continued if there is a clear and worthwhile response.

Many patients with asthma not controlled on inhaled steroids and $\beta_2$-agonists will benefit from a small dose of oral steroids. The aim then is to manage patients on the highest dose of inhaled steroid they can tolerate and the lowest dose of oral steroid. When starting oral steroids it is best to start with a high dose, such as 30 mg daily for 3 weeks, to allow both the patient and the doctor to see how much steroid reversibility is present. The dose should be decreased in an exponential fashion over the next few weeks to determine the minimum dose which maintains maximal improvement, the patient continuing maximum tolerated doses of inhaled steroid during this time. Patients can sometimes be weaned off oral steroids or may benefit from a maintenance dose of as little as 1 mg or 2 mg prednisolone daily. Continuing assessment of steroid dosage is necessary in the future

**Table 4.4.** Management of chronic asthma of increasing severity

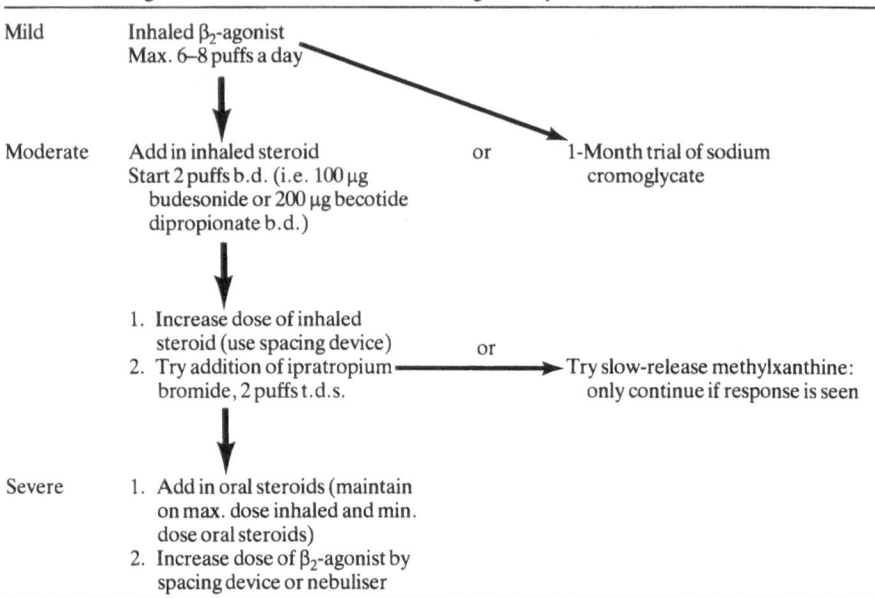

| Mild | Inhaled $\beta_2$-agonist<br>Max. 6–8 puffs a day | | |
|---|---|---|---|
| Moderate | Add in inhaled steroid<br>Start 2 puffs b.d. (i.e. 100 µg<br>  budesonide or 200 µg becotide<br>  dipropionate b.d.) | or | 1-Month trial of sodium<br>cromoglycate |
| | 1. Increase dose of inhaled<br>   steroid (use spacing device)<br>2. Try addition of ipratropium<br>   bromide, 2 puffs t.d.s. | or | Try slow-release methylxanthine:<br>only continue if response is seen |
| Severe | 1. Add in oral steroids (maintain<br>   on max. dose inhaled and min.<br>   dose oral steroids)<br>2. Increase dose of $\beta_2$-agonist by<br>   spacing device or nebuliser | | |

if the patient is going to continue to maintain an acceptable lifestyle and reasonable exercise tolerance without running risks from unnecessarily large doses.

Sensible patients should be encouraged to adjust the dose of oral steroids themselves, using peak flow measurements as a guide, and after careful explanation of the reasons for a low dose of oral steroids overall and the need for a prompt increase when their asthma deteriorates. The common practice of treating exacerbations with a 6-day course of prednisolone, reducing from 30 mg on day 1 to 5 mg on day 6, is far too rapid for most patients with chronic asthma; they merely relapse a few days later. Patients should take a high dose until their asthma is better and the PEF has improved to somewhere near to their usual readings and then reduce gradually, the rate of reduction depending on peak flow rates. In general, the faster the onset of an attack the faster the rate at which it improves.

Patients with severe asthma may have a greater response to a higher dose of $\beta_2$-agonist than is currently recommended for use by metered dose inhaler. Large doses can be given regularly at home by nebuliser, though a spacing device would probably deliver the same dose as effectively and more cheaply. There is currently some disquiet about the use of nebulisers because the optimum dose of $\beta_2$-agonist has not been determined in these patients. With higher doses, side-effects start to appear and in elderly patients they could be dangerous. Until further information is available the lower recommended doses of $\beta_2$-agonists should be given, e.g. 2.5 mg salbutamol or terbutaline t.d.s., unless there is good evidence that higher doses cause greater benefit.

6. *Severe acute asthma.*

a) Outside hospital. Many patients, particularly children, have fairly acute episodes of asthma which if treated promptly are short lived and do not require hospital admission. These attacks respond well to high dose inhaled $\beta_2$-agonist given by spacing device or nebuliser and this is probably as effective and safer than intravenous aminophylline. Peak flow rates should be recorded before and after treatment to monitor the response and ensure that the improvement is maintained. Patients showing only a small response are likely to relapse later. Patients with more severe attacks should be given a short course of prednisolone.

Particular difficulties arise in the occasional patient who deteriorates very rapidly, sometimes over 2 or 3 min. Inhalers are often inadequate and there may be insufficient time to set up and use a nebuliser. The self-administration of adrenaline or terbutaline subcutaneously can be useful, though only adrenaline is available in a prepacked form. A permanent arteriovenous shunt has been inserted for this purpose on rare occasions.

b) Acute severe sustained asthma requiring hospital admission. Some hospitals have a self-admission policy for at-risk patients on lines pioneered in Edinburgh. In the absence of an official policy, patients who are known to deteriorate rapidly must be allowed and encouraged to call an ambulance or go directly to hospital. Patients should be given oral or parenteral steroids prior to the journey if possible.

Patients with severe asthma need careful assessment, including measurement of heart rate, ability to speak, respiratory rate, a measure of airflow obstruction and, in patients sufficiently ill to be admitted to hospital, arterial blood gas estimations. The speed of deterioration is important as well as the absolute level of airflow obstruction. In general, patients with a tachycardia above 120 beats/min, those having difficulty in completing a sentence and patients with a peak flow rate below 160 1/min or an $FEV_1$ below 1 litre are at risk and will almost certainly need active and fairly urgent intervention.

An outline of management is shown in Fig. 4.4. Treatment consists of oxygen, steroids and bronchodilators. All patients should be given oxygen in sufficient concentrations to relieve hypoxaemia. Corticosteroids should be given to all patients with severe asthma and to patients with less severe asthma who have had oral corticosteroids in the fairly recent past or high dose inhaled steroids. This includes virtually all patients ill enough to require admission to hospital. Intravenous hydrocortisone 200 mg 6-hourly has been used traditionally, but prednisolone 40 mg orally is acceptable unless the patient is very ill (see Chap. 18). A $\beta_2$-agonist should be given by nebuliser in the first instance, e.g. salbutamol or terbutaline 2.5 mg 4-hourly. Most patients respond well to nebulised $\beta$-agonists despite severe airways obstruction. Intravenous fluids are required if the attack is protracted.

If the response to initial treatment is poor, additional therapy is required. Nebulised ipratropium is worth adding to the nebulised $\beta$-agonist and an intravenous drug should be tried. The intravenous route ensures that the drug reaches the bloodstream although it carries a greater risk of side effects. The choice between intravenous salbutamol and aminophylline depends on safety and side-effects

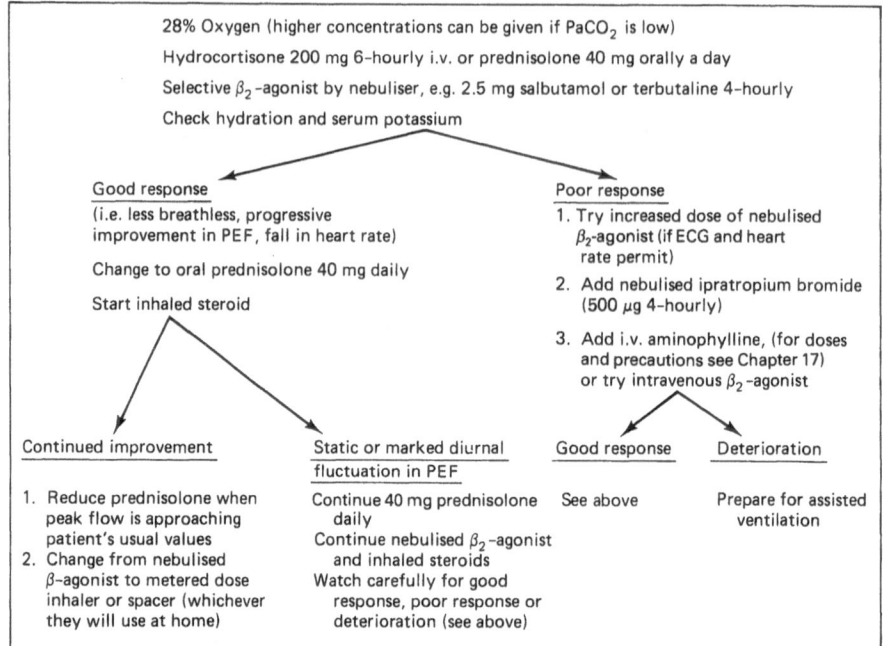

**Fig. 4.4.** Management of acute severe asthma.

since both are effective bronchodilators. More serious side effects have been documented with aminophylline, though this may be because it has been used more extensively. Patients on regular oral theophylline should not be given aminophylline until serum theophylline concentrations are known. They are at particular risk if given aminophylline inadvertently. It is reasonable to try the combination of a nebulised $\beta_2$-agonist and intravenous aminophylline in ill patients, though it has been difficult to document much evidence of benefit in formal studies. When both drugs are given intravenously side-effects are a greater problem.

Patients not responding to intensive therapy need to be considered for assisted ventilation; see Chap. 6. The warning signs are increasing signs of tiredness and deteriorating blood gases, particularly a rising $PaCO_2$ even if within the normal range. Assisted ventilation is difficult and not without risk in these patients which is why all patients with severe asthma should be treated actively and energetically with drugs.

Patients are particularly vulnerable at the time of discharge from hospital. They should be stable prior to discharge and on the same treatment they will be taking at home. It is dangerous to change from nebulisers to inhalers on the day of discharge. Arrangements for monitoring and early follow-up are particularly important when treatment such as steroids is being reduced in an outpatient.

# Asthma Deaths

Apart from the transient increase in asthma mortality in the 1960s, deaths from asthma in Britain have remained at approximately 1500 per annum, though they appear to be increasing slowly at present. The mortality rate is higher than that seen in the United States, though lower than that in Australia and New Zealand, who also shared the increased mortality in the 1960s. There has been a second rise in mortality in New Zealand since the late 1970s so that deaths are now running at four times the level in the United Kingdom. Although several studies have shed light on factors surrounding death both during and between epidemics, the cause of the increased mortality continues to generate heated debate.

## Endemic Deaths

The very large majority of asthma deaths are associated with inadequate assessment and inadequate treatment. In general terms, about a third of patients who die from asthma fail to call for medical help until it is too late. A further third visit a doctor but the severity of their asthma is not appreciated and almost invariably airways obstruction is not assessed. The final third are admitted to hospital, but once again assessment and treatment are grossly inadequate by current standards. Deaths occur most often at night and in patients who continue to show marked diurnal fluctuation and "morning dipping" when apparently recovering from an acute attack.

## Epidemic Deaths

The increase in mortality in asthma in the 1960s and more recently in New Zealand could be due to:

1. An increased prevalence of asthma
2. Increased severity of asthma in those with the disease
3. A direct or indirect effect of treatment

The increased mortality in the 1960s occurred in some countries, but not all. There was concern that the more concentrated preparation of isoprenaline might be implicated, since the sales of this preparation were higher in the countries with the increased mortality and there was a good correlation between isoprenaline sales and mortality in the different states of Australia. Asthma mortality in the United Kingdom and isoprenaline sales fell in parallel once the problem had been recognised. Some believe that the association was causal, others that it was coincidental, both factors being a reflection of severe inadequately treated asthma. It is impossible to obtain a definitive answer now. Several factors related to the changing pattern of treatment of asthma may have been involved. If some of the deaths were due to isoprenaline, the underlying mechanism is also uncertain. The introduction of simple inhalers may have given a false feeling of security, so that patients were less inclined to use other treatment. Alternatively, isoprenaline might have had a more direct adverse effect by causing cardiac arrhythmias or, perhaps less likely, by causing the development of tolerance or resistance to β-agonists (see Chap. 15).

The cause of the more recent increase in mortality in New Zealand is giving rise to similar controversy. The increased use of nebulised $β_2$-agonists and oral theophylline has come under suspicion, though the evidence suggests that the increased use of these drugs followed rather than predated the increase in mortality. Other studies suggest that the prevalence of asthma may have increased. This continuing uncertainty demonstrates the urgent need for continuing longitudinal studies of asthma prevalence.

Trying to determine whether β-agonists may have caused some deaths from asthma is very difficult. There is no doubt that even selective $β_2$-agonists can cause arrhythmias. The middle-aged patient dying from asthma will almost certainly have other arrhythmogenic risk factors — coronary artery narrowing, hypokalaemia from steroids, β-agonists and theophylline, hypoxaemia from asthma and β-agonists, and a direct cardiac effect of other treatment such as theophylline. Asthma deaths are obviously very rare in comparison to the total number of episodes of acute severe asthma and this makes it difficult to determine whether a minority are drug related.

There are certain paradoxes about the pattern of asthma deaths which are unexplained. The first is that mortality in Britain is greater in the more affluent areas where undertreatment is less likely to occur. The second is that despite reduced morbidity, greater awareness of the risks of severe asthma, increased hospital admissions and safer drugs, asthma mortality has not decreased and is in fact slowly increasing. This is in contrast to death from other diseases where death is considered to be preventable such as tuberculosis or appendicitis where mortality has fallen dramatically in the last 20 years. If underdiagnosis, inadequate assessment and undertreatment are the major causes of asthma deaths, then the implication from the continuing rise in asthma mortality is that management is getting progressively worse. This seems unlikely. It is important not to assume that, because patients with asthma often die from inadequate assessment and treatment, the cause of death and changing mortality patterns in asthma is understood. Any patient who dies from a "preventable disease", whether tuberculosis, appendicitis or asthma, must by definition have had inadequate treatment and management in the broadest sense.

# Useful References

Britton J, Tattersfield AE (1986) Does measurement of bronchial hyperreactivity help in the clinical diagnosis of asthma? Eur J Resp Dis 68: 233–238

Burney PGJ (1986) Asthma mortality in England and Wales: evidence for a further increase, 1974–84. Lancet II: 323–326

Crompton GK, Grant IWB, Bloomfield P (1979) Edinburgh Emergency Asthma Admission Service: report on 10 years' experience. Br Med J 2: 1199–1201

Cushley MJ, Tattersfield AE (1983) Sudden death in asthma: discussion paper. J Roy Soc Med 76: 662–666

Davies RJ, Baliney AD (1983) Occupational asthma In: Clark TJH, Godfrey S (eds) Asthma, 2nd edn. Chapman and Hall, London, pp 202–241

Gregg I (1983) Epidemiological aspects In: Clark TJH, Godfrey S (eds) Asthma, 2nd edn. Chapman and Hall, London, pp 242–284

Lewis RA, Lewis MN, Tattersfield AE (1984) Asthma induced by suggestion: is it due to airway cooling? Am Rev Resp Dis 129: 691–695

Pride NB (1983) Physiology. In. Clark TJH, Godfrey S (eds) Asthma, 2nd edn. Chapman and Hall, London, pp 12–56

# 5 Chronic Bronchitis and Emphysema

Chronic bronchitis and emphysema are two distinct pathological processes but they share several common aetiological factors and often co-exist. Patients are frequently described as having "chronic bronchitis and emphysema" because the two cannot be separated clinically with any degree of certainty. Fortunately, from the point of view of management, this is unimportant.

## Definitions

Emphysema is currently defined as "an increase beyond the normal in the size of air spaces distal to the terminal bronchiole with destructive changes in the walls". Chronic bronchitis, in contrast, is usually defined on clinical criteria, the MRC definition being "coughing up sputum on most days for at least 3 months of the year for 2 consecutive years, for which no other cause such as bronchiectasis or tuberculosis is evident". Neither definition is particularly useful to the clinician, since emphysema can only be accurately assessed at necropsy while the definition of chronic bronchitis is too wide for clinical purposes, covering a large number of patients with "smoker's cough", many of whom have no other symptoms and will not develop significant respiratory problems.

The relationship between mucus secretion, atopy, infection and airway narrowing has still not been fully unravelled. Discussion over the last 25 years focused initially on two alternative hypotheses. The "British" view suggested that airway irritants such as cigarette smoke cause mucus hypersecretion, that hypersecretion reduces mucociliary clearance and predisposes to infection, and that infection leads to airway damage and irreversible airways obstruction. The "Dutch hypothesis" suggested that both mucus hypersecretion and airways obstruction result from hypersensitivity of pulmonary airways to a variety of insults and these changes predispose to infection. Neither hypothesis explains all the findings satisfactorily.

A more useful model has emerged from long-term follow-up studies of 792 working men in London by Fletcher and Peto (1977), and of the 20-year mortality of 2718 British men reported by Peto and colleagues (1983). The first study clearly showed an excessive rate of decline in $FEV_1$ in smokers compared to non-smokers. However, the majority of smokers (70%–80%) show a normal or only slightly increased rate of decline in $FEV_1$ (20–30 ml/year) and only 20%–30% have a markedly greater rate of decline (60–80 ml/year) (Fig. 5.1). In the 20-year follow-up, mortality was closely related to initial $FEV_1$, but once this was accounted for there was no independent association with mucus hypersecretion. These studies suggest that there are two separate syndromes.

1.   Hypersecretion of mucus, which predisposes to recurrent chest infections but not to airways obstruction.
2.   The development of progressive airflow obstruction which leads to severe respiratory disability and accounts for the high mortality from chronic bronchitis.

The development of airflow obstruction will often occur in patients with mucus hypersecretion since both have common aetiological factors.

## The Size of the Problem

The prevalence of chronic bronchitis and emphysema varies considerably between countries, with Britain in the invidious position of having the highest

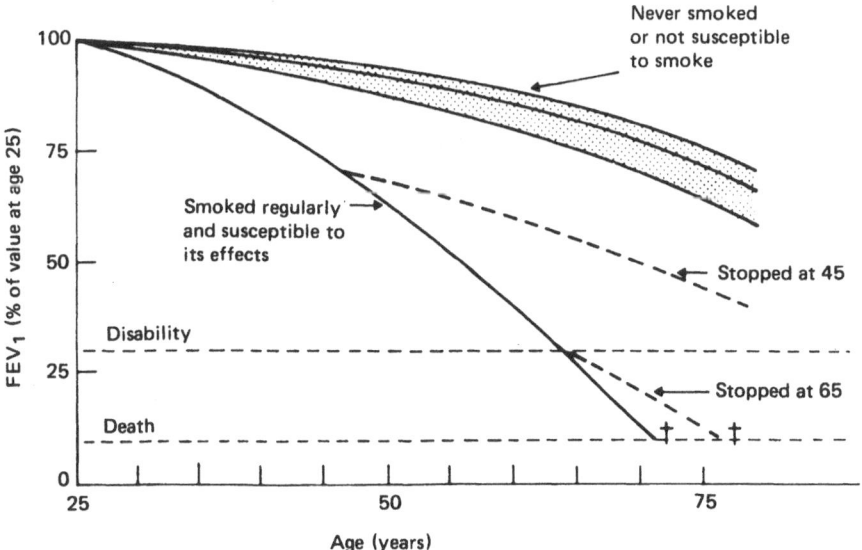

**Fig. 5.1.** $FEV_1$ "glide path" for men, comparing smokers with non-smokers. The effect of stopping smoking at different times is also shown. (Data taken from Fletcher and Peto 1977 with permission.)

reported prevalence. In 1961 the Royal College of General Practitioners found that 17% of men and 8% of women aged 40–64 years were considered to have chronic bronchitis by their general practitioners. Ten per cent of sickness absences from work are classified as being due to chronic bronchitis. Much of the high prevalence in Britain can be accounted for by cigarette smoking, air pollution earlier this century and poor living conditions.

Hospital admissions for bronchitis have fallen over the last decade by at least a third. This is probably due to a reduction in prevalence and also to prompt treatment of infective exacerbations with antibiotics at home. Patients with mucus hypersecretion account for some of the morbidity and absence from work due to chronic bronchitis but the high mortality occurs in the 20%–30% of cigarette smokers who develop progressive airways obstruction. Despite a 50% reduction in mortality over the last 20 years, there are still around 15 000 deaths each year in the United Kingdom. The fivefold greater prevalence amongst men is probably due largely to their greater cigarette consumption in the past, though occupational factors have also contributed.

# Aetiology

### Pathophysiology

It has been known since the 1960s that intratracheal administration of enzymes such as papain and pancreatic elastase to animals would cause degradation of the elastic fibres in the lung and emphysema. Elastase is released by human neutrophils and to a lesser extent by macrophages, and there is now strong circumstantial evidence that elastases released in the lung can in certain circumstances cause emphysema. The action of elastase is normally neutralised by serum protease inhibitors such as $\alpha_1$-antitrypsin ($\alpha_1$PI) and $\alpha_2$-macroglobulin. The importance of $\alpha_1$PI was recognised in 1963 when patients deficient in this glycoprotein were found to be particularly vulnerable to emphysema. These findings over the last 20 years have been pulled together in the protease/antiprotease hypothesis of emphysema which postulates that the balance between the two determines the rate at which emphysema develops (Snider 1981; Stockley 1983; Flenley et al. 1986). The balance may be disturbed by increased levels of proteases or by decreased levels or inactivation of antiproteases. The most important aetiological factor, cigarette smoke, is thought to disturb the balance in several ways.

1.  It stimulates macrophages to release elastases and to release neutrophil chemo-attractants, which in turn cause neutrophils to congregate and release neutrophil elastase, a serine protease.
2.  Oxidants both from cigarette smoke and from neutrophils and macrophages recruited by cigarette smoke appear to inactivate lung elastase inhibitors such as $\alpha_1$PI.
3.  Cigarette smoke may interfere with elastin synthesis.

In patients with $\alpha_1$PI deficiency the reduction in antiprotease activity is the predominant factor. Other protease inhibitors are present in serum and some found in bronchoalveolar lavage fluid are produced locally. Their role in the development of emphysema has not been clarified.

## Aetiological Factors

The development of chronic bronchitis and emphysema depends on the interaction of cigarette smoking and other environmental factors, and on genetic susceptibility. Studies of migrants suggest that, in general, constitutional factors are far less important than environmental factors. Cigarette smoking is two to four times more important than any other risk factor. The large impact of smoking makes it difficult to assess the relative risk of other factors accurately.

### Environmental Factors

1. *Cigarette smoking.* Personal atmospheric pollution by cigarette smoking is the single most important risk factor for both chronic bronchitis and emphysema, and for both mucus hypersecretion and the development of airways obstruction. There is a very strong correlation between mortality from chronic bronchitis and the amount of tobacco smoked. Autopsy studies show that lifetime non-smokers, almost without exception, do not have significant airway disease or emphysema. In a 20-year follow-up study by Doll and Peto (1976) mortality from chronic bronchitis in male doctors was 38 times greater in doctors smoking 25 cigarettes a day than in their non-smoking colleagues. In the other 20-year follow-up study there were 104 deaths from chronic airflow obstruction in 2718 British men, but none of these occurred in the 295 lifetime non-smokers (Peto et al. 1983). Subjects with an $FEV_1$ of more than 2 standard deviations below expected had a more than fiftyfold increased risk of dying from chronic obstructive lung disease.

Long-term follow-up studies of the rate of decline in $FEV_1$ show that this is related to the number of cigarettes smoked, and they also show that the rate is reduced when cigarette smoking is discontinued. In the study by Fletcher and colleagues (1976), none of the 103 lifetime non-smokers had clinically significant airflow obstruction. Studies of young adults both at school and shortly after leaving have demonstrated impaired pulmonary function in smokers compared to non-smokers and it now appears that passive smoking, particularly by young children, may contribute to the risk of developing chronic bronchitis in later life.

The prevalence of mucus hypersecretion is again related to cigarette consumption, mainly to the number of cigarettes smoked, but it is also related to the use of non-filtered cigarettes, relighting, smoking down to a small stub, high tar cigarettes and "drooping", i.e. leaving the cigarette in the mouth between puffs.

2. *Atmospheric pollution*
    a) *Outdoor.* Atmospheric pollution with smoke and sulphur dioxide was an important contributory factor to the high prevalence of and mortality from chronic bronchitis in the United Kingdom until the 1960s. There were 4000 excess deaths in Greater London alone during the December fog of 1952. The Clean Air Acts of 1956 and 1968 account for much of the reduction in

prevalence of chronic bronchitis. Patients studied in the 1970s in Sheffield, where atmospheric pollution had decreased dramatically, showed less breathlessness and phlegm, fewer illnesses and a much lower rate of decline in $FEV_1$ than patients with similar smoking habits studied prior to the Clean Air Acts. Unlike the situation 20 years ago, there is now no correlation between air pollution and mortality from respiratory disease in different parts of the United Kingdom, suggesting that air pollution is not now a significant cause of respiratory symptoms or mortality in this country. The situation may be different in other parts of the world.

b) *Indoor.* Exposure to domestic smoke in poorly ventilated houses is an important cause of chronic bronchitis in Third World countries, affecting women as much or more than men. The importance of indoor pollution in western countries is less clear, though an association between gas cooking and childhood infections has been suggested.

3. *Occupation.* Dusty occupations such as coal mining appear to make a small contribution to the development of chronic bronchitis, but much less than does smoking.

4. *Respiratory illness in childhood.* This is a difficult area to study, but it would appear that pneumonia and bronchitis in early childhood may predispose to the risk of developing chronic bronchitis in later life. These infections are more likely to occur in the first year of life if parents smoke.

5. *Other factors.* The prevalence of chronic bronchitis and emphysema in the United Kingdom is strongly related to social class. Much of this difference can be accounted for by air pollution, occupational factors, cigarette smoking and crowded living conditions.

## Constitutional Factors

Why one cigarette smoker develops emphysema, a second chronic bronchitis and a third no lung trouble at all is not clear. Constitutional factors obviously play a part. The only specific abnormality which has been identified is $\alpha_1$-antitrypsin deficiency. Although rare (occurring in only about 1% of patients with severe airways obstruction), its discovery has led to a much better understanding of the basic mechanisms underlying emphysema and this in turn raises the possibility of more specific preventative measures for a wider group of patients. It is probable that genetic differences in proteases and antiproteases other than $\alpha_1PI$ account for differences in predisposition to emphysema, but none has been identified as yet. The roles of atopy and non-specific reactivity in the development of airflow obstruction are also under investigation.

1. *$\alpha_1PI$ deficiency.* $\alpha_1PI$ is a low molecular weight (54 000 daltons) glycoprotein, manufactured largely by the liver but to a small extent by macrophages. It diffuses from the hepatocyte into the circulation, where it has a half-life of a few days. The amino acid sequence of $\alpha_1$-antitrypsin is determined genetically, the normal gene being PiM and the main problem gene PiZ. More than 20 phenotypes have been identified and classified in the Pi system. In Britain, approximately 0.02% of the population has the ZZ phenotype (around 50 000 people altogether), about 3% the MZ phenotype, and 97% the normal MM phenotype.

The different phenotypes are associated with small changes in the amino acid sequences of $\alpha_1$-antitrypsin glycoprotein; the PiZZ phenotype, for example, involves the exchange of one glutamic acid for lysine. The resulting glycoprotein has normal $\alpha_1$-antitrypsin activity, but abnormal folding of the protein within the hepatocyte impairs its release from the liver. This leads to very low serum levels of $\alpha_1$PI (<40 mg/dl) compared to normal levels of >200 mg/dl. Other rarer phenotypes usually have intermediate activity between those of PiMM and PiZZ, though one extremely rare variant is associated with no serum $\alpha_1$PI activity.

Patients with $\alpha_1$-antitrypsin deficiency have an increased risk of cirrhosis and, in those who smoke, of developing severe progressive emphysema. Cigarette smokers with $\alpha_1$PI deficiency show a rapid decline in $FEV_1$ (>300 ml/year in one study). PiZZ phenotype subjects who do not smoke have a slightly greater decline in $FEV_1$ than non-smoking normal subjects (80 ml/year versus 30 ml/year), but not enough to cause significant problems for the majority. Heterozygotes with PiMZ phenotype in general appear to have no greater risk of developing emphysema than normal PiMM subjects, though an occasional patient has developed disproportionately severe emphysema at a young age.

2. *Atopy.* Although cigarette smokers have increased levels of IgE, prick skin test responses to common allergens are not increased and other indices of atopy have usually been normal or only slightly increased. The increased IgE levels may result from increased airway permeability as a result of mucosal damage. At present the evidence is against atopy being an important factor in the development of airways obstruction in cigarette smokers.

3. *Non-specific bronchial reactivity.* Patients with chronic bronchitis show increased non-specific reactivity to bronchoconstrictor agents such as histamine and methacholine. The degree of hyperreactivity correlates closely with both the number of cigarettes smoked and the degree of airways obstruction. There is much debate about the nature of the relationship. Smoking may increase bronchial reactivity or, alternatively, subjects with increased bronchial reactivity may be more vulnerable to the development of airways obstruction if they smoke. The third alternative is that the increased bronchial reactivity is merely a reflection of airways obstruction, due to changes in airway geometry rather than a true increase in smooth muscle responsiveness in the airways.

# Pathological Findings

## Chronic Bronchitis

The most obvious pathological feature of chronic bronchitis is the marked hypertrophy of mucus-secreting glands in large airways. This is assessed as the thickness of the gland layer relative to that of the bronchial wall (Reid Index). Inflammatory cells are present in the mucosa in between acute exacerbations of bronchitis, predominantly lymphocytes and plasma cells. There may also be some bronchial muscle hypertrophy, but much less than in asthma. Although the obvious pathological changes are seen in large airways, retrograde catheter studies show that the main site of increased resistance is in small bronchi and bronchioles of 3 mm or less. These findings are associated with goblet cell metaplasia, inflammatory cells, mucous plugging and fibrosis resulting in airway distortion and obliteration (Mullen et al. 1985). Asymptomatic smokers dying from other causes often have fairly extensive small airway changes at autopsy.

## Emphysema

There are two important types of emphysema.

1. *Centriacinar (centrilobular) emphysema,* consisting of destruction and dilatation of respiratory bronchioles, often with pathological evidence of chronic bronchiolitis and bronchitis. With increasing severity, there is destruction of adjacent alveoli but the more peripheral parts of the acinus remain intact. It is associated with cigarette smoking and coal dust, both of which cause macrophages to congregate around small airways where they attract neutrophils. Proteolytic enzymes released by these inflammatory cells are thought to cause the destructive changes.

2. *Panacinar emphysema*, which occurs more evenly throughout the acinus and in many patients throughout the lung. It is strongly associated with cigarette smoking and some evidence of chronic bronchitis is usually present. Widespread panacinar emphysema is associated with severe respiratory disability and marked deterioration in lung function. It occurs predominantly in the basal regions in patients with $\alpha_1$PI deficiency, but a similar pattern may be seen in patients with normal $\alpha_1$PI levels.

## Pulmonary Vessels and Heart

Both chronic bronchitis and emphysema are associated with the gradual development of pulmonary hypertension. Destruction of alveolar walls in emphysema causes loss of the capillary bed and obliteration of arterioles, while hypoxaemia causes constriction of pulmonary arterioles. The development of pulmonary hypertension is associated with smooth muscle hypertrophy in pulmonary arterioles, atheroma, pulmonary thromboembolism and right ventricular hypertrophy. Left ventricular hypertrophy also occurs more commonly than in the normal population for reasons which are unclear. Most studies have found left ventricular function to be normal.

# Physiological Consequences of Bronchitis and Emphysema

## Airflow Obstruction

Airflow obstruction is the physiological hallmark of patients with severe disabling chronic bronchitis and emphysema. This is due to pathological changes in airways causing distortion, narrowing and obliteration of smaller airways. It is also due to the loss of lung recoil pressure which results from panacinar emphysema, since lung recoil pressure is a direct determinant of airway calibre. Patients with "pure" emphysema will inevitably develop increasing airflow obstruction as a result of alveolar destruction.

Asymptomatic smokers often have normal values for $FEV_1$ but abnormal values for more sensitive tests of small airways function. Autopsy studies show that patients have fairly extensive abnormalities in small airways before the $FEV_1$ is reduced significantly. Thus anyone with even a modest reduction in $FEV_1$ already has fairly extensive disease. Once the $FEV_1$ is reduced, the rate of decline in $FEV_1$ is the best way to identify patients who are heading for severe respiratory disability.

## Lung Volumes

Vital capacity (VC) is maintained for some time after the $FEV_1$ starts to decline but it too declines as the disease progresses. Absolute lung volumes are usually increased, with the residual volume often increased two to threefold. Total lung capacity is often increased, particularly in patients with emphysema where it may be 2 or 3 litres above the predicted value. Lung volumes measured by dilution techniques such as helium dilution (i.e. available lung volume) show a smaller increase than those measured by plethysmography (total intrathoracic volume), and the difference between the two is sometimes used as a measure of airtrapping.

## Gas Exchange

Emphysema causes extensive loss of gas exchanging surface in the lungs. Pathological changes to both airways and the pulmonary circulation cause ventilation perfusion ($\dot{V}/\dot{Q}$) mismatching. Hyperventilation occurs in some patients, particularly those with predominant emphysema. This allows carbon dioxide to be exchanged adequately, but the $PaO_2$ remains low because the shape of the oxygen dissociation curve does not allow areas with a high $\dot{V}/\dot{Q}$ ratio to increase oxygen transport adequately to compensate for areas of low $\dot{V}/\dot{Q}$. The loss of gas exchanging surface is reflected in low values for carbon monoxide transfer, particularly when corrected for lung volume (KCO).

Patients with chronic bronchitis tend to underventilate. They have a normal or high normal cardiac output so that overall $\dot{V}/\dot{Q}$ ratio is low, causing a physiological shunt and arterial hypoxaemia. The KCO may be normal or slightly impaired. Arterial hypoxaemia is therefore due to a combination of $\dot{V}/\dot{Q}$ mismatching and hypoventilation, the $\dot{V}/\dot{Q}$ mismatching usually making the larger contribution even when hypoventilation is present.

Lung scans of the regional distribution of ventilation and perfusion show matching patchy losses of both ventilation and perfusion in patients with bronchitis and even more so in patients with emphysema, in contrast to the predominant perfusion loss in pulmonary embolus. Using a perfusion scan alone to diagnose pulmonary embolus can be misleading in these patients.

The low $PaO_2$ in patients with chronic bronchitis stimulates erythropoietin production by the kidney, the precise stimulus being renal oxygen tissue tension. The relationship between daytime oxygen saturation levels and red cell mass is less good for patients with chronic bronchitis than for subjects at altitude. This is perhaps not surprising since the relationship is affected by other factors such as change in $O_2$ saturation at night and during exercise, variation in lung function and carboxyhaemoglobin levels.

## Exercise Capacity

Patients with emphysema have a high resting ventilation and can only increase this slightly on exercise. Consequently, oxygen saturation falls and exercise tolerance is very limited. Patients with chronic bronchitis are better able to increase ventilation and so can usually do a greater amount of exercise without a fall in arterial oxygen saturation.

## Fluid Balance

Fluid retention occurs more commonly in patients with hypoxaemia due to chronic bronchitis than in subjects with a similar degree of hypoxaemia at altitude or due to restrictive conditions such as fibrosing alveolitis. The development of oedema is associated with increased arterial $PCO_2$, reduced renal blood flow and increased levels of renin, angiotensin and aldosterone. Although patients often show a raised jugular venous pressure and hepatomegaly with their oedema, total exchangeable sodium has usually been normal and exercise studies show a normal increase in cardiac output. These findings suggest that the main problem is fluid retention rather than true cardiac failure, though the latter can occur with severe pulmonary hypertension.

## Changes During Sleep

Patients with chronic bronchitis, hypoventilation and arterial hypoxaemia are more likely to die at night than patients dying from other causes. This is presumably related to the nocturnal falls in oxygen saturation which frequently exceed 10%. Sleep studies show that the desaturation is related to hypoventilation rather than to episodes of apnoea. The degree of hypoventilation and fall in arterial $PO_2$ are no greater in these patients than in normal subjects or patients with airways obstruction who are not hypoventilating, but the fall in oxygen saturation is much greater because resting arterial $PO_2$ is already reduced and lies on the steep part of the oxygen-dissociation curve. Oxygen (24%) at night has been shown to relieve hypoxaemia and improve sleep quality. Patients with chronic bronchitis do not appear to be particularly vulnerable to the sleep apnoea syndrome, though the coincidence of both has serious consequences.

Patients with carbon dioxide retention are more sensitive to sedatives of any kind, including alcohol.

## Pulmonary Circulation

In patients with chronic bronchitis and emphysema, pulmonary blood volume is reduced due to loss of pulmonary blood vessels. Pulmonary hypertension develops gradually as the underlying disease progresses. Mean values of pulmonary artery pressure in patients with an $FEV_1$ of 1 litre or so are usually around 4 kPa (30 mmHg) and in patients with fairly end-stage disease around 5–6 kPa (40–50 mmHg) at rest. These values are considerably less than those seen in patients with severe mitral stenosis or in subjects living at altitude. However, pulmonary artery pressure increases markedly on exercise, during episodes of hypoxaemia at night and during episodes of acute respiratory failure. It falls during the acute administration of oxygen.

# Clinical Presentation and Diagnosis

The majority of patients with chronic bronchitis give a history of a smoker's cough, some clear phlegm and occasional episodes of acute bronchitis with purulent sputum. Making the diagnosis of chronic bronchitis on the basis of chronic sputum production is easy, though not perhaps particularly useful. Making the diagnosis of airflow obstruction is also easy though it is rarely detected at an early stage in these patients, usually because neither peak flow rate nor spirometry is measured.

The clinical presentation and natural history of patients with chronic bronchitis and emphysema vary considerably, with the ends of the spectrum being defined by the "blue bloater" and "pink puffer" respectively. The "blue bloater" tends to hypoventilate, thus giving the appearance of being less breathless. Central cyanosis is usually marked due to the combination of marked arterial hypoxaemia and polycythaemia. These patients often have hypercarbia, fluid retention and a raised jugular venous pressure, though ankle and sacral oedema are seen less often now with the more liberal use of diuretics. These patients run into problems from respiratory failure and from the complications of their arterial hypoxaemia, particularly secondary polycythaemia and pulmonary hypertension.

"Pink puffers" have a well preserved respiratory drive and tend to hyperventilate to maintain a reasonable $PaO_2$ at rest. Consequently they remain pink but at the cost of being breathless and having a poor exercise tolerance. On examination they are usually thin, have a large, round barrel-shaped chest, use accessory muscles and they may demonstrate pursed-lips breathing. Eventually the patient is unable to maintain a high arterial $PO_2$ and arterial hypoxaemia occurs. Oedema occurs at a relatively late stage. Patients with $\alpha_1$-antitrypsin deficiency develop a predominantly basal form of emphysema at a relatively early age and are often breathless on exertion by the third or fourth decade. In one series of 120 patients, only 16% were expected to reach the age of 60.

Most patients show clinical features in between the extremes of the "blue bloater" and "pink puffer", but the distinction has some relevance to the approach to management.

## Exacerbations of Bronchitis

Upper respiratory tract infections do not occur more frequently in patients with chronic bronchitis and emphysema, but they are more likely to cause a lower respiratory tract infection, and this is more likely to last longer and cause complications such as ventilatory failure. Exacerbations have been related to falls in temperature and increased humidity and are particularly common during influenza epidemics. Evidence of a viral infection has been found in up to 60% of exacerbations, particularly rhinovirus but also parainfluenza and respiratory syncytial virus. The viral infection appears to predispose to secondary bacterial infection, almost invariably *Haemophilus influenzae* or *Streptococcus pneumoniae*.

## Correlation of Clinical, Radiological, Pathological and Physiological Features

Attempts to separate the relative contributions of bronchitis and emphysema to airways obstruction in individual patients are unreliable. The "pink puffer" tends to have more panacinar emphysema at autopsy and the "blue bloater" more bronchitis and less emphysema, but the overlap is considerable and predictions often wrong.

Several prospective studies have related pulmonary function and radiological findings during life to the extent and severity of emphysema at autopsy. For a given degree of airways obstruction, patients found eventually to have extensive panacinar emphysema are more likely to have had a relatively low $PaCO_2$, a low KCO and a high TLC. They are also more likely to have certain radiological features, including a low flat diaphragm, increased retrosternal airspace on the lateral film, long thin heart, and more marked attenuation of pulmonary blood vessels. Patients with less emphysema at autopsy have a higher $PaCO_2$, a smaller reduction in KCO, less of an increase in TLC and fewer of the radiological features described above, though a large heart is often present. Although these findings are significant epidemiologically, the correlation is not good enough to allow accurate predictions in individual patients. CT scanning might allow more accurate quantification of emphysema, and detailed correlations are awaited. It should be emphasised that determining how much emphysema is present is not necessary for clinical management. It would, however, be extremely valuable in assessing the value of drugs designed to reduce the rate of development of emphysema.

## Differential Diagnosis

In clinical practice there is little value in attempting to distinguish between chronic bronchitis and emphysema but it is essential not to miss the diagnosis of asthma. It is misdiagnosed as chronic bronchitis and emphysema frequently enough to justify a trial of oral corticosteroids in all patients with symptomatic airflow obstruction (see Chap. 18).

# Pulmonary Function Testing

The overwhelming priority in patients who smoke is to detect airways obstruction at an early stage so that pressure can be directed towards stopping smoking. Serial measurements of PEF or $FEV_1$ in the same person are more valuable than isolated measurements because of the wide range of predicted normal values; a large fall in $FEV_1$ can occur in some patients before they are two standard deviations below their predicted $FEV_1$. Measurement of $FEV_1$ and vital capacity gives slightly more information than PEF in that a low $FEV_1/VC$ indicates significant airways disease even if $FEV_1$ as a percentage of predicted is normal. The normal decline in $FEV_1$ is 20–30 ml/year. Patients showing a more rapid rate of decline are clearly at risk of developing disabling airflow obstruction.

Other measures of pulmonary function (as listed below) are required for specific indications.

1. *Bronchodilator or steroid response.* The response to a bronchodilator or a steroid trial is the best way to identify patients with asthma.
2. *Exercise study.* This is the most relevant way to assess the effect of treatment such as oxygen. The 6-min or 12-min walk test is a simple test in which the patient is asked to walk as far as he can for 6 or 12 mins at his own speed. Results are reasonably reproducible after one practice walk.
3. *Blood gas analysis.* This is essential for assessing the adequacy of ventilation and gas exchange. Arterial $PCO_2$ measurements will determine whether the patient is underventilating and should be carried out in all patients who are drowsy and confused.

# Prevention of Chronic Bronchitis and Emphysema

Chronic bronchitis and emphysema are irreversible diseases which tend to present at a relatively late stage. Patients usually do not become symptomatic until the $FEV_1$ is reduced by 50%. Preventative measures applied sufficiently early can stop the development of severe airways obstruction (see Fig. 5.1). They will decrease the rate of deterioration in patients with severe disease but their value is clearly greater the earlier the stage of disease at which they are introduced. Great emphasis must be put on early diagnosis.

The earlier that a measure of airways obstruction can be made and the relevance of this explained to the patient, the more likely the patient is to stop smoking. Repeat measurements of $FEV_1$ or PEF will chart the rate of deterioration and identify patients at particular risk.

General measures to reduce atmospheric pollution have clearly been important in the past. They need to be kept in mind in the future, particularly in countries which are now becoming industrialised. Dust levels should be monitored and controlled in certain occupations, such as mining. In the Third World better ventilation of houses is required.

# Management of Patients with Chronic Bronchitis and Emphysema

There is at present no definitive treatment for chronic bronchitis and emphysema. The aims of management and treatment are to treat exacerbations promptly, alleviate symptoms and try to prevent complications. The management of ventilatory failure is discussed in Chapter 6. Recent developments in replacing $\alpha_1 PI$ are discussed on page 67.

## General Measures

In patients with relatively mild symptoms, stopping smoking is of paramount importance. Patients able to do so show a reduced rate of decline in $FEV_1$, reduced morbidity and reduced mortality. Dusty atmospheres should be avoided and overweight patients should be encouraged to lose weight. Exercise should be encouraged. Exacerbations of acute bronchitis should be treated promptly.

In patients with more severe disability, cough and breathlessness may be improved by stopping smoking. In these patients exercise should be encouraged within the patient's capability to maintain general fitness and morale. Unsupervised rehabilitation programmes at home can increase exercise tolerance and general well being. Specific aids, including a lightweight tricycle and a walking frame with wheels, can increase mobility in the severely disabled but often do not translate easily to a home environment. Influenza vaccination is recommended during epidemics but routine vaccination is probably not worthwhile because of lack of specificity of the vaccine.

Patients contemplating air travel may need guidance since aircraft cabins are not pressurised and arterial $PO_2$ will fall. In one study of patients with an $FEV_1$ of around 1 litre, $PaO_2$ fell from 9 kPa to 6.8 kPa (70–50 mmHg). The most useful index of ability to cope with a commercial flight is the patient's exercise tolerance; if this exceeds 50 m there will usually be no problems. Patients often find getting on and off the aeroplane more trying than the flight and most airlines will provide a wheelchair. The airline should be informed if the patient is disabled and hypoxaemic so that oxygen can be made available on the flight if requested.

## Acute Exacerbation of Bronchitis

In the absence of an effective antiviral agent, treatment of acute exacerbations is directed towards the bacterial infection, usually recognised by the development of purulent sputum. These episodes should be treated promptly with a 5- or 7-day course of a suitable antibiotic. Sputum culture is unnecessary in an uncomplicated episode, being often unhelpful and sometimes misleading. Infection may also present with a feeling of "congestion" but no purulent sputum, or with increased cough, particularly at night, and these episodes should also be treated with antibiotics.

The antibiotics of choice are tetracycline, co-trimoxazole, ampicillin or amoxycillin. Most studies with these antibiotics show clearing of sputum purulence in about 70% of patients by 7 days. Patients with airways obstruction or recurrent episodes of acute bronchitis should keep a supply of antibiotics at home with instructions to take them promptly when an exacerbation occurs, or be told to contact their doctor at the first sign of a chest infection. Treating exacerbations promptly is better than routine long-term chemoprophylaxis, except in a few selected patients. The general use of chemoprophylaxis may cause problems with resistant organisms. Physiotherapy is not necessary for most patients who cough up sputum easily. It may be helpful when sputum is tenacious and is essential when the patient is drowsy. Drowsiness or confusion complicating any infection is an indication for admission to hospital.

An oral vaccine of killed *Haemophilus influenzae* is under trial. In early studies it has caused a marked reduction in the number of clinical episodes of acute bronchitis in patients with chronic airflow obstruction.

## Chronic Symptoms

### Cough and Phlegm

The amount of phlegm will usually decrease when the patient stops smoking. Cough is common but rarely a problem and many patients consider it a normal event. The recent development of cough suggests a new development such as an infection requiring antibiotics or, more rarely, a carcinoma. If cough continues to be a problem, an inhaled $\beta_2$-agonist or antimuscarinic drug should be tried, and if these fail, an innocuous antitussive agent such as simple linctus. Other cough medicines are rarely indicated since the drugs most likely to be effective, such as linctus codeine, may depress ventilation and precipitate respiratory failure (see Chap. 22).

Mucolytic agents have been advocated for patients with tenacious sputum but have been disappointing in practice. Although three recent studies have shown a reduction in infective episodes in patients taking acetylcysteine for several months, further studies are needed to balance the relatively small benefit against the cost and possible side-effects of a drug taken regularly for many years. Present evidence does not justify the routine use of mucolytic agents but they may be tried in patients with particularly viscous or sticky sputum.

### Ankle Oedema

Ankle oedema usually responds to a thiazide diuretic initially, such as bendrofluorazide 5 mg daily, but a stronger diuretic such as frusemide or bumetamide may be needed as fluid retention increases. Digoxin is not indicated since oedema is usually due to excess fluid retention rather than heart failure and patients with chronic bronchitis appear to be more prone to digoxin-induced arrhythmias such as atrial tachycardia.

## Breathlessness

β-Adrenoceptor agonists, antimuscarinic drugs and theophyllines all cause some bronchodilatation in patients with chronic bronchitis and emphysema though considerably less than that seen in patients with asthma. Treatment should be started with an inhaled drug — either a $\beta_2$-agonist or an antimuscarinic drug. In general, the increase in $FEV_1$ or peak flow is similar with the two types of drug when given in standard doses. The combination of a $\beta_2$-agonist and ipratropium has caused a greater increase in $FEV_1$ in most studies, but the actual magnitude of this increase is small. It is probably only worth trying in patients with severe disability. The addition of an oral theophylline usually causes minimal additional bronchodilatation and does not normally justify the use of these potentially toxic drugs in these patients.

The place of steroids in the management of patients with chronic bronchitis and emphysema is still debated. The majority of patients with chronic bronchitis show no benefit from a steroid trial in which prednisolone 30 mg or 40 mg daily is given orally for 2 or 3 weeks. A few patients show a small increase in $FEV_1$ which would not in itself justify long-term steroid therapy. A trial of steroids should be carried out in any patient with significant symptoms and in any with a large response to a β-adrenoceptor agonist, variability in their airways obstruction, or blood or sputum eosinophilia. If the patient shows a good response (a 20% improvement in $FEV_1$ or PEF), an inhaled steroid should be added and the prednisolone reduced to the minimum dose needed to maintain the improvement. Whether these patients should be described as having late onset asthma or an allergic element to their chronic bronchitis is of some academic interest but does not affect management.

A few patients with chronic bronchitis and emphysema have a large bulla or bullae which can occasionally be helped by resection or plication. Unfortunately, breathlessness in these patients is usually due more to their generalised emphysema that to the bulla, and when this is the case the effects of surgery are disappointing. Detailed investigations are needed to try to assess the contribution of the bulla to the patient's symptoms. Patients with a relatively well preserved $FEV_1$ appear to benefit most from surgery.

## Severe Breathlessness

This is the most distressing symptom in patients with end-stage chronic bronchitis and emphysema. Attempts to alleviate it include the following:

1. *High dose nebulised $\beta_2$-agonists.* Large doses of a $\beta_2$-agonist can be given on a regular basis by nebuliser to patients at home. There have been few studies of

this treatment in patients with chronic bronchitis except to show that it is better than placebo and can be administered without too much difficulty. Patients appear to gain some benefit, though it is relatively small and in some instances may be a placebo effect. These ex-smoking patients have an increased risk of having coronary artery disease so doses of $\beta_2$-agonists should be kept on the low side of those recommended. The potential development of arrhythmias or tolerance to the effects of the drug might be anticipated but in a severely breathless patient the risk is worth taking.

2. *Domiciliary oxygen.* Oxygen is often prescribed at the request of the patient in the hope that it will alleviate breathlessness. The symptomatic benefit to most patients is unfortunately small, mainly because breathlessness is due in large part to factors other than hypoxaemia. Nocturnal oxygen may improve sleep quality. An attempt should be made to assess whether oxygen is going to give symptomatic relief before prescribing it for use at home. This requires a single-blind comparison of oxygen with air, since controlled studies have shown a fairly marked placebo effect for both exercise tolerance and breathlessness. Oxygen, whether taken before or during exercise, usually causes a small further increase (10%–20%) in exercise tolerance with some relief of breathlessness. Patients need oxygen at times of maximal activity such as getting dressed, going to the lavatory and eating meals, and in practice it is difficult to administer oxygen on these occasions from a single cylinder. Portable oxygen circumvents this problem to some extent but the extra effort needed to carry the apparatus tends to offset the advantage gained from the oxygen itself. When patients with domiciliary oxygen were asked whether, given the choice, they would prefer to keep their salbutamol inhaler or oxygen, most chose salbutamol despite the fact that they had chronic bronchitis for which the benefit from a β-agonist was unlikely to be large.

3. *Drugs to relieve breathlessness.* Recent attempts have been made to identify drugs which would relieve the sensation of breathlessness without depressing ventilation. Most drugs unfortunately reduce the two in parallel. The limited studies so far have usually looked at single doses of each drug and more studies are needed. A drug such as promethazine or dihydrocodeine can be tried in patients who are extremely breathless if symptoms warrant the risk entailed and care is taken with dosage.

4. *Experimental procedures.* The poor results with conventional attempts to relieve severe breathlessness have led to more experimental approaches such as right-sided vagotomy and radiotherapy to the emphysematous lung. Neither has been shown to be of benefit.

## Treatment of Complications

Polycythaemia and pulmonary hypertension inevitably develop as chronic airflow obstruction becomes more severe. It is unclear to what extent they independently affect morbidity and prognosis and to what extent they merely reflect the severity of the underlying disease. This is important since it influences the enthusiasm with which the complications are identified and treated as separate problems.

*Polycythaemia*

Red cell mass in patients with chronic bronchitis correlates reasonably well with daytime arterial oxygen saturation. Patients with polycythaemia have a higher incidence of right ventricular hypertrophy, right heart failure and symptoms of somnolence, lethargy and headache. Some of these findings are thought to be due to polycythaemia and others to the underlying disease. Animal studies suggest that more severe polycythaemia has a disadvantageous effect on oxygen delivery, the advantages of increased oxygen carrying capacity being more than offset by the increased blood viscosity which causes increased pulmonary and systemic vascular resistance and a fall in cardiac output. In patients with haematocrit values above 60%, a reduction of haematocrit to below 50% by venesection has usually been associated with a reduction in pulmonary artery pressure and pulmonary vascular resistance and an increase in exercise capacity. Symptoms of lethargy and headache have improved, possibly as a result of increased cerebral blood flow. The risks and morbidity attached to untreated polycythaemia have not been clearly established, but in view of the symptomatic improvement, it is recommended that patients with a haematocrit above 60% should be treated with the aim of reducing it to around 50%.

Various forms of treatment for polycythaemia have been tried, including venesection, exchange transfusion, erythrapheresis, long-term oxygen and drugs.

1. Venesection is the most widely used method. Between 300 ml and 500 ml blood are removed every 48 h until the desired haematocrit is obtained. Simple venesection can cause over-rapid fluid depletion and may lead to a temporary increase in some clotting factors. Exchange transfusion has been advocated, replacing half of the volume of blood removed with plasma or dextran 40 in 5% dextrose immediately, and giving the remainder over the next 8–12 h. Up to 3 litres of blood can be removed at one time so the total reduction in red cell mass can be achieved in one session. The fall in cardiac output and tissue oxygen delivery which follows venesection alone has not been seen following exchange transfusion, but anaphylactic reactions to dextran can occur. More recently, erythrapheresis has been recommended, and again the total reduction in red cell mass can be achieved in one session. The volume of the removed red cells is replaced by plasma. Patients having red cells removed must not be allowed to become iron deficient and may require iron treatment.

2. Although continuous oxygen treatment when given in hospital for 6 weeks will reduce polycythaemia and produce symptomatic improvement, two recent studies of long-term domiciliary oxygen for 18 h a day showed only a small reduction in red cell mass at 6 months. In a smaller study, red cell mass decreased in subjects whose carboxyhaemoglobin values fell but not in those who continued to smoke.

3. Radioactive phosphorus and combinations of drugs such as dapsone to reduce red cell survival and pyrimethamine to reduce erythropoiesis have been used to reduce red cell mass, but their side effects (over-correction anaemia, thrombocytopenia and folate deficiency) make them less acceptable than venesection.

At present venesection, exchange transfusion, or erythrapheresis if facilities are available, are the treatments of choice. Polycythaemia usually recurs in 3 to 6 months, though the time can vary from weeks to years. Packed cell volume should be checked every 2 to 3 months.

## Pulmonary Hypertension

Several studies have shown that long-term domiciliary oxygen when taken for 15 hours a day reduces pulmonary hypertension and causes a small reduction in mortality in patients with chronic bronchitis. This can be managed by patients going out to work but it obviously requires considerable co-operation and adaptation. In the MRC study (1981), benefit was apparent after 500 days of treatment. The benefit has to be balanced against the cost, inconvenience and disruption of normal life for these patients. We only use it in highly selected, relatively young patients who have stopped smoking and who recognise that they must adhere to the number of hours of oxygen a day for the rest of their lives.

The short-term oxygen studies demonstrate that part of the pulmonary hypertension in patients with chronic bronchitis and emphysema is reversible, and raise the relatively unexplored possibility that it might be modified by pharmacological intervention. Drugs which cause systemic vasodilatation, such as $\alpha$-methyl dopa, hydralazine, nifedipine, $\beta$-agonists and diazoxide, usually cause a fall in pulmonary vascular resistance. However, large doses can reduce cardiac output and blood pressure and the drugs appear to have a fairly small therapeutic window in patients with pulmonary hypertension. They cannot be recommended for routine use at present.

Pulmonary embolism and thrombosis are not uncommon findings at necropsy in patients with chronic bronchitis and emphysema, and will accentuate the development of pulmonary hypertension. Diagnosis can be difficult since small additional losses of perfusion are not easily detected in these patients with abnormal ventilation perfusion scans. Anticoagulants should be considered when the condition is strongly suspected on clinical grounds.

## Future Developments

Increased understanding of protease/antiprotease balance in the lung and the isolation and ability to manufacture $\alpha_1$PI protein have already led to exciting developments and new approaches to the prevention of emphysema. These aim to reduce the rate at which emphysema develops by tilting the balance between proteases and protease inhibitors in the lung. So far, attempts to increase production or release of $\alpha_1$PI from the liver have not been very successful. Both danazol and tamoxifen have caused small increases in serum $\alpha_1$PI levels in some patients but not enough to be likely to be clinically effective. Attempts are now being made to replace $\alpha_1$PI in deficient patients. It has been obtained from pooled human plasma with 60% purity and is now being administered on a weekly basis to selected patients. Serum levels remain above those considered necessary to neutralise elastase in the lung. Long-term protection by this route is not practicable and is undesirable because of the risk of bloodborne infections. Recombinant

DNA techniques have therefore been used to produce an aglycosylated protein with the same amino acid sequence as $\alpha_1$PI. Unfortunately, the absence of the carbohydrate group results in a much shorter half-life, measured in hours rather than days as with human $\alpha_1$PI. Manipulation of the amino acid sequence is now being attempted to produce a molecule with similar activity against elastases but a longer half-life. Elastase inhibitors other than $\alpha_1$PI are also being investigated. These developments are likely to provide effective therapy for patients with $\alpha_1$PI in the next few years and perhaps to a wider group of patients with emphysema at a later date. It must be emphasised, however, that no treatment will ever be anywhere near as effective as prevention, and chronic bronchitis and emphysema are almost completely preventable.

# Useful References

Cohen AB (1986) Unravelling the mysteries of alpha$_1$-antitrypsin deficiency. N Engl J Med 314: 778–779

Doll R, Peto R (1976) Mortality in relation to smoking: 20 years' observations on male British doctors. Br Med J II: 1525–1536

Editorial (1985) Treatment for alpha$_1$-antitrypsin deficiency. Lancet II: 812–813

Flenley DC, Downing I, Greening AP (1986) The pathogenesis of emphysema. Bull Eur Physiopathol Resp 22: 245s–252s

Fletcher C, Peto R (1977) The natural history of chronic airflow obstruction. Br Med J 1: 1645–1648

Fletcher C, Peto R, Tinker C, Speizer FE (1976) The natural history of chronic bronchitis and emphysema. Oxford University Press, London

Harrison BDW, Stokes TC (1982) Secondary polycythaemia: its causes, effects and treatment. Br J Dis Chest 76: 313–339

Holland WW (1982) Beginnings of bronchitis. Thorax 37: 401–403

Janoff A (1985) Elastases and emphysema. Current assessment of the protease–antiprotease hypothesis. Am Rev Resp Dis 132: 417–433

Medical Research Council Working Party (1981) Long term domiciliary oxygen therapy in chronic hypoxic cor pulmonale complicating chronic bronchitis and emphysema. Lancet I: 681–685

Mullen JBM, Wright JL, Wiggs BR, Pare PD, Hogg JC (1985) Reassessment of inflammation of airways in chronic bronchitis. Br Med J 291: 1235–1239

Peto R, Speizer FE, Cochrane AL, Moore F, Fletcher CM, Tinker CM, Higgins ITT, Gray RG, Richards SM, Gilliland J, Norman-Smith B (1983) The relevance in adults of airflow obstruction, but not of mucus hypersecretion, to mortality from chronic lung disease. Am Rev Resp Dis 128: 491–500

Snider GL (1981) The pathogenesis of emphysema — twenty years of progress. Am Rev Resp Dis 198: 321–324

Stockley RA (1983) Proteolytic enzymes, their inhibitors and lung diseases. Clin Sci 64: 119–126

Stradling JR, Lane DJ (1981) Editorial. Development of secondary polycythaemia in chronic airways obstruction. Thorax 36: 321–325

Warren PM, Flenley DC (1983) Chronic bronchitis and emphysema. In: Flenley DC, Petty TL (eds) Recent advances in respiratory medicine. Churchill Livingstone, Edinburgh, pp 173–191

# 6 Respiratory Failure and Sleep-related Breathing Disorders

## Definition

Respiratory failure is defined in terms of arterial blood gases — a low $PO_2$, a high $PCO_2$ or a combination of the two. The working definition of the normal limits for oxygen and carbon dioxide is loosely set ($PaO_2$ >8 kPa, 60 mmHg; $PaCO_2$ <7 kPa, 50 mmHg). A stricter definition would include so many patients as to be clinically meaningless.

Hypoxaemia frequently occurs in the absence of carbon dioxide retention, but carbon dioxide retention is almost invariably accompanied by hypoxaemia.

## General Approach to the Patient in Respiratory Failure

The mechanisms producing blood gas abnormalities must be identified and treatment directed at them and at the primary disease. Low arterial oxygen tension almost always reflects failure of gas exchange in the lung, while high arterial carbon dioxide tension usually reflects abnormality of ventilatory control or ventilatory mechanisms. It is useful to consider hypoxaemia and carbon dioxide retention separately.

### Hypoxaemia

In broad physiological terms hypoxaemia may be due to:

1. low inspired oxygen
2. inadequate ventilation
3. impairment of gas exchange in the lung
4. anatomical shunting through a right-to-left shunt.

Low inspired oxygen is a very rare cause of hypoxaemia, but the possibility must be borne in mind in the highly artificial situations of mechanical ventilation during anaesthesia or in the intensive care unit when gases may be wrongly identified and low oxygen mixtures given in error. Underventilation is a more important cause of hypoxaemia. A rise in alveolar $PCO_2$ inevitably causes a fall in alveolar and arterial $PO_2$, but its effect is not great unless the rise in $PCO_2$ is considerable. The most important cause of hypoxaemia is failure of gas exchange and this almost invariably complicates respiratory failure whatever its primary cause. Although anatomical right-to-left shunts cause marked hypoxaemia, in practice they are rare.

Failure of gas exchange is due to mismatching of ventilation and blood flow, with an increased proportion of alveoli underventilated relative to their blood flow. It usually results from factors which cause patchy reduction in ventilation. There is no ventilation in the consolidated or atelectatic lung and if perfusion continues, the capillaries function as anatomical shunts. Interstitial oedema or lung infiltration makes alveoli stiff so that they are relatively poorly ventilated. Change in airway resistance, as in asthma, or secretion retention reduces ventilation of the distal segment. Abnormalities of distribution of perfusion are of lesser importance, but they make a large contribution to hypoxaemia in pulmonary embolism. Cardiac output becomes important when gas exchange impairment is severe. Arterial $PO_2$ is then increasingly dependent on mixed venous $PO_2$, which is largely determined by cardiac output.

Impairment of gas exchange is quantitated by measurement of either the alveolar–arterial oxygen tension difference ($A–aDO_2$), or the shunt ratio. Both measurements take into account inspired oxygen tension, arterial $PO_2$, and arterial $PCO_2$. The $A–aDO_2$ expresses the abnormality in terms of a notional pressure drop for oxygen between the alveolus and the arterial blood, and the shunt ratio in terms of a notional proportion of cardiac output which bypasses the lungs. The normal values for $A–aDO_2$ rise from 1 kPa (7 mmHg) in young adults to 4 kPa (30 mmHg) at 70 years, and the shunt ratio from 5% to 10%.

## Carbon Dioxide Retention

The normal control of ventilation is set to maintain a broadly constant $PaCO_2$ in the face of wide variations in carbon dioxide production. Its efficacy depends on an intact central sensing mechanism, and a normally functioning effector mechanism — neuromuscular pathways, respiratory muscles, chest wall, airways and alveoli. Failure of ventilatory control may have a single specific cause such as respiratory depression in drug overdose, but its cause is more often multifactorial and it rarely remains uncomplicated for any length of time. Patients with apparently straightforward central respiratory depression from drug overdose quickly develop problems from secretion retention, atelectasis and infection; patients with severe airways disease usually develop problems with central control mechanisms, and gas exchange is often also abnormal; respiratory muscle fatigue is a common complication of respiratory failure, whatever its cause.

Once carbon dioxide retention is established, central respiratory sensitivity is blunted and the ventilatory response to a further rise in arterial $PCO_2$ is depressed. Other mechanisms such as the hypoxic drive become increasingly important in ventilatory control.

# Effects of Hypoxaemia and Carbon Dioxide Retention

## Hypoxaemia

For hypoxaemia the situation is complex. Tissue oxygen delivery is more important than any particular level of arterial $PO_2$. Oxygen delivery depends primarily on tissue perfusion and is more dependent on cardiac output and blood flow than on arterial oxygen content or pressure. Arterial oxygen content is a function of the amount and quality of the haemoglobin and its oxygen saturation, the last being the only factor directly influenced by the $PO_2$. The normal response to inadequate oxygen delivery is vasodilatation and an increase in cardiac output. Severe anaemia and hypoxaemia are usually tolerated with little evidence of impairment of tissue function, but problems arise when cardiac output or tissue blood flow cannot be increased, as is often the case in acutely ill patients. The only available method to compensate for hypoxaemia in this situation is to increase oxygen extraction. Tissue damage from oxygen lack is likely to be produced first and most severely in tissues such as the brain which require a high $PO_2$ and cannot increase oxygen extraction. Hypoxaemia itself rarely produces hypoxic tissue damage; it is almost always the result of inadequate perfusion, either from a low cardiac output or local reduction in tissue blood flow.

There is no good index of overall adequacy of tissue oxygenation. Arterial $PO_2$ and saturation are easy to measure, but have limited significance. Mixed venous oxygen saturation is probably the single most useful index of the overall adequacy of tissue perfusion. However, even a normal mixed venous oxygen level does not exclude severe hypoxia in individual poorly perfused tissues since their lack of perfusion ensures that they are ill-represented in mixed venous blood. Measures of anaerobic metabolism such as lactic acidosis or metabolic acidosis are more readily available, but only become abnormal when tissue hypoxia is severe and widespread. There are no useful indicators for hypoxia in individual tissues. Progressive intellectual impairment, the classical clinical sign of hypoxaemia, is of little practical value. Evidence of failure of other organs such as the liver with rise in circulating enzyme levels is similarly of little help in patient management.

## Carbon Dioxide Retention

Carbon dioxide retention of itself rarely produces major problems unless it is severe (PaCO$_2$ >9 kPa, 70 mmHg). The main physiological response to a rise in arterial $PCO_2$ is an increase in cardiac output and peripheral vasodilatation. Neither is of major consequence, except in patients with organic neurological disease and increased intracranial pressure, when increased formation of cerebrospinal fluid may promote brain oedema. At high levels ($PCO_2$ >10 kPa, 75 mmHg) CNS function starts to be depressed, with lowering of the level of consciousness and depression of respiration and cough. In the spontaneously breathing patient this can initiate a vicious cycle of deteriorating lung function. In the anaesthetised patient with adequate oxygenation, levels of $PCO_2$ over 16 kPa (120 mmHg) have been tolerated without major problems.

# Assessment of the Patient in Respiratory Failure

It is helpful to consider the factors influencing carbon dioxide excretion and oxygen uptake separately. If the $PaCO_2$ is elevated, a cause of overall ventilatory failure should be sought. If the $PaCO_2$ is low and the A–a$DO_2$ increased, a cause of failure of gas exchange should be sought. An attempt must be made to identify both the primary cause and its complications.

### Causes of Ventilatory Failure

Central respiratory depression by drugs is common. The drugs may have been used therapeutically — anaesthetic agents, analgesics and sedatives — or they may have been taken in overdose — barbiturates, benzodiazepines, opiates etc. Respiratory depression from organic disease affecting the respiratory centre is much less common. The most extreme example is respiratory arrest from medullary coning due to increased intracranial pressure. Lesser increases in intracranial pressure or vascular lesions can produce changes in the pattern of breathing or respiratory depression. When neurological disease affects the brain stem it may involve not only the respiratory centre, but also the laryngeal reflexes. Airway protection is then impaired and the risks to the lung are greatly increased.

Modern intensive care owes much to the epidemic of poliomyelitis of the early 1950s. Today, ventilatory failure from neurological or muscle disease affecting the respiratory muscles is relatively rare. Prolonged postoperative action of the neuromuscular drugs given during anaesthesia is now the commonest neuromuscular cause of ventilatory failure. Most patients with extensive neurological or neuromuscular disease eventually die a respiratory death, but only a few patients are treated by mechanical ventilation. In the United Kingdom it is usually reserved for patients with a potentially reversible condition such as polyneuritis. Assessment of the cause and prognosis of the underlying neurological disease is essential before mechanical ventilation is undertaken.

Two types of chest wall lesion are common causes of respiratory failure: the flail chest of trauma with multiple rib fractures, and the grossly deformed chest of the patient with severe kyphoscoliosis.

The single condition most often associated with inadequate ventilation is severe chronic airway obstruction ($FEV_1 < 1.2$ l). These patients often have mild chronic underventilation and develop major problems with ventilatory failure in the course of a complicating illness such as an acute respiratory infection or a surgical procedure. Ventilatory failure due to extensive alveolar disease is rare but is seen in the adult respiratory distress syndrome or severe left ventricular failure when it is due to a combination of stiff lungs and increased physiological dead space.

### Causes of Gas Exchange Failure

Impairment of gas exchange in respiratory failure is due to abnormalities which increase the number of underventilated alveoli: atelectasis or consolidation with continuing perfusion; airway obstruction by secretions or bronchoconstriction; alveoli made uncompliant by interstitial oedema due to infection, heart failure or capillary damage. The role of oedema in the lung is particularly important. The fluid balance of the lung is normally fairly delicate. Pulmonary venous capillary pressure is higher than in systemic capillaries and tissue pressure, like intrathoracic pressure, is negative. Both tend to cause movement of fluid into the lung. Any rise in left atrial pressure, lowering of oncotic pressure or increase in capillary permeability will tend to cause lung oedema with increasing impairment of gas exchange.

# The General Objectives of Treatment

Treatment is directed at four objectives:

1. curing the primary abnormality
2. improving lung function
3. maintaining an adequate oxygen supply
4. maintaining adequate ventilation for carbon dioxide excretion.

Recovery depends on success in dealing with the primary cause and in maintaining or improving lung function. Maintenance of oxygen supply and carbon dioxide excretion are essentially supportive measures. The vigour with which these objectives are pursued depends greatly on the underlying condition. For the patient with an acute, completely reversible illness, complete recovery is the only acceptable outcome, while in patients with advanced and essentially irreversible disease a much more limited objective is clearly appropriate. An explicit decision on these limitations should be made at an early stage in treatment.

### Management of the Primary Cause

This is considered in the more detailed sections on pages 76–82.

## Improving the Function of the Lungs

Good secretion management is essential; secretion retention is almost invariable and atelectasis is common. Infection must be treated by secretion drainage and antibiotics. If there is any reversible component to airway obstruction, broncho-dilators should be given. As the lungs are liable to become oedematous, fluid balance should be carefully watched and fluid retention should be treated. These apparently not very dramatic measures are essential for all patients in respiratory failure and play a large role in determining the outcome. Meanwhile gas exchange must be maintained.

## Oxygen Supply

As oxygen supply depends mainly on cardiac output, maintenance of cardiac output must have high priority in treatment. Adequate haemoglobin levels are also important ($>10$ g/100 ml). Gas exchange function of the lung will improve with treatment of infection, drainage of secretions, relief of airways obstruction and removal of fluid overload.

In the short term, oxygenation of arterial blood may be improved by increasing the inspired oxygen concentration. Oxygen therapy is supportive, not curative. It may prevent death or serious damage from hypoxaemia, but if carelessly given, particularly in patients with ventilatory failure, it can do much harm. Oxygen is almost invariably given, and its use requires detailed consideration.

The objective of oxygen therapy is to achieve a "safe" arterial $PO_2$. The "safe" or "adequate" level varies under different conditions, but an attempt to define it is essential. For patients without preceding respiratory disease a $PaO_2 > 8$ kPa (60 mmHg), corresponding to an oxygen saturation greater than 90%, is acceptable. In patients with severe chronic respiratory disease, lower levels of $PaO_2$ are usu-ally appropriate, possibly as low as 6 kPa (45 mmHg). Many of these patients are accustomed to living with a low arterial $PO_2$ and have adapted to it. They are remarkably tolerant of hypoxaemia provided that cardiac output is maintained. They often also have ventilatory failure with impaired carbon dioxide sensitivity and their ventilation is dependent on a hypoxic drive. They require particular care with oxygen therapy, as inappropriately vigorous pursuit of high arterial oxygen tensions may lead to serious progressive underventilation.

If respiratory control is normal, as evidenced by a normal $PaCO_2 < 6$ kPa (45 mmHg), inspired oxygen can generally be increased to attain a "safe" $PaO_2$ and hence an "adequate" arterial oxygen content without problems. If inspired oxygen concentrations greater than 40%–50% are required, lung function is seriously impaired and mechanical ventilation should be considered. It is usually an effec-tive and relatively easy method of improving gas exchange. If high inspired oxygen concentrations are required ($F_IO_2 \geq 0.5$) in a ventilated patient, the use of positive end-expiratory pressure (PEEP) should be considered. PEEP maintains alveolar patency and improves gas exchange at the expense of an increase in intrathoracic pressure which tends to reduce venous return and may lower cardiac output. A balance has to be struck between these opposing effects to achieve optimum increase in oxygen delivery. In the spontaneously breathing patient, continuous positive airway pressure (CPAP) has a similar effect but its application is less easy.

If respiratory control is impaired, as evidenced by a high $PaCO_2$, particularly if the acid–base values suggest that carbon dioxide retention is chronic, much more care is required with oxygen therapy. Enough oxygen must be given to relieve dangerous hypoxaemia, but not enough to cause a dangerous increase in under-ventilation. The use of oxygen in these patients is considered in more detail on page 79.

## Carbon Dioxide Excretion

Measurement of arterial $PCO_2$ provides a simple assessment of the overall adequacy of ventilation and carbon dioxide excretion. It does not measure the work of breathing nor the oxygen cost of ventilation, both of which may be considerably increased in patients with stiff lungs or high airway resistance, and which, like muscle fatigue, may be important limiting factors. They are difficult to measure, but should be assessed subjectively when evaluating the spontaneously breathing patient. Great respiratory effort or fatigue as well as a rising $PaCO_2$ suggest a need for mechanical ventilation.

In general, mechanical ventilation is indicated when there is an acute elevation of $PaCO_2$. It is not a particularly difficult undertaking and provides effective short-term support with the added advantages of access for secretion drainage and usually improvement in gas exchange. Initially there are few drawbacks, but when mechanical ventilation is prolonged, secondary infection and hypersecretion are almost invariable, and muscle wasting is rapid. When the primary disease is advanced and there is no well defined reversible precipitating cause of the acute episode, the complications of ventilation can easily outweigh the benefits, and major difficulties may be encountered when weaning is attempted. Prolonged ventilation of the patient with end-stage respiratory disease is not generally regarded as appropriate in the United Kingdom, although it is sometimes used in North America. In patients with advanced disease a more conservative approach is required. Carbon dioxide retention is not of itself particularly harmful provided that the $PaCO_2$ does not reach narcotic levels. If mechanical ventilation is thought to be contraindicated, particular care should be taken to limit the rise in $PaCO_2$. This almost always involves a more cautious approach to oxygen therapy.

The alternative approach for underventilation is the use of respiratory stimulants (see Chap. 20). Their role is limited. Central respiratory depression is not often a specific problem and there is as yet no really effective specific respiratory stimulant. Even if such a drug were available, the response to it might be less than expected, as the cost of the increased ventilation in patients with abnormal lungs and airways may be high. Treatment directed exclusively to respiratory depression has a role in the management of opiate overdose where a specific antagonist is available, and a limited role in the management of progressive respiratory depression following oxygen therapy in patients with severe chronic chest disease. Respiratory stimulants may also have a limited place in the treatment of post-operative respiratory failure.

# Respiratory Failure in Specific Diseases

The common causes of respiratory failure are as follows:

1. *Postoperative.* Central respiratory depression from anaesthetics and analgesics and ventilatory impairment from persisting muscle relaxant action and wound pain. Most often occurs in patients with chronic chest disease, electrolyte or acid base disturbances.
2. *Drug overdose.* Mainly central depression.
3. *Trauma.* Mechanical chest wall problems with contused, oedematous and hypersecreting lung.
4. *Chronic bronchitis.* Ventilatory failure from chronic airway obstruction often with infection and always with secretion problems.
5. *Asthma.* Acute unevenly distributed airway obstruction with hypoxaemia, ventilatory failure and often low cardiac output.
6. *Pulmonary oedema due to left ventricular failure.* Oedematous and stiff alveoli.
7. *Adult respiratory distress syndrome (ARDS).* A syndrome of diffuse capillary damage with prominent pulmonary manifestations.

These more common conditions are considered in detail.

## Postoperative Respiratory Failure

Inadequate restoration of spontaneous ventilation in the immediate postoperative period is most common in patients who are generally unwell and have other problems such as hypokalaemia, metabolic acidosis or hypothermia. Respiratory depression is due to persisting effects of anaesthetic or analgesic agents together with inadequate or delayed reversal of muscle relaxant drugs. The respiratory pattern may be diagnostic, with slow or shallow breathing from persisting analgesic or anaesthetic action, or jerky irregular breathing with a tracheal tug from the persisting muscle relaxant effect.

A clear airway should be maintained and the patient should be kept well oxygenated. The patient should be re-intubated promptly and ventilated if there is any doubt about his or her ability to maintain ventilation. Inadequate reversal of non-depolarising block should be treated with a further dose of atropine and neostigmine, and persisting opiate action reversed by naloxone. Fresh frozen plasma should be given for persisting neuromuscular block due to depolarising agents. Metabolic acidosis and hypokalaemia should be corrected. Unless there is an unequivocal reponse to these measures, continuation of ventilation is to be preferred to the repeated use of pharmacological antagonists. It is usually required for 12–18 h. The abnormal responses to anaesthetics, analgesics and muscle relaxants wear off within 12 h, and during that time acid–base, electrolyte and temperature abnormalities can be corrected. The action of most of the antagonists is short lived and they are not entirely free from side-effects.

Late postoperative respiratory failure tends to occur in patients with chronic chest disease who have a poor cough and usually a painful upper abdominal wound. It should be treated by vigorous physiotherapy to clear secretions, antibiotics if infection is present, and extra oxygen if the $PaO_2$ is <8 kPa (60 mmHg). Minitracheostomy may give adequate access for secretion control. Mechanical ventilation may occasionally be required, but unless there is a specific reversible cause of deterioration the results are usually poor.

## Respiratory Failure in Drug Overdose

In drug overdose, central depression of respiration is common, but many drugs also lower metabolic rate and oxygen requirements and this has a "protective" effect. Respiration is rarely affected alone, and other autonomic functions such as temperature control (benzodiazepine and phenothiazine overdose) and circulatory control (barbiturate, opiate and phenothiazine overdose) are often depressed. With the exception of the use of naloxone in opiate overdose, there are no specific antagonists. Non-specific "antagonists" should not be used as primary therapy as their side-effects can be troublesome and they usually do more harm than good.

Adequate fluid should be given so that cardiac output and urine flow are maintained. Hypothermic patients should be slowly rewarmed. When unconsciousness is prolonged, respiratory tract care and secretion management are of great importance; aspiration or atelectasis is likely to lead to infection. Oxygen should be given to maintain an adequate $PaO_2$. Provided that oxygenation is maintained and that the patient's condition is clinically stable, it is safe in drug overdose to accept moderate underventilation ($PaCO_2$ up to 8 kPa, 60 mmHg). For more severe underventilation mechanical ventilation is indicated. As cardiovascular reflexes are usually depressed, adequate volume replacement is essential to prevent hypotension with intermittent positive pressure ventilation (IPPV). Ventilation will have to be continued for a variable period until the drug involved is cleared, perhaps for several days with the currently fashionable benzodiazepines. Measures aimed at increasing drug excretion such as inducing brisk diuresis are of no value.

## Respiratory Failure in Chest Injury

Chest injuries cause multiple interacting problems. Lung contusion produces hypersecretion and stiff lungs with impairment of gas exchange. Rib fractures, pneumothorax or haemothorax cause problems with ventilation. Pain and analgesics tend to depress respiration, and an unstable chest wall impairs secretion clearance. Treatment has to be directed at all of these problems. Adequate analgesia is essential and morphine is often required. Intercostal block may be helpful. Oxygen should be given for hypoxaemia and the circulating volume should be adequately restored. If there is a significant pneumothorax or haemothorax, an intercostal drain should be inserted. Cough should be encouraged, but may not be effective.

Mechanical ventilation may be required. The decision to ventilate should be made on clinical grounds. In some patients it is required urgently for obvious acute ventilatory problems. In others the indications, persisting respiratory distress, persisting severe hypoxaemia, failure of secretion clearance and gross chest wall instability, are less urgent. Some patients appear to cope well initially, but lung function deteriorates and increased respiratory effort is required. They become exhausted, paradoxical chest wall movement becomes marked and respiratory failure develops rapidly.

Any pneumothorax must be dealt with before ventilation is started as IPPV can produce a tension pneumothorax with frightening rapidity. When mechanical ventilation has been started it has to be continued until the condition of the underlying lung improves and rib fractures have healed sufficiently to stabilise the chest wall. In young adults this takes 10–14 days, but in older patients it may take over 3 weeks. Tracheostomy may be required.

## Acute Respiratory Failure in Chronic Bronchitis

When airways obstruction is severe ($FEV_1$ <1.2 l), a proportion of patients with chronic bronchitis fail to maintain normal respiratory control and develop chronic underventilation. Underventilation and accompanying abnormalities of gas exchange cause hypoxaemia and this combination is often associated with polycythaemia, fluid retention and pulmonary hypertension. Obesity and nocturnal underventilation may be complicating factors. The commonest precipitating cause of acute respiratory failure is an acute respiratory infection, but it often occurs postoperatively in these patients, and may present unexpected problems if the severity of the underlying chronic chest disease has not been recognised. Acute episodes or respiratory failure have a high mortality (around 20% in the best centres) and the long-term prognosis is also poor.

Infection should be treated vigorously, and good secretion drainage is essential. Although reversibility of airways obstruction is limited, the greatest possible bronchodilatation should be achieved. Fluid retention should be treated with diuretics. There is little specific treatment for underventilation. Although in the chronic state underventilation may be seen as a worthwhile physiological adaptation to severe airways obstruction, the respiratory control mechanisms cope poorly during an acute exacerbation and $PaCO_2$ may reach high and potentially narcotic levels (11 kPa, 80 mmHg). Cardiac output is usually normal or increased, haemoglobin levels are high and there is peripheral vasodilatation as a result of carbon dioxide retention so that oxygen delivery tends to be well maintained despite severe arterial hypoxaemia. It may be difficult to find evidence of tissue impairment other than confusion and drowsiness, which may owe more to hypercarbia than hypoxia.

Correct use of oxygen therapy is important since patients can die from anoxia almost certainly, but they can also die from poorly managed oxygen therapy. Judgement of what constitutes "dangerous" hypoxaemia is empirical. It takes into account arterial $PO_2$ and $PCO_2$ levels and the severity of the underlying chest disease and it involves assumptions about cardiac output and haemoglobin levels. In these patients, in whom carbon dioxide sensitivity is impaired and hypoxic drive important in maintaining ventilation, reduction of hypoxaemia may lead to progressive underventilation. The risk is difficult to predict but is to some extent related to the level of $PaCO_2$. At higher levels of $PaCO_2$, sensitivity to carbon dioxide is more depressed, and dependence on hypoxic drive is more likely. If elevation of $PaCO_2$ is not marked ($<8$ kPa, 60 mmHg), underventilation with oxygen therapy is unlikely to be marked, and its consequences are unlikely to be severe. If the $PaCO_2$ is very high (11 kPa, 80 mmHg), underventilation is not only more likely but its consequences are more likely to be serious since the narcotic level ($>12$–13 kPa, 90–100 mmHg) will be reached with only a small rise in $PaCO_2$. There is little doubt that a $PaO_2$ $>7$ kPa (50 mmHg) is both "safe" and "normal" for many of these patients, giving an oxygen saturation of above 80% and an oxygen supply $>700$ ml/min. With a $PaO_2$ $<5$ kPa (40 mmHg), oxygen saturation is less than 60% and the oxygen supply less than 600 ml/min. Tissue oxygen is liable to be at dangerously low levels, and supplemental oxygen is necessary. When mechanical ventilation is considered to be contraindicated, potentially narcotic rises in $PaCO_2$ must be avoided and a very cautious approach to oxygen therapy is required. A more aggressive approach may be adopted if mechanical ventilation is available to supply a "safety net".

Controlled low concentrations of oxygen should be used either 24% (inspired $PO_2$ = 23 kPa, 170 mmHg) or 28% (inspired $PO_2$ = 27 kPa, 200 mmHg). These concentrations are most effectively delivered by Venturi masks. There should be a target for the arterial $PaO_2$ (6 kPa, 45 mmHg), and the lowest oxygen concentration producing it should be used. If $PaCO_2$ is above 8 kPa (60 mmHg), the initial oxygen concentration should be 24%, with 28% being used only in exceptional circumstances. When oxygen is given it should be given continuously. It is normally required for a relatively short period (up to 72 h), during which time other treatment should produce sufficient improvement in the underlying problem to permit its discontinuation.

If adequate oxygenation cannot be achieved with 28% oxygen, or if there is a rise of $PaCO_2$ with impairment of conscious level, the optimum treatment is mechanical ventilation. It is usually easy to start, but in patients with advanced disease restoration of spontaneous ventilation is difficult and there may be major problems in weaning. It is clearly essential to treat any reversible episode, but it is equally important to recognise that respiratory failure often complicates end-stage chronic chest disease and that in these patients mechanical ventilation has no part in treatment. Criteria for selection for ventilation are based on deteriorating blood gases, and on an assessment of the patient's functional capacity between exacerbations. This appears to be the best predictor of the feasibility of weaning. Ventilation is normally contraindicated in the housebound respiratory cripple and in patients with an exercise tolerance of less than 18 m (20 yards). Ventilation and weaning usually present no problems in those who are able to work, or undertake equivalent physical activity. When the patient's capabilities lie between these extremes, individual judgement is required.

With mechanical ventilation, hypoxaemia can be promptly corrected by increasing inspired oxygen concentrations; a target value for $PaO_2$ of 8 kPa (60 mmHg) is now reasonable. $PaCO_2$ should be reduced over a 24-h period to around

7 kPa (50 mmHg). Lower values are not appropriate. Excessive reduction of $PaCO_2$ may cause problems from reduced cerebral blood flow and will create great problems on weaning. The endotracheal tube allows adequate access for secretion removal, and control of infection is easier in the short term. There are rarely problems in maintaining cardiac output. Ventilation normally has to be continued for 3–5 days. During this time infection should be controlled, adequate clearance of secretions and full bronchodilatation should be achieved, and fluid retention should be dealt with. Weaning should be approached with care. The $PaCO_2$ should be maintained between 6 kPa and 7 kPa (45 mmHg and 50 mmHg) and $PaO_2$ around 7 kPa (55 mmHg) for 24 h before weaning is started. A variety of techniques are available for weaning such as intermittent short spells of spontaneous ventilation and intermittent mandatory ventilation. The period of spontaneous ventilation should be progressively increased over 2–3 days and the patient extubated when adequate spontaneous ventilation has been maintained for 24 h. Weaning may have to be prolonged and tracheostomy, which almost always makes weaning easier, may then be necessary. In patients with chronic chest disease it is better to aim for a short period of ventilation. Secondary infection, hypersecretion and respiratory muscle wasting are inevitable complications of prolonged ventilation, making restoration of spontaneous ventilation much more difficult.

If the patient develops carbon dioxide narcosis and mechanical ventilation is felt to be contraindicated, respiratory stimulants should be used to lower the $PaCO_2$ to "safe" levels. At the moment the drug of choice appears to be doxapram given by continuous intravenous infusion in a dose of 1–2 mg/min (see Chap. 20).

## Respiratory Failure in Asthma

Hypoxaemia increases with increasing severity of asthma. Overventilation is common in the earlier stages, but in severe attacks there is eventually a rise in $PaCO_2$ with a consequent further deterioration in arterial $PO_2$. The ventilatory response in children is less predictable and elevation of $PaCO_2$ may occur in relatively mild attacks. In asthma, unlike chronic bronchitis, cardiac output is usually low. Dehydration reduces circulating volume and increased alveolar pressure reduces left atrial filling. Oxygen delivery is therefore markedly impaired, and metabolic acidosis as a result of anaerobic metabolism is not uncommon in severe attacks. Poor peripheral perfusion makes cyanosis difficult to detect, although hypoxaemia may be severe.

The treatment of respiratory failure in asthma is the standard treatment of severe asthma — steroids, bronchodilators, fluids and oxygen (see Chap. 4). If severe metabolic acidosis is present, it should be partially corrected with bicarbonate to bring the pH above 7.2. If treatment is prompt, most patients respond quickly. Ventilation should be considered if the patient deteriorates despite treatment, or if a previously low $PaCO_2$ rises significantly. In severe asthma, ventilation is not easy and timing of intervention is difficult. Occasionally respiratory arrest forces the issue. If the airways are tightly constricted, very high airway pressures ($>60$ cmH$_2$O) will be required. It is usually possible to improve oxygenation but it may be difficult to achieve sufficient improvement in ventilation to lower the

$PaCO_2$ to normal levels. Initially it is reasonable to accept a moderate reduction in $PaCO_2$ (to around 8 kPa, 60 mmHg), provided that oxygen levels are satisfactory. When exhaustion is the cause of the rising $PaCO_2$, ventilation is usually less difficult.

An "elective" decision to ventilate requires good facilities and skilled operators. It may be difficult to suppress the patient's own respiratory drive and achieve synchronisation with the ventilator. Ineffective respiratory effort not only wastes oxygen supply on the muscles of respiration but it also increases intrathoracic pressure and further reduces venous return and cardiac output. Sedation and paralysis should be adequate to prevent spontaneous ventilation, although this may aggravate the problems of maintaining cardiac output in the volume-depleted patient. The distribution of airways obstruction is always uneven and there is an increased risk of alveolar rupture with pneumothorax or mediastinal emphysema. The ventilator settings require careful adjustment and compromises. A low inspiratory flow rate minimises the rise in airway pressure, but a longer inspiratory time is required to achieve adequate ventilation; excessive prolongation of inspiratory time tends to reduce cardiac output. When ventilation is difficult the priority should be adequate oxygenation rather than reduction in $PaCO_2$.

During the period of intubation and ventilation, secretion control is important. Bronchial lavage to remove mucous plugs enjoyed some popularity, but probably makes little contribution. Other treatment such as the use of ether and halothane, has been described, but has little place in management.

Following mechanical ventilation, improvement is usually rapid, with falling airway pressures and improving gas exchange. Even in the most severely ill the attack usually reverses within 48–72 h. Weaning is rarely a problem.

If patients with asthma are seen and treated appropriately at an earlier stage, many of the more severe attacks requiring mechanical ventilation could be prevented. For most patients the need for ventilation represents a failure of management.

## Left Ventricular Failure

Hypoxaemia is invariable in left ventricular failure and often severe, but it is rarely diagnosed because peripheral vasoconstriction makes detection of cyanosis virtually impossible. It usually responds to conventional treatment with opiates, diuretics and oxygen. If there is delay in response and the patient is very ill, or if exhaustion is a problem, mechanical ventilation is a most useful temporary supportive measure. Hypoxaemia is readily relieved, and the patient spared the work of ventilating stiff oedematous lungs. The mean increase in intrathoracic pressure reduces venous return and is probably beneficial. Left atrial pressure is elevated and left heart filling is usually well maintained despite ventilation. Adverse effects on cardiac output are unusual. Ventilation can normally be discontinued in 24–48 h without problems.

## Sepsis, Shock and Adult Respiratory Distress Syndrome (ARDS)

Diffuse capillary damage complicates several acute illnesses. The most prominent manifestations of this syndrome are in the lung — the adult respiratory distress syndrome, a triad of hypoxaemia, decreased lung compliance and diffuse shadowing on the chest X-ray occurring in the absence of raised left atrial pressure. It is associated with septic states, particularly gram-negative septicaemias, and a wide variety of other conditions: extensive trauma, after massive blood transfusion (>20 units); in prolonged shock states; in fat embolism and in pancreatitis. ARDS is associated with sequestration of neutrophils in the lung, with release of toxic oxygen radicals and other potentially damaging agents. A similar picture restricted to the pulmonary capillaries is seen in smoke or irritant inhalation.

The clinical and radiographic picture may be indistinguishable from that of pulmonary oedema from left heart failure. The pattern of impairment of lung function is also similar — overventilation initially and hypoxaemia. In more severe cases gas exchange becomes so disorganised that carbon dioxide retention may occur despite maintenance of high minute volumes, and hypoxaemia cannot be corrected by high inspired oxygen concentration and PEEP. The problems of increased capillary permeability are made worse if the patient is hypoalbuminaemic with low oncotic pressure, or if left atrial pressure is elevated either by cardiac failure or overtransfusion. The fully developed syndrome has a high mortality (60%–70%), but more transient and completely reversible forms are seen, and some patients survive with irreversible fibrotic changes in the lung. It is not at the moment possible to predict outcome, although mortality is highest in patients with evidence of continuing low cardiac output, persisting metabolic acidosis or renal failure. Continuing or progressive damage is presumably due to persistence of mediators in the circulation, or continuing mediator release from cells infiltrating the lung. The only "specific" therapy appears to be prompt treatment of infection where ARDS is due to sepsis.

There is agreement about many aspects of treatment. Prevention is clearly important. Prompt control of major gram-negative sepsis is essential. When massive transfusion is required the blood products used should be in good condition. Filtration of blood products to remove cellular debris has been recommended, but evidence of its efficacy is lacking, as it is for warming of blood and other infusion fluids. Care should be taken to prevent both hypotensive episodes and overtransfusion with left atrial overload. Inspired oxygen concentrations must be high enough to produce an adequate arterial $PO_2$ (>8 kPa, 60 mmHg), despite the risk of pulmonary capillary damage from high alveolar oxygen tension. Mechanical ventilation is required in most patients. PEEP is often required to maintain adequate gas exchange, but it may reduce cardiac output and a compromise between arterial oxygen levels and cardiac output is necessary. High minute volumes are often necessary to maintain ventilation in the face of an increased physiological dead space, and it may not be possible to maintain a normal $PCO_2$. Albumin should be given to maintain an adequate oncotic pressure, but it is difficult to maintain an adequate albumin level in the face of the generalised increase in capillary permeability, hypercatabolism or high external protein losses which are common in these patients.

There is little specific therapy. At present the only approach is to continue maximum supportive treatment until the patient either recovers or dies. Complete recovery is possible after many weeks, although treatment for this period of time is a formidable undertaking. Controversy continues about the role of high dose steroids, usually given as three doses of methyl prednisolone 500 mg i.v. 12 h apart — the so-called shock pack. There is an unconfirmed suggestion that this minimises pulmonary capillary damage, but if it is to be effective it must be given early, preferably prophylactically. So far attempts to demonstrate benefit in clinical trials have not been successful. There is no place for long-term steroid therapy and its side-effects are likely to be harmful. Extracorporeal membrane oxygenators have been used to provide temporary support, but the oxygenators themselves tend to produce pulmonary capillary damage and they do not have a place in the management of ARDS.

Survivors may make a complete recovery with complete clearing of functional and radiological abnormality, or there may be persisting fibrosis. The outcome cannot be predicted by any of the available techniques such as the cellular content of lavage fluid or the mediators it contains. Lung biopsy may be useful in excluding diffuse cryptogenic infection; it demonstrates the extent of fibrosis, but it does not appear to provide prognostic information. It is not without risk.

# Sleep-related Breathing Disorders

### Respiration and Sleep

There is a fall in tidal volume and minute ventilation in normal subjects during slow wave and rapid eye movement sleep (REM), with a rise in arterial $PCO_2$ of more than 0.5 kPa (2–3 mmHg) and a reduction in $PaO_2$ of approximately 2 kPa (15–25 mmHg). However, the fall in oxygen saturation is usually less than 2% because resting arterial $PO_2$ is high. The same reduction in ventilation occurs in patients with chronic respiratory problems, with a similar fall in $PaO_2$, but because resting $PaO_2$ is lower there is a greater fall in oxygen saturation (see Chap. 5).

In addition to hypoventilation, some normal subjects have occasional apnoeic periods during REM sleep (an apnoeic period being defined as complete cessation of air flow at the mouth and nose for at lease 10 s). When apnoeic periods occur frequently during the night they are associated with other symptoms such as daytime hypersomnolence. This constitutes the sleep apnoea syndrome.

### Sleep Apnoea Syndrome

Although some of the features of the sleep apnoea syndrome were first described 100 years ago, it is only since the late 1970s that the syndrome has been clearly recognised, the underlying mechanisms investigated and treatment given. The syndrome is arbitrarily defined as being present when there are more than 40 apnoeic periods during 7 h of sleep. It is usually present in patients with normal lungs and spirometry, and sometimes with normal daytime arterial blood gas tensions. The patients are characteristically male, middle aged and overweight, and the two commonest presenting symptoms are daytime hypersomnolence and snoring at night. Patients with more frequent and prolonged apnoeic episodes have more severe symptoms, including mental deterioration, personality changes, early morning headaches and impotence. A minority of patients develop Pickwickian features — daytime hypercapnia and hypoxaemia, polycythaemia and heart failure. Observation of the breathing pattern during sleep reveals a very characteristic and rather dramatic pattern with gradually increasing depth of snoring over a few seconds followed by a period of apnoea with silence lasting for a variable time, occasionally as long as 90 s. Respiratory efforts increase during this period until apnoea terminates with an explosive snort and a few big breaths before the cycle restarts. Arterial oxygen saturation falls steadily during the period of apnoea and rises rapidly when the apnoeic period ends.

## Physiological Changes

The discovery of the sleep apnoea syndrome as a "new disease" has stimulated intensive investigation in these patients. The syndrome was initially divided into central (arrhythmic) and obstructive groups, but it is now clear that the two are closely linked and the differentiation may be less real than was supposed. There are three important elements in the development of apnoea: a sleep-related imbalance between diaphragmatic and pharyngeal muscle activity; the size of the pharynx; and the resistance to airflow proximal to the pharynx (Fig. 6.1). Normally, inspiratory phasic activity in pharyngeal muscles is synchronous with diaphragmatic contraction so that the development of negative pressures in the upper airways during inspiration is balanced by the stabilising effect of pharyngeal muscle contraction. Sleep reduces phasic activity of the upper airway muscles to a

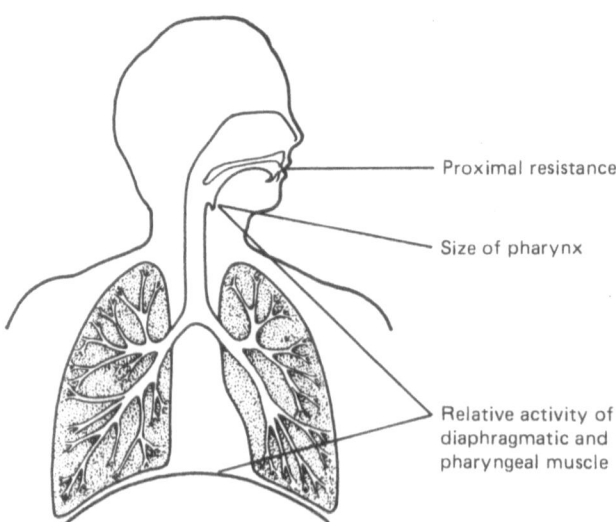

Proximal resistance

Size of pharynx

Relative activity of diaphragmatic and pharyngeal muscle

**Fig. 6.1.** Factors contributing to upper airways obstruction in the sleep apnoea syndrome.

**Table 6.1.** Factors predisposing to the sleep apnoea syndrome

| | |
|---|---|
| Nose | Allergic rhinitis |
| | Deviated nasal septum |
| Pharynx | Obesity |
| | Myxoedema |
| | Acromegaly |
| | Enlarged tonsils and adenoids |
| | Micrognathia |
| | Macroglossia |
| | Retropharyngeal masses |
| Brain stem | Alcohol and sedation |
| problems | Hypoxaemia |
| | Brain stem disease, e.g. polio |

greater extent than to the diaphragm. This effect is accentuated by alcohol, sedation or brain-stem problems. It is also increased by the hypoxaemia which results from the episodes of apnoea, thus initiating a vicious cycle. The tendency to develop pharyngeal obstruction during inspiration is increased if the pharynx is small, or if it is reduced in size for any reason such as obesity, myxoedema or macroglossia. Increased proximal resistance to airflow in the nose or from large tonsils and adenoids necessitates a greater inspiratory effort to generate a more negative pressure in the pharynx and this increases the tendency to obstruction.

The conditions associated with the sleep apnoea syndrome are shown in Table 6.1. The commonest factor is obesity: two-thirds of the patients are at least 30% overweight. Other relatively common associations are nasal problems such as nasal polyps, enlarged tonsils and adenoids in children, and myxoedema and acromegaly in adults. Primary brain-stem problems such as encephalitis and poliomyelitis are less common causes, but can lead to the late development of the syndrome.

## Diagnosis and Investigation

Diagnosis is difficult because the patients present with a wide variety of vague symptoms which often fail to arouse the suspicion of an underlying sleep-related problem. It is common for patients to have had symptoms for many years before the diagnosis is made. Diagnosis is difficult when patients with chronic respiratory problems also have sleep apnoea syndrome (overlap syndrome — see Chap. 5); polycythaemia or hypoventilation which is disproportionate for the degree of airways obstruction is an indication for sleep studies.

Once suspected, the diagnosis is easily confirmed by recording arterial oxygen saturation with an ear oximeter during sleep and observing the patient. If it is unclear whether the patient is apnoeic or hypopnoeic, ventilation should be monitored by a thermistor or $PCO_2$ probe at the nose and mouth. Electroencephalographic recording of sleep phases is not required for clinical diagnosis and, like other more detailed physiological investigations, does not usually affect management. Investigations should concentrate on the underlying cause; ENT abnormalities should always be looked for.

## Management

The extent to which treatment is pursued depends on the severity of the symptoms and assessment of the risk to the patient if no treatment is given. The majority of patients will show some response to one or more of the approaches outlined below.

1. Obese patients must lose weight.
2. Sedation and alcohol should be avoided.
3. Any source of upper airways obstruction should be treated. Surgery should be considered for nasal polyps or enlarged tonsils and drugs should be given for allergic rhinitis.
4. Nocturnal oxygen therapy is of help to some patients. It appears to work by relieving the secondary adverse effects of hypoxaemia on respiratory control during the apnoeic periods.
5. The tricyclic antidepressant protriptyline produces improvement in some patients. It probably acts by reducing REM sleep. Other drugs have been tried and may be useful, including medroxyprogesterone and strychnine, but they have not been evaluated fully. Naloxone, methylxanthines, almitrine and bromocriptine do not have a useful effect.
6. The most innovative approach has been the use of nasal continuous positive airway pressure (nasal CPAP). A nose mask moulded to fit closely onto the patient's nose is worn at night, connected to a biased airflow of 20–40 l/min with a downstream resistance. The positive pressure produced effectively splints the nose and pharynx during inspiration and expiration. Pressures between 3 $cmH_2O$ and 16 $cmH_2O$ have been effective in eradicating sleep apnoea and improving daytime well being. Some patients find the device unacceptable, but many can tolerate it in long-term use.
7. Surgical removal of redundant tissue round the pharynx (uvulopalatopharyngoplasty) has been advocated for patients with a small pharynx. Results are variable and the operation often leads to nasal regurgitation and nasal speech.
8. Tracheostomy is a highly effective, but rather extreme treatment. It is indicated in patients with incapacitating symptoms in whom other treatment has been ineffective and who are prepared to tolerate the social and medical consequences of a permanent tracheostomy, and in patients in whom sleep apnoea syndrome is associated with dangerous arrhythmias or refractory pulmonary hypertension.

# Useful References

Andreadis N, Petty TL (1985) Adult respiratory distress syndrome. Problems and progress. Am Rev Resp Dis 132: 344–346

Bushnell SS (1973) Respiratory intensive care nursing. Little Brown, Boston

Douglas NJ (1984) Editorial review, Control of breathing during sleep. Clin Sci 67: 465–471
Editorial (1983) The treatment of obstructive sleep apnea. Am Rev Resp Dis 128: 583–586
Editorial (1986) Adult respiratory distress syndrome. Lancet I: 301–303
Flenley DC (1980) Editorial. Hypoxaemia during sleep. Thorax 35: 81–84
Hedley-Whyte J, Burgess GE, Feeley TW, Miller GM (1976) Applied physiology of respiratory care.
    Little Brown, Boston
Kinnear WJM, Shneerson JM (1985) Assisted ventilation at home: Is it worth considering? Br J Dis
    Chest 79: 313–351
MacNee WN (1985) Treatment of respiratory failure. A review. J R Soc Med 78: 61–71
Morrison ML (ed) (1979) Respiratory intensive care nursing, 2nd edn. Little Brown, Boston
Petty TL (1985) Editorial. Indicators of risk, course, and prognosis in adult respiratory distress syn-
    drome (ARDS). Am Rev Resp Dis 132: 471
Sykes MK, McNicol MW, Campbell EJM (1976) Respiratory failure, 2nd edn. Blackwell Scientific,
    Oxford London Edinburgh
Tinker J, Rapin M (1983) Care of the critically ill patient. Springer, London
Warren PM, Flenley DC (1983) Chronic bronchitis and emphysema. In: Flenley DC, Petty TL (eds)
    Recent advances in respiratory medicine. Churchill Livingston, Edinburgh

# 7 Lower Respiratory Tract Infections

## Acute Infections

The main acute infections of the lower respiratory tract — pneumonia and acute bronchitis — are usually both acquired and treated outside hospital. Admission to hospital occurs when the infection is severe or the patient is otherwise unwell. The same general principles of diagnosis and treatment apply whether the patient is managed in hospital or outside. Attempts to identify the causative organism are rarely made outside hospital and even in hospital positive identification is usually not possible in the first 48 h. Antibiotics are the only specific treatment, and if these are to be effective they should be started promptly as soon as the infection is diagnosed. The choice of antibiotic is determined by clinical diagnosis of the underlying infection and a judgement of the most likely organism responsible. The patient should therefore be assessed: (a) to determine clinically whether a lower respiratory tract infection is present; (b) to determine the type of infection, whether pneumonia or acute bronchitis; and (c) to decide, on the basis of the information available, which organism is likely to be causing the infection and which antibiotic or antibiotics are likely to be effective.

### General Approach

Infection usually reaches the lower respiratory tract via the upper airways, either by inhalation of pathogenic organisms or by aspiration of infected material. The organisms responsible for bronchitis differ from those causing pneumonia, but these in turn differ depending on whether pneumonia is acquired in the community or in hospital, and whether it occurs in patients who were previously fit, have underlying chest problems, or are generally debilitated or immunosuppressed.

Since the antibiotic susceptibilities of the organisms responsible for acute bronchitis and pneumonia differ, it is important to determine which is present. Patients with acute bronchitis are often afebrile, and respiratory symptoms predominate with sputum production being a prominent feature. In pneumonia illness is often more severe, "toxic" features more common and fever and leucocytosis are more marked. Sputum may not be present initially. Pleuritic pain in a patient with chest infection is strongly suggestive of pneumonia, and the finding of signs of consolidation confirms the diagnosis. In patients admitted to hospital the clinical diagnosis should be supported by a chest X-ray.

In the lower respiratory tract it can be difficult to distinguish bacterial from viral infections. In an uncomplicated viral infection sputum is normally mucoid; when it is purulent or contains numerous pus cells it is reasonable to assume that bacterial infection is present. A polymorphonuclear leucocytosis is suggestive of bacterial infection, but it is often absent in acute bronchitis. Fever is much more common in pneumonia than in bronchitis, but it can be present in both bacterial and viral infections.

Pneumonia is usually due to bacterial or *Mycoplasma pneumoniae* infection. Acute bronchitis following an upper respiratory tract infection with mucoid sputum is usually viral in origin. The majority of patients admitted to hospital with bronchitis have underlying chronic chest disease and in these patients secondary bacterial infection has usually supervened. Particular problems in diagnosing infection and in differentiating between viral and bacterial infection arise in patients with pre-existing chronic chest disease. The presence of cough and sputum may then not be helpful and deterioration in respiratory function, although often associated with bacterial infection, is not specific to infection.

### Investigation

Investigation of the patient with an acute lower respiratory tract infection is designed to identify the causative organism and to assess the extent of the infection. Many of the techniques available to culture or identify the presence of a specific organism take several days or, in some instances, weeks to provide a result and treatment usually needs to be started immediately. The extent to which investigations are carried out varies enormously, depending on how ill the patient is, whether treatment occurs in or outside hospital, whether the infection was acquired in or outside hospital and whether the patient has other medical problems. The range of investigations normally carried out in and outside hospital are shown below.

1.  The majority of patients with acute lower respiratory tract infection acquired and treated outside hospital have no laboratory investigations, and this appears to be a reasonable firstline policy.
2.  Patients with infection acquired outside hospital but considered ill enough to be admitted to hospital will normally have a chest X-ray and sputum examination in addition to routine blood tests. Patients with pneumonia should also have a blood culture and blood for serological studies.
3.  For immunocompromised patients and those with hospital-acquired infection, the pathogen is much more likely to be an antibiotic resistant or unusual organism. It is very important that the infecting organism is identified and, unless the patient is very ill, it is better to withhold treatment until the organism has been isolated. Procedures such as tracheal aspiration and

fibreoptic bronchoscopy with bronchial aspiration, washing, brushing or transbronchial biopsy may be required to isolate the pathogen.

## Bacteriology

Bacteriological examination of sputum is less helpful than might be expected because some pathogens are difficult to identify and grow and because sputum is often contaminated by upper respiratory tract organisms which overgrow on culture. A stained smear of a fresh specimen of sputum may help to discriminate between infection and contamination on the basis of numbers of organisms, but the distinction is not easily made. Sampling of lower respiratory tract secretions by transtracheal aspiration or fibreoptic bronchoscopy obviates this problem, but these approaches are not normally justified.

## Serology

In some patients with pneumonia the causative organism can only be determined by finding high or rising titres of specific antibodies.

## Radiology

A chest X-ray should be taken and interpreted carefully in patients admitted to hospital. The distribution of consolidation and other radiological features may point towards a particular microbiological diagnosis (Table 7.1), but there is considerable overlap. The chest X-ray may also indicate underlying problems such as bronchial carcinoma.

## Microbiology

There are wide variations in the frequency with which positive bacteriology has been obtained in patients with lower respiratory tract infections, and some variation in the range of pathogens isolated. These to a large extent represent the enthusiasm and skill with which investigation is pursued.

## Viral

Viral pathogens are common. They are a frequent cause of acute tracheobronchitis but a rare cause of primary pneumonia. They disrupt the defence mechanisms and predispose to secondary bacterial infection. The viruses commonly involved are respiratory syncytial and influenza virus. In children, respiratory infections are also caused by measles and varicella viruses. In measles a tracheobronchitis is compounded by a general depression of immunity, predisposing to more serious respiratory infection.

There is no specific therapy for viral respiratory infection save that in an influenza epidemic secondary staphylococcal pneumonia is common and anti-staphylococcal cover should be given to all patients with pneumonia. For patients

**Table 7.1.** Clinical features of specific bacterial pneumonias

| Organism | Incidence | Clinical features |
|---|---|---|
| *Pneumococcus* | 75% of primary pneumonia | Acute onset, pleurisy, "rusty sputum", herpes, fe WBC + +, clinical signs + + <br> CXR — lobar or major segment consolidation |
| *Mycoplasma* | <10% <br> Case clusters | Young adults, insidious onset, myalgia, malaise, l sputum, few signs <br> ESR + + <br> CXR — patchy consolidation |
| *Legionella* | <10% <br> Sporadic <br> Case clusters <br> Outbreaks | All ages, not directly infectious, insidious, malaisi cough, few signs <br> CXR — patchy to lobar consolidation <br> Severe cases — renal and hepatic failure |
| *Staphylococcus* | Uncommon <br> Infants, debilitated <br> post-influenza | Usually acute, fever, WBC +, cough, sputum pui poor signs <br> CXR — multiple patchy consolidation, abscesses tension cysts, pneumo- or pyothorax |
| *Klebsiella* | Uncommon <br> Older with intercurrent disease <br> Chronic bronchitis <br> Alcoholics | Subacute, cough, sputum + +, purulent + + <br> Signs variable <br> CXR — localised, often in upper lobe, breakdow single abscess common |

aCIE, countercurrent immunoelectrophoresis.

with other severe viral pneumonias, careful bacteriological monitoring is required
to detect significant secondary infection at an early stage.

### Bacterial

In patients with chronic obstructive lung disease, acute bronchitis is most likely to
bé due to *Haemophilus influenzae*. Table 7.1 lists the organisms likely to cause
pneumonia according to the type of infection and the nature of the breakdown in
defence mechanisms. The nature of the organism causing pneumonia varies
depending on whether the infection is community acquired or hospital acquired
and whether it occurs in a previously fit patient, one with modest impairment of
lung defence mechanisms as in chronic bronchitis or in a patient with major
depression of immunity.

# Pneumonia

### Primary Community-acquired Pneumonia

The main surveys on the range of infecting agents in community-acquired
pneumonia are summarised in Table 7.2. Of the bacterial pathogens, the most
common and most important is *Streptococcus pneumoniae* — the pneumococcus.
When an exhaustive search is made, the pneumococcus is usually found to be
responsible for more than 50% of primary community-acquired pneumonias, and
in some series for as many as 90%. It must be regarded as the most likely cause of
any extensive pneumonia with a lobar or major segmental pattern of distribution.

The frequency with which other agents are identified varies widely but it is
unusual for a specific pathogen other than the pneumococcus to be responsible for
more than 10% of patients admitted to hospital with pneumonia. The variability
in the reported incidence of other common causative organisms is probably
related mainly to the effect of season and locality. Other important pathogens in
primary pneumonia are *Mycoplasma pneumoniae* and *Legionella* species. *H.
influenzae* may produce a pneumonic illness, as can a wide variety of other
organisms such as *Chlamydia psittaci*. Tuberculosis may occasionally present with
a pneumonic illness, a possibility which must be borne in mind in vulnerable
groups or if response to treatment is slow.

Pneumonia following a viral infection in patients with previously normal lungs
is usually due to mixed upper respiratory tract flora, though infections with *Strep.
pneumoniae* or *Staphylococcus aureus* may also occur. Staphylococcal infection is
particularly associated with severe influenza virus infections. In patients with pre-
existing chronic chest disease the most likely pathogen is *H. influenzae*.

### Secondary Pneumonia

Secondary pneumonia, in which upper respiratory tract organisms are aspirated,
occurs most often in debilitated patients and those with poor oral hygiene. Outside

**Table 7.2.** Aetiology of community-acquired pneumonia

| Author[a] | Year | Total cases | Percent-age with bacterial diagnosis | Percentage of diagnosed cases due to: | | | | |
|---|---|---|---|---|---|---|---|---|
| | | | | *Strep. pneumo-niae* | *Legion-ella pneumo-phila* | *Myco-plasma pneumo-niae* | *Haemo-philus influ-enzae* | *St o a* |
| Humphrey | 1948 | 351 | 85 | 93 | | | | ? |
| Bath | 1964 | 140 | 62 | 54 | | | 17 | 1⁴ |
| Sullivan | 1972 | 292 | 57 | 61 | | | 9 | 1] |
| Spencer | 1973 | 76 | 50 | 40 | | | 18 | ? |
| Dorff | 1973 | 148 | 83 | 64 | | 5 | 4 | { |
| Burns | 1976 | 222 | 32 | 69 | | | 16 | ? |
| Garb | 1978 | 35 | 100 | 43 | | | 20 | |
| White | 1981 | 210 | 49 | 23 | 2 | 29 | 4 | { |
| Macfarlane | 1982 | 127 | 98 | 78 | 15 | 2 | 3 | ? |
| Kennedy | 1983 | 96 | 56 | 16 | 20 | 14 | 7 | |
| McNabb | 1984 | 80 | 64 | 78 | | | 6 | |
| Allen | 1984 | 502 | 19 | 42 | | | | |
| Shann | 1984 | 83 | 61 | 20 | | | 30 | |

[a]References at end of chapter.

hospital the organisms usually consist of mixed upper respiratory tract commensals and may include anaerobes.

## Hospital-acquired Pneumonia

Gram-negative organisms, including *Pseudomonas*, *Klebsiella* and coliform species, are more likely to be found in hospital in-patients, particularly those who have already received antibiotics which select out resistant organisms of relatively low virulence. When antibiotic use has been very heavy, relatively low-grade but often multiply resistant pathogens or yeasts may colonise and invade the respiratory tract. The colonising organisms tend to be specific to each hospital. At present *Pseudomonas* and gram-negative organisms are found most often under these conditions, with staphylococcal infection occurring occasionally and with a tendency to be invasive. If vomit has been aspirated, alimentary tract organisms including anaerobes may be causing infection.

## Pneumonia in Immunocompromised Patients

Patients who are immunocompromised for any reason, e.g. due to cytoxic drugs following transplant surgery, lymphoproliferative disorders or the acquired immune deficiency syndrome (AIDS), are particularly vulnerable to pneumonia from a wide range of bacteria and opportunistic organisms. The list of causes includes the bacteria mentioned above and particularly the multiply resistant gram-negative 'commensals' of the *Pseudomonas* and *Klebsiella* species. It also includes *Mycobacterium tuberculosis* and atypical mycobacteria, yeasts and fungi such as *Aspergillus*, protozoa such as *Pneumocystis carinii* and viruses such as cytomegalovirus. Patients with AIDS are particularly vulnerable to *P. carinii*.

## Pneumonia as a Consequence of Extrathoracic Infection

The lung is occasionally involved as part of a septicaemic illness or, even more rarely, as a result of direct spread from sepsis elsewhere such as a subphrenic abscess or from a penetrating injury. The type of organism depends on the source of infection and is not usually difficult to predict.

## Clinical Features

### Community-acquired Pneumonias

*Pneumococcal Pneumonia.* Most extensive primary pneumonias are pneumococcal. The clinical features are the classic ones of an acute pneumonia, sudden onset, fever, pleuritic chest pain, and cough productive of small amounts of sputum which is initially not purulent but "rusty" from the characteristic haemorrhagic pulmonary oedema. Physical signs of consolidation are usually conspicuous at the peak of the illness but crepitations may be prominent at an early stage or during resolution. The lower lobes are affected rather more often than the upper lobes. Radiologically there is usually uniform lobar or major segmental consolidation, reflecting the intense inflammatory oedema which spreads via interalveolar communications until restricted by lobar boundaries. With cure, the exudate liquefies and is reabsorbed, with restoration of normal appearance and normal function to the lobe. The pleural surface is almost invariably involved, and some degree of pleural inflammation is very common, often with a small effusion. Large effusions or empyema are rare.

Diagnosis is usually based on sputum culture and blood culture, since septicaemia is common in the more acutely ill patients. Many cases are undiagnosed because the pneumococcus is highly susceptible to antibiotics and many patients have received antibiotics before admission to hospital. Other techniques may lead to positive identification, including direct smear of the sputum which may show the organisms even when they can no longer be cultured. Pneumococcal capsular antigens can be detected in sputum, serum or urine by countercurrent immunoelectrophoresis when cultures are negative.

Pneumococci can be classified by their capsular antigens into 84 different serotypes. One serotype — type III — is associated with severe infections and a high mortality which appears to be little influenced by antibiotic treatment. Other factors associated with high mortality are intercurrent illness, age and the extent of consolidation.

*Legionella Pneumonia.*    *Legionella pneumophila* has only been recognised as an important primary pathogen relatively recently. There has been a tendency to associate the diagnosis with more extreme clinical complications such as fluid and electrolyte disturbance, renal failure and jaundice. These features are manifestations of any severe pneumonia and recent studies suggest they are not related specifically to *L. pneumophila*.

Legionella infections are spread by aerosol from infected water, and are not directly infectious from patient to patient. Clustering of cases has been common in reports thus far, but sporadic cases also occur. In general, legionella pneumonia shows no specific clinical features. Clinical features vary from low-grade systemic symptoms of fever, malaise and muscle aches to a minority with a fulminating illness with fatal outcome. Respiratory symptoms other than cough are rather less common; sputum is usually non-purulent. The radiological distribution of consolidation is usually patchy but extensive consolidation may occur. The diagnosis is confirmed by high or rising antibody titres. The organisms can be cultured or detected by direct immunofluorescent antibody staining but with considerable difficulty and the diagnosis is seldom made in this way.

*Mycoplasma Pneumonia.*    There is considerable variation in the frequency with which mycoplasma pneumonia is diagnosed, mainly due to secular variations in incidence. Cases tend to cluster and there is an undoubted seasonal effect, with an increased number of cases in autumn and early winter. Young adults are most often affected, and the disease tends to occur in small outbreaks. General symptoms are often prominent, malaise and myalgia in particular. Apart from cough, which can be troublesome, respiratory symptoms are not conspicuous. Sputum is usually non-purulent and physical signs of consolidation are not marked. Radiologically the distribution of consolidation tends to be patchy and irregular. Cold agglutinins are often present, producing a very marked elevation of the ESR. Other immunological problems occur and can cause complications such as haemolytic anaemia. Mycoplasma pneumonia occasionally presents with these complications rather than as a primary respiratory illness. The clinical course tends to be rather protracted.

### Other Specific Primary Pneumonias

Pneumonia due to staphylococcal infection occurs more commonly in influenza epidemics and is seen particularly in small children. It shows a marked tendency to breakdown, with formation of multiple abscesses or tension cysts which may rupture into the pleura to cause pneumothorax or empyema. Resolution of the abscesses is slow and marked radiological changes may persist long after apparent clinical recovery. These abnormalities almost invariably resolve completely over the following months. Pneumonia due to *Klebsiella* species usually affects the upper lobes and is more common in alcoholics, and in generally debilitated and immunosuppressed patients. It also tends to breakdown, but the abscesses are usually fewer and larger than in staphylococcal pneumonia; resolution again is slow but often surprisingly complete. The affected lobe may enlarge as a result of oedema, shown radiologically by bulging fissures.

### Pneumonia in Immunocompromised Patients

Pneumonia in immunocompromised patients often lacks distinctive clinical features and respiratory symptoms and signs may be absent. The patient may show signs of general deterioration, with increasing hypoxaemia. A wide variety of abnormalities may be found on the chest X-ray. Other features are often masked by the underlying illness or its treatment. Many of the organisms causing pneumonia in these patients are unresponsive to broad-spectrum antibiotics so it is important to identify the causative organism before starting treatment, using more invasive techniques if necessary. With the gram-negative organisms, the problem is to decide whether the bacteria are invasive and producing infection or merely colonising the respiratory tract. There is no easy answer.

## Complications

*Pleural Effusion and Empyema.*   A small pleural effusion is a common accompaniment of pneumonia and requires no treatment. Empyema and lung abscess occur less frequently. Lung abscess is particularly associated with staphylococcal and klebsiella infections but can occur with any pneumonia.

*Impaired Respiratory Function.*   Pneumonia impairs gas exchange. Consolidated alveoli cannot contribute to gas exchange, and since they continue to be perfused to some extent, hypoxaemia is inevitable.

*"Toxic" Complications.*    More severe pneumonia is associated with "toxic" features, e.g. the exotoxic shock of staphylococcal infection. Some degree of depression of cardiac function is not uncommon in iller patients, particularly those with type III pneumococcal pneumonia. In the very ill there is often evidence of widespread tissue damage with abnormal liver function tests. These complications are more likely in the old, and in those with extensive pneumonia.

Elevation of blood urea as a result of dehydration is common. Renal failure may complicate any severe pneumonia, but is more likely in pneumonia due to *Strep. pneumoniae* and *L. pneumophila*, and with some of the rarer causes such as *Chl. psittaci*. It may be due to acute tubular necrosis or occasionally an immune complex nephritis. Although it is essentially completely reversible, it is associated with a poor prognosis since it tends to accompany more severe illness.

## Treatment

Treatment of pneumonia depends on instituting appropriate antibiotics, secretion drainage and general support of respiration and circulation as necessary.

### The Appropriate Antibiotic

In this section, antibiotic choice is approached first in terms of specific organisms and then in terms of clinical diagnostic categories. The effectiveness of an antibiotic depends on the sensitivity of the organism, the blood level of antibiotic achieved and the extent of tissue penetration by the antibiotic. Tissue penetration is rarely a problem with pneumonia, and the effectiveness of treatment can be assumed to be related to the appropriate choice of antibiotic and the blood levels obtained. The situation is different in more chronic forms of sepsis such as lung abscess, and when trying to eradicate persistent infection in patients with chronic bronchitis and bronchiectasis where tissue and secretion penetration are of greater importance, and antibiotic levels in airway secretions may determine the success of treatment.

Prompt administration of antibiotics is essential for patients with community-acquired pneumonia. A disturbing feature of almost all reports of death from pneumonia is the long delay following admission to hospital before treatment was given. Delays of up to 8 h between prescription and administration of antibiotics have been described in patients admitted to hospital and particularly in those who died. The first dose of antibiotic should be given as soon as the diagnosis is made. Treatment must not be delayed whilst the patient is investigated.

When considering antibiotic choice, the possibility of drug resistance must be taken into account. The pattern of resistance varies with different organisms and in different communities, hospitals and countries, so the local pattern must be known. The minimum inhibitory concentrations of antibiotics given in Tables 7.3–7.5, with expected peak and trough concentrations and plasma half-life, are those generally applicable.

**Table 7.3.** The penicillins

|  | Benzyl penicillin | Ampicillin | Amoxycillin | Flucloxacillin | Carbenicillin |
|---|---|---|---|---|---|
| Dose | 300–600 mg q.i.d. | 250–500 mg q.i.d. | 250–500 mg t.d.s. | 250–500 mg q.i.d. | 5 g q.i.d. |
| Route | i.m., i.v. | o, i.m., i.v. | o, i.m., i.v. | o, i.m., i.v. | i.m., i.v. |
| Peak level ($\mu$g/ml) | 8 | 3–10 | 4 | 5–15 |  |
| Half-life (h) | 1.5 | 1.5 | 1.5 | 1 | ·1.5 |
| Protein binding (%) | 65 | 20 | 20 | 95 | 50 |
| Excretion | Renal | Renal +/− hepatic | Renal | Renal | Renal + hepatic |
| MIC ($\mu$g/ml) for |  |  |  |  |  |
| *Streptococcus pneumoniae* | 0.02 | 0.05 | 0.05 | 0.25 | 1.25 |
| *Haemophilus influenzae* | 0.5+ | 0.25 | 0.25 | 12.5 | 0.25 |
| *Staphylococcus aureus* | R | R | R | 0.1 | R |
| Oral anaerobes | S | S | S | R | S |
| *Klebsiella* | R | R | R | R | 250 |
| *Pseudomonas* | R | R | R | R | 50 |
| *Legionella* | R | R | R | R | R |
| *Mycoplasma* | R | R | R | R | R |
| *Chlamydia* | R | R | R | R | R |

R, resistant; S, sensitive.

**Table 7.4.** The cephalosporins

|  | Cephalexin | Cephaloridine | Cephalothin | Cefuroxime | Cefotaxime |
|---|---|---|---|---|---|
| Dose | 250 mg q.i.d. | 0.5–1.0 g t.d.s. | 1 g q.i.d. | 750 mg t.d.s. | 1 g b.d. |
| Route | o | i.m., i.v. | i.m. | i.m., i.v. | i.m., i.v. |
| Peak level ($\mu$g/ml) | 18 | 40 | 20 | 35 |  |
| Half-life (h) | 0.8 | 1.5 | 0.6 | 1.1 |  |
| Protein binding (%) | 15 | 20 | 65 | 30 |  |
| Excretion | Renal | Renal | Renal | Renal | Renal |
| MIC ($\mu$g/ml) for |  |  |  |  |  |
| *Streptococcus pneumoniae* | 2 | 0.03 | 0.06 | 0.03 | 0.06 |
| *Haemophilus influenzae* | 32 | 8 | 8 | 0.5 | 0.5 |
| *Staphylococcus aureus* | 2 | 4 | 0.5 | 1 | 2 |
| Oral anaerobes |  |  |  |  |  |
| *Klebsiella* | 8 | 4 | 4 | 4 | 0.1 |
| *Pseudomonas* | R | R | R | R | R |
| *Legionella* | R | R | R | R | R |
| *Mycoplasma* | R | R | R | R | R |
| *Chlamydia* | R | R | R | R | R |

R, resistant.

**Table 7.5.** Other antibiotics

| | Erythromycin | Tetracycline | Co-trimoxazole | Gentamicin | Chlor-amphenicol |
|---|---|---|---|---|---|
| Dose (mg) | 250–500 q.i.d. | 250–500 q.i.d. | 960 b.d. | 80–120 t.d.s. | 500 q.i.d. |
| Route | o, i.v. | o, i.v. | o, i.v. | i.v. | o, i.m., i.v. |
| Peak level (μg/ml) | 1.5 | 3 | | 8 | 8–15 |
| Half-life (h) | 1.5 | 9 | | 2 | 2.5 |
| Protein binding (%) | 70+ | 25 | 45 | 25 | 60 |
| Excretion | Hepatic | Renal + hepatic | Renal | Renal | Renal + hepatic |
| MIC (μg/ml) for | | | | | |
| *Streptococcus pneumoniae* | 0.25 | 0.8 | 1.25 | 2 | 2 |
| *Haemophilus influenzae* | 0.5–8 | 1.6 | 0.1–1 | 0.5 | 0.5 |
| *Staphylococcus aureus* | 0.1–2 | 3.2 | | 0.03–0.12 | 2 |
| Oral anaerobes | | | | | |
| *Klebsiella* | R | 50 | 0.5–2 | 0.25–1 | 1–8 |
| *Pseudomonas* | R | 200 | 12 | 0.25–2 | R |
| *Legionella* | S | S | R | R | R |
| *Mycoplasma* | S | 1.6 | R | R | R |
| *Chlamydia* | S | 2 | R | R | R |

R, resistant; S, sensitive.

## Choice of Antibiotic by Infecting Organism

*Streptococcus pneumoniae.*  This organism is usually very sensitive to benzyl penicillin, to which resistance has rarely been reported. Bacteriocidal concentrations are readily obtained by conventional doses. The pneumococcus is about five times less sensitive to the "broad-spectrum" penicillins such as ampicillin or amoxycillin. Although these are not the preparations of choice, they are still effective and adequate blood levels are obtained with conventional dosage. Sensitivity to more specialised penicillins, such as methicillin, flucloxacillin, and carbenicillin, is less (by a factor of more than 10), and they should not be regarded as providing adequate cover. Many other antibiotics are active against *Strep. pneumoniae* (sulphonamides, trimethoprim, tetracycline, cephalosporins, erythromycin, aminoglycosides, etc.), but none is as satisfactory.

Penicillin resistance has been reported in southern Africa and SE Asia where penicillin has been used extensively for prophylaxis, but penicillin-resistant strains do not yet appear to have spread widely. Sensitivity to ampicillin is retained in southern Africa, but has been lost in the resistant strains in SE Asia. For the "older" antibiotics, other than penicillin, resistance is a significant problem — as high as 30% for the tetracyclines.

*Legionella pneumophila.*  The antibiotic of choice is erythromycin. The organism is also sensitive to rifampicin and in the ill or poorly responding patient erythromycin and rifampicin should be given in combination. Although the organisms may be sensitive in vitro to other antibiotics, none has a worthwhile clinical effect. The difference between in-vitro sensitivity and clinical effectiveness is probably related to intracellular survival and multiplication of the organisms in man.

*Mycoplasma pneumoniae.*   These organisms are sensitive to tetracycline and erythromycin, and to virtually no other antibiotic.

*Staphylococcus aureus.*   The penicillinase-resistant penicillins flucloxacillin and methicillin are the drugs of choice. Combination antibiotic therapy is desirable to prevent the emergence of resistant strains. The choice of the second antibiotic should be dictated by knowledge of local sensitivity patterns. Fucidin is normally effective and compatible with the penicillins. Many other antibiotics have worthwhile antistaphylococcal activity, including the aminoglycosides and cephalosporins, and may be used as a second antibiotic in combination chemotherapy but should not be used alone.

*Klebsiella.*   Antibiotic resistance is likely to be a problem so combined antibiotic therapy should be used, and sensitivities carefully monitored. In general the organisms are sensitive to aminoglycosides and cephalosporins.

*Pseudomonas aeruginosa.*   Antibiotic resistance is a major problem with *Ps. aeruginosa*. It is difficult to find an effective antibiotic regimen, despite the apparent sensitivity of the organisms in vitro to several antibiotics — carbenicillin, azlocillin, ticarcillin, gentamicin, tobramycin or amikacin. For patients with significant infection, combined antibiotic therapy should be used. The choice of antibiotics depends on the laboratory sensitivities and previous antibiotic therapy. Careful laboratory monitoring is needed to ensure adequate drug concentrations and continuing sensitivity of the organism. For patients who have had several different antibiotics in the recent past, the best result may be obtained by stopping all antibiotic therapy.

*Haemophilus influenzae.*   This organism is usually sensitive to ampicillin, amoxycillin, cotrimoxazole and the cephalosporins. It is quite often sensitive to tetracyclines. For severe or resistant infections, chloramphenicol is the antibiotic of choice despite its potential toxicity.

*Chlamydia psittaci.*   These organisms are sensitive to tetracycline and erythromycin, but to virtually no other antibiotics.

*Upper Respiratory Tract Flora Including Oral Anaerobes.*   The majority of buccal organisms are sensitive to benzyl penicillin. Many oral anaerobes are sensitive to both penicillin and metronidazole. For patients in hospital where there is a significant possibility of colonisation with gram-negative organisms, ampicillin or amoxycillin is a more satisfactory first choice, with the addition of an aminoglycoside in the more seriously ill. Local knowledge of sensitivity patterns is important for the hospitalised patient.

## Choice of Antibiotic by "Clinical" Presentation

When faced with a patient with community-acquired pneumonia, treatment must be started before laboratory confirmation of the underlying organism is available. It may in some patients be possible to guess the underlying organism with a high probability of being correct, as in the young patient with lobar consolidation and circumoral herpes where *Strep. pneumoniae* is almost certainly the organism responsible. There is, however, considerable overlap between the clinical presentations of pneumonia due to different organisms, and in an ill patient it is wise to cover all the more likely organisms. In a patient who is not unduly ill and in whom the clinical picture strongly suggests a particular organism, it is reasonable to treat with the most appropriate antibiotic and only widen the antibiotic cover if progress is not satisfactory. For patients who have more severe infection it is recommended that they should be covered by an antibiotic regimen which would cover all the most likely organisms, i.e. *Strep. pneumoniae*, *L. pneumophila*, *M. pneumoniae* and *H. influenzae* for community-acquired pneumonia. This is achieved with a combination of amoxicillin/ampicillin plus erythromycin, or alternatively by penicillin plus erythromycin. For patients sensitive to the penicillins or unable to take erythromycin, a cephalosporin and either tetracycline or rifampicin, depending on the likely organism, are reasonable alternatives.

In immunocompromised patients, bacterial infections including tuberculosis are treated conventionally. Specific therapy is needed for opportunistic infections. Fungal infections are usually treated with amphotericin B. *Pneumocystis carinii* can be treated with high dose intravenous cotrimoxazole or intramuscular pentamidine. Patients with AIDS appear to require more prolonged treatment (3 weeks) and can expect more side-effects from cotrimoxazole than other patients. The response rate (85%) and incidence of side-effects are similar with the two drugs. The high incidence of side-effects limits the value of these drugs as prophylactic agents for *Pneumocystis* infections in patients with AIDS.

The most appropriate antibiotics for different clinical presentations of pneumonia are shown in Table 7.6.

## Secretion Drainage

Drainage of secretions is important in any chest infection and all patients should be encouraged to cough effectively. It is particularly important in patients with chronic chest disease and chronic suppurative conditions such as bronchiectasis. If the patient is weak or unwell or secretion volumes are large, the assistance of the physiotherapist using posture and forced cough is valuable. If cough fails, intubation for effective secretion drainage may be needed.

## Supportive Therapy

In pneumonia good general supportive therapy may be essential to permit survival while antibiotics deal with the infection. Dehydration is common in the iller patient and hypoxaemia almost universal. The acutely ill febrile patient has high water losses and may not be able to drink enough to maintain adequate hydration.

**Table 7.6.** Antibiotic treatments for different clinical presentations of pneumonia

| *Primary pneumonia* | |
|---|---|
| Primary pneumonia with lobar or major segmental distribution, probably pneumococcal | Benzyl penicillin |
| Patchy primary pneumonia p/c during mycoplasma and legionella epidemics | Erythromycin |
| Patchy primary pneumonia with multiple abscess formation — staphylococcal | Flucloxacillin + fucidin |
| Pneumonia complicating influenza — pneumococci and staphylococci | Cover with penicillin and flucloxacillin |
| Pneumonia with large single abscess — probably *Klebsiella* | Aminoglycoside + second antibiotic depending on local sensitivity pattern |
| *Secondary or complicated pneumonia* | |
| "Aspiration pneumonia" secondary to upper respiratory infection — mixed upper respiratory tract flora | Benzyl penicillin or ampicillin/amoxycillin |
| "Aspiration pneumonia" with significant risk of having aspirated vomit | Gentamicin and metronidazole |
| In patients with chronic bronchitis — *H. influenzae* must be covered | Amoxycillin or cephalosporin |
| Bronchitis/"aspiration pneumonia" in hospitalised patients | Amoxycillin or cephalosporin, possibly aminoglycoside |
| Exacerbation of infection in severe bronchiectasis — cover *H. influenzae* and pneumococcus | Amoxycillin, cephalosporin or cotrimoxazole |
| Consider possibility of resistant gram-negative organisms | Aminoglycoside + penicillinase resistant or antipseudomonal penicillin or anaerobes — metronidazole |
| *Pneumonia in immunocompromised patients* | |
| Bacterial infections and *M. tuberculosis* | Conventional treatment |
| *Pneumocystis carinii* | Cotrimoxazole or pentamidine |
| Fungal infections | Amphotericin B |

In the penicillin-sensitive patient substitute erythromycin or a cephalosporin

The requirements of patients with pneumonia are often underestimated and fluids may have to be given intravenously. Oxygen should be given for significant hypoxaemia ($PO_2$ <8 kPa, 60 mmHg). If hypoxaemia is refractory, high concentrations can usually be given without problems unless the patient has severe chronic bronchitis, where arterial $PCO_2$ levels need to be monitored.

Intubation and mechanical ventilation should be considered in patients unable to clear secretions, for those who are persistently hypoxaemic despite oxygen, and for patients who are becoming exhausted. Treatment should be very energetic. Pneumonia is potentially completely reversible, and both extensive radiological changes and a very sick patient are compatible with complete recovery.

Cardiac function may be impaired and cardiac output poorly maintained, especially in patients requiring mechanical ventilation. Volume depletion is common, requiring volume replacement though careful monitoring is necessary since pulmonary oedema is an undesirable added burden for the patient with pneumonia. Inotropic drugs may be needed. There is no specific therapy for renal failure complicating pneumonia. If sufficiently severe, it should be managed by peritoneal or haemodialysis on the assumption that the renal lesion is potentially completely reversible. Liver failure should be treated symptomatically.

Certain precautions are needed for patients with AIDS, although the risk of cross-infection is very small. The main requirement is for suitable labelling and disposal of blood and excretions. Bronchoscopies require particular care both to protect the bronchoscopist and to ensure that the bronchoscope is adequately sterilised after use.

## Treatment of Complications

Empyema should be treated by repeated aspiration with adequate antibiotic cover. Surgical drainage is virtually never required. Lung abscess requires secretion drainage and prolonged antibiotic therapy with careful bacteriological monitoring. The possibility of a pneumothorax in patients with staphylococcal pneumonia must be borne in mind and facilities must be available for prompt treatment.

## Response to Treatment

### Normal Response

If pneumonia is bacterial in origin and an appropriate antibiotic has been given, there should be unequivocal evidence of response within 72 h. The patient's temperature should be falling and toxic symptoms starting to disappear. Resolution tends to be slower in patients with infection due to gram-negative organisms, *Legionella pneumophila* and *M. pneumoniae* and in some patients with pneumococcal pneumonia, particularly when due to type III organisms.

Most patients treated with the appropriate antibiotic recover completely both clinically and radiologically. Radiological resolution may, however, be considerably delayed and even in pneumococcal pneumonia may take several months. In extensive pneumonia the chest X-ray is virtually never normal at the time the patient has recovered sufficiently to permit discharge from hospital. In staphylococcal and klebsiella pneumonia where abscess formation is common, radiological improvement is slower and may take up to a year to be complete. Permanent fibrotic scarring or bronchiectasis develops in a few patients, usually those in whom appropriate treatment was delayed or where other factors such as failure to clear secretions or persisting atelectasis were present. It is rare however, and even quite grossly abnormal radiological appearances will usually return to normal given time.

### Delayed Response — Is a Change of Antibiotic Required?

In the first instance, the accuracy of the microbiological diagnosis should be reassessed. If this is thought to be wrong, then a more appropriate antibiotic should be substituted. If the evidence suggests that the right organism is being treated, the possibility of antibiotic resistance should be considered. It is difficult to give hard and fast guidance about antibiotic change, but on the whole antibiotics are probably changed too frequently. When a second choice antibiotic is given, local information about likely patterns of antibiotic sensitivity should be borne in mind.

A change of antibiotics must be considered if there is no evidence of a response at 72 h, though in the acutely ill patient review at 48 h may be required. The nature of the infecting organism will influence these decisions. Most pneumococcal pneumonias respond promptly and unequivocally, though a few serotypes run a more protracted course. If there is microbiological evidence of pneumococcal infection, antibiotic change is not worthwhile unless there is strong evidence to suggest antibiotic resistance.

When a change of antibiotic is considered advisable in patients with primary community-acquired pneumonia, erythromycin should normally be used. It will provide cover against the majority of likely organisms, including the pneumococcus, *L. pneumophila* and *M. pneumoniae*. When infection is likely to be due to mixed upper respiratory tract flora, a different "broad-spectrum" antibiotic should be considered, ampicillin/amoxycillin, a cephalosporin, cotrimoxazole or a tetracycline. The addition of a second drug may be helpful for infections due to *Staph. aureas* or an organism likely to show a poor response to antibiotics, such as gram-negative bacteria or *L. pneumophila*.

However, it is well to be cautious in reappraising treatment requirements. The timescale of resolution of any extensive lower respiratory tract infection is slow and most doctors tend to be too optimistic. Antibiotics may eradicate the infecting organism quickly, but the patient takes time to get better. The extreme example is type III pneumococcal pneumonia, where the patient may be gravely ill despite bacteriological "cure".

## Delayed Response — When to Investigate Further

If there is an inadequate response to a second course of antibiotics, careful reappraisal is needed. Fibreoptic bronchoscopy should be considered, both to obtain specimens to confirm the microbiological diagnosis and to exclude bronchial obstruction. If the patient is improving clinically but radiological clearing is delayed, bronchoscopy can be delayed for 3 months. If major abnormality persists at 3 months, fibreoptic bronchoscopy should be carried out to exclude underlying carcinoma and sputum culture to exclude tuberculosis. Earlier investigation is advisable in smokers, or in any patient with other reasons to suspect an obstructive endobronchial lesion.

## Prophylaxis Against Pneumonia

Secondary infection with antibiotic-resistant organisms may be a problem with long-term antibiotic prophylaxis and when antibiotics are given early in a viral infection in an attempt to prevent secondary bacterial infection.

There is a case for prophylaxis against pneumococcal pneumonia in clearly defined, at-risk groups using the specific narrow spectrum antibiotic, benzyl penicillin. These include immunosuppressed patients who have had a splenectomy and patients with homozygous sickle cell disease. It is important to note that penicillin prophylaxis in SE Asia has led to the emergence of a penicillin-resistant pneumococcus.

A small group of patients run a particularly high risk of developing pneumococcal pneumonia and the pneumonia, when it occurs, is often fulminant and carries a high mortality. Patients at risk include any who have had a splenectomy or who have splenic dysfunction, as in homozygous sickle cell disease, and patients with either hypogammaglobulinaemia or complement deficiencies. Pneumococcal vaccine is effective in these patients. When elective splenectomy is being considered the vaccine should be given two weeks or more prior to splenectomy. The vaccine is less effective if given after splenectomy or in the immunosuppressed, but is still worthwhile. It is not used as widely as it should be. Adverse reactions are rare for the first vaccination, but more likely thereafter, so revaccination is not recommended at present.

### Acute Bronchitis

Acute bronchitis following an upper respiratory tract infection in otherwise fit people will usually resolve in a few days without treatment. In patients with chronic obstructive lung disease it should be treated promptly with an antibiotic which will cover the usual organism, *H. influenzae* (see Chap. 4). Secretion drainage is not usually a problem but if it is the patient should be admitted to hospital. With effective treatment for tracheobronchitis, a reduction in sputum purulence and perhaps sputum volume would be expected by 72–96 h.

## Chronic Infections

### Bronchiectasis

Antibiotics have revolutionised the clinical picture of bronchiectasis so that the classic appearance of gross putrid bronchiectasis is no longer seen. Infective episodes are easily treated in the vast majority of patients and hospital admissions in the United Kingdom have declined markedly. It also seems likely that the incidence of bronchiectasis is falling. This is probably due to earlier and better treatment of chest infection in childhood, the reduction in whooping cough and measles as a result of vaccination and the great reduction in primary tuberculosis.

There is still a group of patients, however, including those with cystic fibrosis, in whom generalised bronchiectasis is associated with increasingly severe symptoms and deteriorating lung function, and management of these patients still poses major problems. Secretion drainage appears to be at least as important as antibiotics in these patients and effective secretion drainage by patient, parent or therapist is essential. Many of these patients have some response to bronchodilators and a smaller proportion have a worthwhile response to corticosteroids. All patients with symptoms or evidence of airways obstruction should have their bronchodilator response to $\beta_2$-agonists assessed. Patients with more severe airways obstruction should undergo a formal steroid trial (see Chap. 18). Corticosteroids do not appear to cause particular problems in patients with bronchiectasis, despite the infection, and some patients undoubtedly benefit from their use.

The management of secondary bacterial infection is difficult. The common "problem" organism in the 1960s, *Staph. aureus*, is largely controlled by effective antistaphylococcal drugs. The main "problem" organisms now are gram-negative bacteria, particularly the *Pseudomonas* species. Repeated use of antibiotics in conjunction with the disordered anatomy and stagnant secretions pave the way for colonisation and infection by resistant organisms. When treatment is needed consideration has to be given to both the potential pathogens and the resident flora. In general, antibiotics are reserved for exacerbations of infection presenting as episodes of increased sputum volume and purulence and general malaise. The antibiotic used should cover the common respiratory pathogen — *H. influenzae* — and other colonising organisms known to be present.

Normal doses of antibiotics will not eliminate all the pathogenic organisms in these patients. This can be achieved by higher doses of antibiotic and recent evidence suggests that this may be worthwhile. The long-term effect of intermittent courses of high doses of antibiotics given orally, intravenously or by inhalation is currently being evaluated. It is too soon to say whether they will retard the deterioration in lung function in these patients or whether the development of resistant organisms will prove to be a problem as in the past.

The role of long-term antibiotics in patients with severe bronchiectasis is more difficult. In general, prophylaxis has had little place but its role is currently being reassessed in conjunction with that of high-dose antibiotics. There are some patients with recurrent infective exacerbations in whom long-term antibiotic therapy appears to maintain a reduction in sputum volume and purulence and for whom prophylaxis may be worthwhile.

Patients with bronchiectasis often have recurrent haemoptyses. They should be advised to rest at home unless bleeding is severe. If recurrent haemoptyses are large or troublesome, further investigations may be needed. The source of the haemoptysis must be accurately identified in patients with widespread disease, preferably by carrying out bronchoscopy at the time of bleeding. If a bleeding point can be identified, cautery may cure the problem. Other procedures are not without hazard in these patients but lobectomy, pneumonectomy, bronchial artery embolisation and radiotherapy have a role in carefully selected patients.

# Useful References

Bryan CS, Reynolds KL (1984) Bacteremic nosocomial pneumonia. Am Rev Resp Dis 129: 668–671
Editorial (1983) How common is Legionnaires' disease? Lancet I: 103–104

Gransden WR, Eykyn SJ, Phillips I (1985) Pneumococcal bacteraemia: 325 episodes diagnosed at St Thomas's Hospital. Br Med J 290: 505–508

Gruer LD, McKendrick MW, Geddes AM (1984) Pneumococcal bacteraemia — a continuing challenge. Q J Med 210: 259–270

Levison ME (1984) The pneumonias. John Wright, Boston

Macfarlane JT (1983) Legionnaires' disease: update. Br Med J 287: 443–444

Macfarlane JT, Miller AC, Roderick Smith WH, Morris AH, Rose DH (1984) Comparative radiographic features of community acquired Legionnaires' disease, pneumococcal pneumonia, mycoplasma pneumonia, and psittacosis. Thorax 39: 28–33

Neild JA, Eykyen SJ, Phillips I (1985) Lung abscess and empyema. Q J Med 57: 875–882

Noah ND (1974) Mycoplasma pneumoniae infection in the United Kingdom — 1967–73. Br Med J II: 544–546

Walzer PD, Perl DP, Krogstad DJ, Rawson PG, Schultz MG (1974) *Pneumocystis carinii* pneumonia in the United States. Ann Intern Med 80: 83–93

Woodhead MA, Macfarlane JT (1985) The protean manifestations of Legionnaires' disease. J R Coll Physicians Lond 19: 224–230

## References for Table 7.2

Allen SC (1984) Lobar pneumonia in northern Zambia: clinical study of 502 adult patients. Thorax 39: 602–606

Bath JCJL, Boissard GPD, Calder MA, Moffat MAJ (1964) Pneumonia in hospital practice in Edinburgh 1960–62. Br J Dis Chest 58: 1–16

Burns MW, Devitt L, Bryant DH (1976) Pneumonia in a city hospital. Med J Aust: 787–791

Dorff DJ, Rytel MW, Farmer SG, Scanlon G (1973) Etiologies and characteristic features of pneumonias in a municipal hospital. Am J Med Sci 266: 349–358

Garb JL, Brown RB, Garb JR, Tuthill RW (1978) Differences in aetiology of pneumonias in nursing home and community patients. JAMA 240: 2169–2172

Humphrey JH, Joules H, Van der Walt ED (1948) Pneumonia in north-west London 1942–4: I — bacterial pneumonias. Thorax 3: 112–121

Kennedy DH, Boreland W (1983) How common is Legionnaires' Disease. Lancet I: 360–361

Macfarlane JT, Finch RG, Ward MJ, Macrae AD (1982) Hospital study of adult community-acquired pneumonia. Lancet II: 255–258

McNabb WR, Williams TDM, Shanson DC, Lant AF (1984) Adult community acquired pneumonia in central London. J R Soc Med 77: 550–555

Shann F, Germer F, Hazlett D, Gratten M, Linneman V, Payne R (1984) Aetiology of pneumonia in children in Goroka Hospital in Papua New Guinea. Lancet II: 537–541

Spencer RC, Philip JR (1973) Effect of previous antimicrobial therapy on bacteriological findings in patients with primary pneumonia. Lancet II: 349–351

Sullivan RJ, Dowdle WR, Marine WM, Hierholzer JC (1972) Adult pneumonia in a general hospital. Etiology and host risk factors. Arch Intern Med 129: 935–942

White RJ, Blainey AD, Harrison KJ, Clarke SKR (1981) Causes of pneumonia presenting to a district general hospital. Thorax 36: 566–570

# 8 Tuberculosis

## Introduction

Tuberculosis is caused by infection with *Mycobacterium tuberculosis*. It is a disease of considerable antiquity, well known in the ancient Indian and Greek worlds. Evidence of bone tuberculosis has been found in Chinese, Egyptian and pre-Columbian mummies. Tuberculosis has tended to be a disease of urbanisation and poverty. The conditions produced in the West by the Industrial Revolution were particularly favourable to its spread among an overcrowded and poorly nourished population. It was always one of the more common causes of death and in the 19th century it became one of the most important. In this century amongst the developed nations, with improvement in housing and nutrition, its incidence and mortality have declined. In England and Wales in the decade 1890–99 it caused 60 000 deaths/year. The notification rate in 1912 was 270/100 000, with a mortality rate of 50%. By 1980 the notification rate had fallen to 18/100 000; there were 9145 cases and 608 deaths. In the Third World there has been little or no change. The incidence remains very high and in some areas such as north-east Africa it is even increasing. Under these conditions mortality of sputum-positive tuberculosis remains high (about 50%) and tuberculosis is still a major cause of death. In the 1970s the annual risk of infection in Africa ranged between 2% and 5%, with 500 000 new cases of sputum-positive cases each year. The World Health Organisation estimated that in 1980 tuberculosis caused 1.25 million deaths — 5% of the total mortality, almost all in underdeveloped countries.

## Bacteriology

*Mycobacterium tuberculosis* was first demonstrated by Koch in 1882. It is a member of the large group of mycobacteria, most of which are non-pathogenic saprophytes. A few non-saprophytic strains are pathogenic to man or other species. They may be capable of protracted survival outside the body, but they multiply only in relation to their host. The main human pathogen is *M. tuberculosis*. The human strain and the closely related variant *M. africanum* are the only significant cause of human disease. Bovine organisms (*M. bovis*) were previously an important source of infection in Western Europe and North America, but since tuberculosis in cattle has been eradicated they are rarely involved in human disease. Infection with other mycobacterial strains does occasionally occur, with widely varying clinical manifestations (see page 122).

The mycobacteria are bacillary in form and are closely related to the corynebacteria. They are strict aerobes and the human strains multiply only at around body temperature. Mycobacteria have one major distinguishing characteristic from which almost all of their unusual features are derived — a complex waxy outer layer beyond the cell membrane. They have been described as being "wrapped in a fur coat", and it is the "fur coat" which determines much of their behaviour. The outer layer of the mycobacteria is a highly organised structure containing peptides, waxes and mycolic acid. It confers resistance to staining by ordinary techniques and the resistance to decolorisation which is the source of "acid-fastness". The need to produce this layer probably in part accounts for the relatively slow rate of multiplication of the organism and it also creates specific metabolic requirements. It accounts for the resistance of the organisms to dehydration and chemical agents. The outer layer provides both protection and a store of nutrients, and is almost certainly the basis of the organism's ability to survive in a dormant phase both within and outside the body. It offers some protection against lysozymal enzymes and inhibits macrophage action. The outer protective layer, by preventing access to the bacterial cell, confers resistance to the action of most antibiotics. It is also the source of the antigenic properties of the organism.

The mycobacteria do not secrete toxins, nor have endotoxins been identified in them. The exact mode of their pathogenicity is uncertain. They appear to be pathogenic only when ingested by macrophages, and the damage they produce probably depends on release of lysozymal enzymes from the macrophages.

Special staining techniques are required to demonstrate the organisms which are resistant to ordinary dyes. They can be stained by the use of hot carbol-fuchsin and then are resistant to decolorisation by either dilute acid or alcohol — hence the term acid- and alcohol-fast bacilli (AAFB). More recent techniques using auramine with fluorescence microscopy permit quicker scanning of smears. The organisms grow slowly (6–12 weeks). Culture requires preliminary sterilisation of the samples to destroy other organisms, and the use of specific media containing their preferred metabolic substrates (e.g. Löwenstein-Jensen). Human, bovine and other strains are identified by their appearance in culture and their biochemical characteristics. Phage typing permits identification of different strains of the organism. Sensitivity testing against antituberculous drugs requires careful standardisation; in the United Kingdom it is carried out in reference laboratories which also type the organisms.

*M. tuberculosis* is a strict aerobe and optimal conditions for its growth in the body are found only in the lung, particularly in the walls of cavities. Large numbers of organisms may be found in sputum from patients with cavitated lung disease, but at other sites organisms are relatively scanty and are more difficult to find either on direct smear or culture.

# Natural History and the Immune Response

There is both natural general immunity against tuberculosis and specific immunity, and there are racial and individual differences in susceptibility. In each individual nutritional state and general health are important, particularly the absence of diseases such as diabetes or recurrent infections which lower immunity. The initial response to infection in an individual without specific immunity differs from the subsequent response to infection. The first episode — the primary infection — is often silent and not associated with overt illness, but it is usually the source of the organisms which cause the subsequent episodes of the disease.

The common route of infection is the lung, susceptible subjects inhaling the bacillary aerosol generated by a sputum-positive case. Other routes of primary infection are rare and of little clinical importance. The inhaled bacilli lodge in the lung, usually in the mid or lower zones where ventilation is greatest. There is local serous exudation and cellular infiltration, and the organisms are rapidly taken up by macrophages. Some organisms persist locally but many are removed to the regional lymph nodes in the lung hilum. The characteristic lesion involving the regional lymph nodes and the lung then evolves. The macrophages modify into epithelioid cells, and these cluster together and may form giant cells. Round the outside of these clusters there is some aggregation of lymphocytes. This lesion, the "tubercle", is characteristic of tuberculosis. Aggregation of these microscopic tubercles forms the macroscopic tubercles which can be seen with the naked eye in many forms of the disease. If the number of organisms is large, lyzosome release within the macrophages leads to cell death and breakdown — caseation. Around the tubercle a fibrous reaction eventually develops. In the primary infection the lesions in the lymph nodes are much more conspicuous than the lesion in the lung. The two together form the "primary complex". If general immunity is good, this lesion has a marked tendency to heal. It is usually not associated with symptoms and regresses undiagnosed. The caseous material is reabsorbed, the fibrous reaction increases and often eventually calcifies to leave the characteristic combination of a small peripheral calcified focus with calcification in the hilar lymph nodes. This response is usually adequate to prevent the development of clinical disease, but it is not adequate to kill all of the bacilli.

At the time of the primary infection, when there is no specific immunity, haematogenous spread of tubercle bacilli is very frequent, possibly universal. Most of the organisms are filtered out in the lung, but they also settle in other tissues. These haematogenously spread organisms are usually initially dormant, but like the organisms in the "healed" lesions of the primary complex, they remain viable. Their subsequent activation is the cause of most adult postprimary tuberculosis.

In the 6–8 weeks following primary infection, cell-mediated immunity develops. The response to subsequent infection is much more prompt, and in animals virtually all organisms in a subsequent infection are destroyed. In man the evidence concerning response to re-infection is not clear cut. It is probable that most re-infecting organisms are killed as promptly as they are in animals and that most postprimary disease is due to reactivation of latent organisms rather than re-infection, but examples of re-infection have been documented. The acquisition of immunity is associated with the development of hypersensitivity to tuberculin, intradermal injection of tuberculin now producing a characteristic delayed local response with induration and erythema. Allergic manifestations such as erythema nodosum and phlyctenular conjunctivitis may appear at this stage. The relationship between immunity and hypersensitivity to tuberculin is complex (see below).

The primary infection is most often acquired in adolescence or early adult life and there is a general pattern to the subsequent development of disease. Miliary tuberculosis and tuberculous meningitis tend to occur very early, being the result of progression of the bacteraemia of the primary infection. Tuberculous pleural effusion usually occurs within a few months of primary infection, while postprimary pulmonary disease and bone disease develop within the next 2 to 5 years. Renal disease tends to occur later, usually after 5 years. The earlier primary infection is acquired, the greater are the risks of serious complications. In reported series of primary infection before the age of 5 years, the incidence of miliary tuberculosis and tuberculous meningitis ranges between 2.6% and 16%.

Most adult tuberculosis is postprimary disease due to reactivation in subjects who already have some specific immunity. It is characterised locally by a more fibrous and cellular reaction with less lymph node involvement. Caseation is less common than in primary infection but breakdown does occur, and in the lung caseous lesions drain into the bronchial tree, producing the "open" case of sputum-positive pulmonary disease. Postprimary lung lesions are found in upper lobes or the apical segment of the lower lobes where oxygen tensions are high and the conditions are most favourable for bacterial multiplication. The numbers of organisms in cavitated lung lesions are very high, and they perpetuate the chain of infection. Breakdown may occur at other sites of settlement of organisms from the bacteraemia at the time of primary infection. Lymph node and abdominal tuberculoses are probably mainly due to haematogenous spread, but may also be affected by direct involvement in a primary complex associated with swallowing rather than inhalation of tubercle bacilli.

## The Tuberculin Test

Acquired immunity is associated with a positive tuberculin test (Mantoux, Heaf or Tine), a typical delayed cell-mediated response. It results either from previous primary infection with tubercle bacilli or immunisation with BCG vaccine. The antigen is protein from tubercle bacilli. The response to tuberculin can be expressed in a semiquantitative fashion (Table 8.1).

The association between tuberculin hypersensitivity and immunity is indirect. A negative or non-specific reaction usually indicates lack of immunity (no previous primary infection or BCG vaccination) but may occasionally be due to loss of reactivity from depression of cell-mediated immunity. The optimum response is associated with a definitely but not strongly positive reaction (Mantoux 5–10 mm or Heaf II). Very strong responses do not indicate increasing immunity. Follow-up

**Table 8.1.** The tuberculin test

|  | Mantoux (10 TU) (mm induration) | Heaf (grade) |
|---|---|---|
| Negative | 0 | 0 |
| Non-specific | <5 | I |
| Positive | 5–10 | II |
| Strong positive | >10 | III–IV |

of those with strong positive reactions shows them to have a disease incidence about twice that of positive reactors. The cause of the increased incidence of disease in the strongly positive reactors is not clear.

A positive tuberculin test is evidence of previous primary infection or BCG vaccination. Although the correlation between tuberculin status and outcome is valid for large groups, in the individual it is dangerous to attempt to read too much into the result of the tuberculin test, either in diagnosis or prognosis. Only when a known negative reactor converts to a positive reaction can a definite diagnosis of recent primary infection be made.

Numerous attempts have been made to demonstrate circulating antibodies to *M. tuberculosis* but none has been successful, and the tuberculin test, despite its limitations, remains the only available immunological test.

# Clinical Features

Symptoms are variable and may be few. When tuberculosis is common, primary infection is almost universal before adult life is reached. It is not usually associated with symptoms and is self-healing in a high proportion of people. Minor systemic disturbance may occur, and there are occasionally pulmonary complications, usually from the enlarged hilar nodes which can compress or perforate the bronchi producing either atelectasis or bronchogenic spread. Pleural effusion usually occurs shortly after the primary infection and produces characteristic symptoms. Postprimary lung disease is associated with cough and sputum. Haemoptysis from bronchial arteries eroded in lung cavities used to be a common and ominous event. When the number of organisms is large, signs of systemic toxic illness are common, with fever, weight loss and general malaise. In partially immune subjects chronic pulmonary disease can persist for many years, with indolent fibrotic lesions in the lung. Disease at other sites usually has the characteristic features of infection in these locations, although the tuberculous infection may be "cold", lacking the heat and redness and sometimes the pain classically associated with infection.

The ability of dormant organisms to reactivate after many years (40+ years) is well documented. In the majority of cases the factors leading to breakdown cannot be identified, although depression of immunity by wasting disease, diabetes and steroid therapy are well recognised causes.

# Diagnosis

The diagnosis is based on the combination of a compatible clinical picture and confirmatory investigation. In Third World countries direct sputum smear may be the only confirmatory test available; it is cheap and reliable, and it identifies the infectious cases. In developed countries X-rays and tuberculin testing are almost always used, and attempts are made to culture the organisms. In pleural effusion, biopsy is easily carried out using an Abram's needle and is almost invariably positive. In non-pulmonary disease it may be necessary to seek confirmation of diagnosis by biopsy and histological or bacteriological examination of the affected tissue, but formal surgical procedures are of little therapeutic value and tend to be complicated by infection at the operation site. They should not be undertaken unless confirmation of diagnosis is essential and they should always be done under cover of antituberculous chemotherapy.

# Treatment

### The Historical Background

Until the 1950s no specific treatment was available. The early approach depended on non-specific measures such as rest and improvement of nutrition in order to improve general resistance. By the end of the 19th century these ideas had been formalised into the concept of the sanatorium regime. Over the next 40 years this rigid approach dominated treatment. It was supplemented by collapse therapy which was introduced following the observation that pulmonary tuberculosis tended to remit after spontaneous pneumothorax. The techniques of collapse therapy became established in the first 20 years of this century but its rationale remains somewhat obscure despite its widespread application. It probably depended for its success on cavity closure. The lining of cavitating lung lesions provides an ideal site for bacterial multiplication; closure of cavities reduced the bacterial burden and tilted the balance in favour of healing. Sanatorium treatment and collapse therapy were vigorously applied to combat the considerable increase in tuberculosis which followed the 1914–1918 war. With improvement of surgical and anaesthetic techniques, various attempts at surgical treatment were made, but none other than thoracoplasty — a form of permanent surgical collapse therapy — was really successful. Thoracoplasty was a mutilating procedure, but it avoided the risk of tuberculous wound infection which, in the era before antituberculous chemotherapy, often complicated disastrously the more radical surgical approaches.

Patients clinically "cured" by sanatorium therapy, rest or collapse therapy continued to harbour viable organisms and relapse was always possible. The diagnosis of tuberculosis tended to involve a lifetime of follow-up with the ever-present risk of recurrence. The mortality from sputum-positive disease was very high — 50% within 2 years of diagnosis.

Despite the fact that neither medical nor surgical treatment was particularly successful, there was a steady decline in the incidence and mortality of tuberculosis. This decline was due to improvement in the general health and living standards of the population, mainly improvement in nutrition and housing. None of the medical measures can be shown to have had any impact on incidence of disease or mortality.

The activity of streptomycin against *M. tuberculosis* was recognised by Waksman in 1944 and the first clinical trials were reported in 1945. The quantities of the drug available were limited and relatively short-term treatment was used. Good initial responses were seen, but even in the early clinical trials, subsequent relapse was often noted, and by 1947 the problem of acquired resistance had been encountered. In 1946 the antituberculous activity of para-amino salicylic acid (PAS) was recognised, and in 1948 the MRC commenced a comparison of streptomycin with PAS and streptomycin alone. The reduction in resistance on combined therapy was such that a preliminary statement stressing the importance of combined chemotherapy was made in 1950 before completion of the trial. The first clinical trial of isoniazid was carried out in 1952. It was potent, relatively non-toxic and cheap, and it rapidly became the most important drug. A series of controlled trials of chemotherapy subsequently laid the foundations of modern chemotherapy. By the late 1950s, effective antituberculous chemotherapy was generally available. The concept of bacteriological as opposed to clinical cure was established by 1960. Classical chemotherapy using 18 months isoniazid and PAS with an initial 3 months of streptomycin was a highly effective regimen, despite its unpalatability and relatively high incidence of side-effects. Isoniazid is an outstandingly effective drug and it probably accounted for much of the success of the early treatment regimens.

A large number of other drugs were subsequently found to have antituberculous activity. In the mid-1960s ethambutol replaced PAS. It was equally effective but much better tolerated. By 1974 the great efficacy of rifampicin had been clearly established. Together with isoniazid it is now the mainstay of current chemotherapeutic regimens. A new role had been established for pyrazinamide and streptomycin. Sterilisation of the lesions with elimination of all viable bacilli is now a realistic objective of treatment and should be almost universally attained.

With the advent of effective chemotherapy it was realised that there was little or no place for other forms of therapy and they have largely been abandoned.


## Principles of Antituberculous Chemotherapy

In recent years, understanding of response to treatment has been supplemented by work on experimental tuberculosis in mice. The activity of antituberculous drugs is assessed in three ways: by their activity against cultures of *M. tuberculosis* in vitro; by their activity in experimental tuberculosis in animals (usually the mouse); and by their efficacy in controlled clinical trials in patients with sputum-positive pulmonary tuberculosis in whom progress of disease can be closely monitored both by sputum examination and radiologically. All antituberculous drugs in sufficient concentration kill *M. tuberculosis* growing in culture medium, although there are wide variations in the rate at which they act and the optimum conditions for their activity. When the drugs are used in the treatment of patients the pattern of activity is different and cannot be explained on the basis of drug activity in vitro. Other factors are clearly important in the patient. These factors are reflected in experimental tuberculosis in the mouse in which the pattern of drug activity is similar to that seen in human disease. Some drugs cure the disease and at subsequent post-mortem no viable organisms are found. They are said to possess high sterilising activity, and this correlates well with the ability of the drugs to eliminate organisms from the sputum of patients with pulmonary disease. Other drugs arrest the development of disease, but organisms can still be cultured from the animals. They have weaker sterilising activity. The ability to prevent the emergence of drug resistance in experimental tuberculosis also varies and is not directly associated with sterilising activity. Some drugs with weak sterilising action are highly effective "resistance preventers".

In tuberculosis there are several different populations of organisms. They may be intracellular or extracellular. Some are actively dividing, some are relatively dormant, dividing only infrequently, and a few are totally dormant, dividing not at all. Antituberculous drugs are active only against actively multiplying organisms. They eliminate relatively dormant organisms much more slowly, and are ineffective against completely dormant organisms. Differences in drug activity are related to differences in action against these different populations and in their efficacy against intracellular organisms. The outstanding efficacy of rifampicin is due to its ability to kill both actively multiplying and relatively dormant organisms, and to its efficacy intracellularly. Isoniazid is less effective against relatively dormant organisms and intracellular organisms. Streptomycin is highly effective against extracellular organisms, but ineffective in the acid intracellular environment in which pyrazinamide has its major action. During the initial phase of chemotherapy, actively dividing organisms are eliminated relatively quickly. In the first 2 weeks of treatment there is a 90% fall in the number of viable organisms in the sputum in patients treated with rifampicin, isoniazid, streptomycin and pyrazinamide, but a prolonged follow-up phase of chemotherapy is necessary to deal with the remaining 10% of relatively dormant organisms. The normal body defences cannot be relied upon to eliminate the remaining tubercle bacilli. In all cases of tuberculosis there appear to be a few completely dormant organisms which are not affected by chemotherapy. In experimental tuberculosis treated by apparently curative drug combinations which give sterile organ cultures at post-mortem in control groups, relapse can be provoked by major immunosuppression and a similar problem is seen in patients given major cytotoxic chemotherapy who are liable to reactivate apparently adequately treated tuberculous lesions. These relapses are thought to be due to reactivation of totally dormant organisms which were not affected by chemotherapy. Their numbers are small, and they are unlikely to cause relapse under normal conditions or to be found at post-mortem organ culture.

In devising regimens for antituberculous chemotherapy the general principles are as follows:

1. The objective of treatment is the killing of all the tubercle bacilli in the body. After treatment it should not be possible to culture the bacillus from any secretion, or surgical or post-mortem specimen. In the whole patient, proof of cure ideally requires negative cultures and absence of relapse. Currently in developed countries a relapse rate below 5% in a 5-year follow-up is regarded as acceptable.

2. Prolonged treatment is necessary to ensure the elimination of all tubercle bacilli. The defence mechanisms cannot be assumed to be capable of killing tubercle bacilli and antituberculous drugs must be given to do so. A prolonged period of treatment is required to eliminate persisting relatively dormant mycobacteria. Continuation of treatment is essential to prevent relapse.

3. Drugs should always be used in combination. Bacillary populations are always liable to contain naturally occurring drug-resistant mutants. Combined therapy prevents the emergence and overgrowth of resistant strains during treatment. Ideally, drugs should be given combined in a single tablet, so that either all or none are taken.

4. Intermittent dosage is more effective in eliminating the organisms. Daily treatment is better than twice daily, and twice weekly better than daily. It is possible that weekly treatment would be more effective still, but its application is limited, mainly by drug side-effects.

Drugs with major sterilising activity are regarded as the first line drugs. Other less effective drugs are mainly used in combination with first line drugs as resistance preventers, or in reserve regimens for treatment of patients with resistant organisms or in patients in whom first line drugs are contraindicated. A regimen which includes more than one first line drug is likely to be highly effective, producing quicker clinical response and more rapid elimination of viable organisms. When three drugs with high sterilising activity are used (rifampicin, isoniazid and pyrazinamide), not only is response more rapid, but it is possible to shorten the follow-up phase of chemotherapy. With combinations of drugs with high sterilising activity, acceptably low relapse rates are achieved by treatment for 6 months. A regimen which includes only one first line drug is usually effective, producing a similar final cure rate but requiring a longer continuation phase (at least 9 months). Cure is less certain if the regimen is entirely dependent on second line drugs and even more prolonged treatment is required (at least 18 months).

The main first line sterilising drugs are rifampicin and isoniazid. Pyrazinamide and streptomycin have good sterilising activity, but under more limited conditions. The remaining drugs have little sterilising activity and must be regarded as second line drugs, normally to be given as resistance preventers.

These principles were derived experimentally and from the treatment of pulmonary tuberculosis in man. They are extrapolated to extrapulmonary disease. Bacterial populations outside the lung are smaller, but there is no evidence that they behave differently or that there are differences in the numbers of latent organisms or accessibility to the drugs. Such comparative trials as have been undertaken confirm that there is no difference in behaviour of the organisms in sites other than the lung.

## Antituberculous Regimens

The regimens used in antituberculous chemotherapy should be:

1. Effective — <5% relapse in 5 years.
2. Safe — no major toxic reactions.
3. Acceptable — side effects few and minor and unlikely to reduce compliance.
4. Unlikely to produce drug resistance. Given satisfactory compliance, the drugs used should prevent the emergence of drug resistance during treatment; when relapse occurs the organisms should remain sensitive.
5. Quick. More rapid elimination of the organisms from the sputum shortens the period of infectivity. Shorter durations of chemotherapy are likely to improve compliance.
6. Cheap. Cost is a major consideration in underdeveloped countries where tuberculosis is common.

By these criteria the "classical" chemotherapy of the 1960s with isoniazid and PAS with an initial phase including streptomycin is no longer satisfactory. Continuation chemotherapy used only one drug (isoniazid) with high sterilising activity. PAS has poor sterilising activity, and was not a particularly good resistance preventer. Although the regimen was effective, sputum conversion was relatively slow. Prolonged treatment was required, side-effects were common, the medication was unpalatable and there were problems with compliance. When relapse occurred there was a tendency to the development of resistance, particularly to isoniazid. The substitution of ethambutol for PAS was a significant advance. It did not shorten the duration of chemotherapy and efficacy was unchanged, but acceptability was considerably increased, and side-effects were lessened.

With the introduction of rifampicin, shortening of the duration of treatment became possible as two sterilising agents were now being used. With ethambutol as a third drug in the initial phase of chemotherapy, 9 months chemotherapy was as effective as 18 months of isoniazid and PAS. Interest in further shortening the duration of chemotherapy prompted the re-evaluation of pyrazinamide and streptomycin. Pyrazinamide used for 2 months in the initial phase of chemotherapy was found to be both highly effective and relatively non-toxic, producing a more rapid clinical response, and much more rapid disappearance of viable organisms from the sputum. Streptomycin in the initial phase of treatment also confers some benefit, but its use is not without problems — injections are required and hypersensitivity and toxic reactions are not uncommon. It is not possible to show improvement in the results from the addition of ethambutol.

The most recently available trials show that 6 months of isoniazid–rifampicin with an initial phase including 2 months pyrazinamide and either streptomycin or ethambutol gives results as good as those achieved with 9 months therapy. In the continuation phase, isoniazid and rifampicin can be given either daily or three times a week with similar efficacy. If intermittent therapy is used, the total number of doses is much smaller but it is very important that all the doses are taken. The taking of each dose should be supervised.

Current U.K. standard chemotherapy comprises either:
isoniazid–rifampicin (9 months)
with pyrazinamide (initial 2 months)

*or*

isoniazid–rifampicin (6 months)
with pyrazinamide + streptomycin/ethambutol (initial 2 months)

Prolonged follow-up is not normally required. When relapse does occur it tends to do so early, the organisms usually remain sensitive and the disease responds to retreatment with the same drugs. Patients with a good result can be discharged at the end of treatment. If the result clinically or radiologically is not good or if there is suspicion about compliance, a relatively short period of follow-up of 6 months is adequate to detect most relapses.

**Short Course Chemotherapy**

In the last 10 years there has been great interest in shortening the duration of anti-tuberculous chemotherapy. Many of the problems of treatment for tuberculosis, particularly those of compliance, are problems of continuation chemotherapy and this period requires good organisation if treatment is to be successful. The ideal duration of treatment would be no longer than the period of ill-health and would overcome these problems, but unfortunately such a short course of treatment would not eliminate many of the dormant organisms and the risk of relapse would be unacceptably high. With 2 months of quadruple chemotherapy the cure rate is about 60%, which is impressive but unacceptable. With 4 months treatment the relapse rate is still significantly in excess of 10%. With the drugs available at present, shortening of the duration of therapy to less than 6 months seems unlikely. It may be feasible if another drug with additional bacteriocidal activity against relatively dormant organisms is identified.

One attraction of short course intermittent chemotherapy is that the continuation phase of treatment requires only 50 doses of the drugs given three times weekly and it may then be possible to supervise the administration of all of the doses. Problems of compliance can be greatly reduced, although the problems of ensuring attendance for treatment remain.

# Treatment of Non-pulmonary Tuberculosis

There is no ground for believing that the behaviour of *M. tuberculosis* is greatly affected by the tissue in which it is producing disease, save that large bacterial populations are uncommon except in cavitating lung lesions. The general principles of chemotherapy which have been evolved for pulmonary tuberculosis apply to disease elsewhere. Information from clinical trials in bone and lymph node tuberculosis suggests that the response is identical to that in lung disease, despite the common clinical belief that the behaviour of lymph node tuberculosis is different, with a higher tendency to relapse and a need for longer periods of chemotherapy. This impression is probably based on the ease with which superficial lymph nodes can be palpated, the variety of causes for their enlargement, and the lack of standards for objective assessment. At present it seems that this belief is ill-founded and that a normal period of standard chemotherapy is effective at all sites.

# Infection with Other Strains of Mammalian Tubercle Bacilli

*Mycobacterium africanum* and *Mycobacterium bovis*, like *Mycobacterium tuberculosis*, are pathogenic in man and other mammals. They produce disease like classic tuberculosis although the organisms differ from *M. tuberculosis* in their cultural characteristics, metabolic requirements, susceptibility to agents such as hydrogen peroxide and in their phage types.

*M. africanum* is a strain commonly found in East Africa and is therefore usually isolated in East African or Indian patients. It produces a disease identical to that produced by *M. tuberculosis* and has a similar sensitivity to antituberculous drugs. The main significance of its identification is epidemiological.

The reservoir for *M. bovis* is in animals, which are much more susceptible to it than man. Infection with *M. bovis* is transmitted from animal to man, and much less commonly directly from person to person. In cows it caused a tuberculous mastitis and infection was spread to man by drinking infected unpasteurised milk. The clinical features were similar to those of disease due to *M. tuberculosis*, except that the commonly involved sites were cervical nodes and the abdomen. The disease has been virtually eliminated in the United Kingdom by pasteurisation of milk and tuberculin testing of cattle with slaughter of infected animals. A few sporadic cases still occur. The organisms are usually sensitive to isoniazid and rifampicin, but may show differences in susceptibility to other antituberculous drugs.

# Prevention

## Case Finding

The single most important preventative measure is the prompt diagnosis and effective treatment of the infectious case — the patient with a positive sputum smear. Any case finding programme should concentrate on identifying these individuals so that the chain of spread of the disease can be broken.

## BCG Vaccination

The second widely used preventative measure, BCG vaccination, attempts to provide the specific immunity normally acquired by primary infection. The vaccine is an attenuated avirulent strain of tubercle bacilli, incapable of producing disease, but retaining antigenic properties. It is injected intradermally. A small local lesion develops, then heals within 2 months. In the period immediately after vaccination there is depression of immunity and exposure to tuberculosis should be avoided, but thereafter the tuberculin reaction converts to a positive reaction, and relative immunity is acquired. The only contraindication to vaccination is severe immunodeficiency. Side-effects of vaccination are few, other than abscess formation which results if the vaccine is injected subcutaneously. The abscesses heal on treatment with isoniazid.

BCG vaccine is cheap and has been widely used in an attempt to establish community immunity. The immunity conferred by BCG slowly declines, but persists for several years. In the 7-year period following vaccination it has been shown to provide 75% protection against the development of tuberculosis in British adolescents. However, similar efficacy has not been demonstrated elsewhere, and unequivocal evidence of community wide protection other than in the United Kingdom is difficult to find. There is much variation in the use of BCG. In the UK, vaccination is given to tuberculin-negative reactors to cover the period of greatest risk of infection, normally adolescence, hence the vaccination programme in 13-year-old children. It is also given to tuberculin-negative reactors at high occupational risk such as nurses and medical students starting clinical work. In areas with high immigrant populations and a significant incidence of tuberculosis in children, neonatal vaccination is used.

Other than abscess formation, which should not occur if the technique of vaccination is adequate, the disadvantages of BCG vaccination are the loss of the tuberculin test as a diagnostic test, and the need to organise a large-scale service for tuberculin testing and vaccination. The loss of the tuberculin test as a diagnostic test is a small penalty to pay if protection is substantial and the risk of developing tuberculosis is high. The incidence of tuberculosis in western countries is declining so rapidly that the value of the adolescent vaccination programme is now in doubt. The number of cases prevented is now so small as to make it difficult to justify the continuation of widespread vaccination. When routine BCG vaccination is discontinued it may still be worthwhile to continue tuberculin testing of adolescents so that positive reactors may be investigated and given chemotherapy. Despite some doubts about the efficacy of BCG in underdeveloped countries where the incidence of tuberculosis is high, it seems reasonable at the moment to continue to use the vaccine.

There are few other useful preventative measures. While the decline in tuberculosis in the western world has clearly been the result of improvement in standards of living, attempts to reduce the incidence of tuberculosis by social change are expensive, have a long timescale, and are not likely to be available to the countries whose need is greatest.

# Chemoprophylaxis

The combination of efficacy and relative freedom from significant toxicity of current chemotherapy makes it feasible to give treatment to patients who have been infected but who do not appear to have active disease. The objectives are to prevent the serious complications of primary infection and to eliminate the risk of development of postprimary disease. There is general agreement that asymptomatic children with primary infection should be treated. A similar approach may be justified in adults in high risk groups such as immigrants from areas with a high incidence of tuberculosis. Prophylaxis is worthwhile if the incidence of tuberculosis is above 1%. If the incidence is lower, the benefits of prevention of tuberculosis have to be set against the risks of drug toxicity, and prophylaxis as a general measure is probably not justified. Its selective use may become more important as the incidence of tuberculosis declines. Chemoprophylaxis for tuberculin-positive adolescents may replace BCG vaccination of negative reactors, as is already the practice in North America.

There is no certainty about the optimum treatment regimen. In tuberculin-positive reactors without clinical evidence of disease, the numbers of organisms are usually small. Most trials of prophylactic chemotherapy have used isoniazid given alone for 1 year and this appears to confer about 70% protection against development of tuberculosis in the following 5 years. Six months' treatment achieves about 60% protection. Isoniazid is probably not the ideal drug as its activity against the relatively dormant organisms likely to be present in these patients is not great. Rifampicin-containing regimens have not yet been assessed.

Chemoprophylaxis should be reserved for patients with no clinical or radiological evidence of disease. Patients with an abnormal chest X-ray should be given full chemotherapy.

# Drug Resistance

Resistance is described as primary when the patient is infected with a strain which is already resistant to antituberculous drugs, or secondary when resistance emerges during the course of chemotherapy. In every patient a few naturally resistant mutant organisms are present, but their numbers are small (usually $<1$ in $10^6$) and they are not detected by conventional sensitivity testing. Secondary resistance arises during treatment with single drugs or inappropriate drug regimens. If single drugs are given, the sensitive organisms are eliminated and the resistant mutants become dominant. The use of combined drug regimens prevents their emergence in significant numbers so that resistance should not be a problem in treatment. However, resistant organisms may emerge if the regimen is badly chosen, the drug dose inadequate or the patient non-compliant. In general, the incidence of drug resistance is a measure of the standards of chemotherapy. It is a major problem in Far Eastern countries where antituberculous drugs are freely available in retail pharmacies but are relatively expensive and tend to be taken in short courses. Self-medication with short courses of single drugs may achieve symptom control but the organisms are not eliminated and resistant strains emerge. Primary drug resistance is the result of infection from a patient with resistant organisms.

Primary resistance is a relatively rare problem in the United Kingdom. Serial surveys over the years have shown it to be <5% for the main drugs and <1% for multiple resistance. The incidence of resistance is not increasing. These findings reflect a reasonably good standard of therapy, with appropriate choice of drugs and adequate supervision of their administration. The situation is similar in most of Western Europe, but in some countries, notably the Eastern countries, primary resistance is much more common, as high as 20% of strains in Hong Kong.

# Treatment of Tuberculosis in Developing Countries

In developing countries where tuberculosis is common, there is usually little money for health care and services are relatively poorly developed. The overriding emphasis of tuberculosis control programmes must be on cheapness and efficacy. Good case finding is essential. Programmes should be based on screening of sputum smears from symptomatic individuals. Isoniazid, which is both effective and cheap, is the mainstay of treatment. Discussion centres on the accompanying drugs both for initial phase and continuation chemotherapy. Where money is available, a 2-month initial phase of triple chemotherapy with isoniazid–rifampicin and pyrazinamide is the ideal. Regimens such as isoniazid + thiacetazone which are both cheap and effective are used for continuation chemotherapy. Where cost does not permit the use of rifampicin, an initial phase with isoniazid, streptomycin and thiacetazone followed by continuation isoniazid + thiacetazone for 1 year probably represents the cheapest reasonably effective combination. The initial phase with streptomycin requires moderately well developed medical facilities so that intramuscular injections can be given.

Good organisation of the control programme is essential, with particular emphasis on case finding and supervision of continuation chemotherapy. A BCG vaccination programme should also be continued.

# Other Mycobacterial Infections

The other mycobacteria are saprophytes, common environmental contaminants which rarely produce human disease when tuberculosis is common (<1% of cases of "tuberculosis"), but which appear to be more important as the incidence of tuberculosis declines. The organisms have widely differing cultural characteristics and metabolic requirements. A variety of descriptions have been used for these organisms — such as "anonymous mycobacteria", photochromogens and scoto-chromogens. These descriptions were mainly based on characteristics on culture and are not clinically relevant. Laboratory identification requires detailed characterisation if it is to be accurate. In the United Kingdom all isolates of mycobacteria are examined in reference laboratories where standardised techniques permit accurate classification.

Infection occurs from the environment, and is virtually never transmitted from patient to patient. Some mycobacteria, such as *M. kansasii*, *M. avium*, *M. intracellulare* and *M. xenopi*, usually produce pulmonary disease. Pre-existing abnormality in the lungs, such as bronchiectasis, old tuberculous scars or pneumoconiosis, may predispose to pulmonary infection. The organisms are often found as contaminants and they should only be regarded as pathogenic if they are repeatedly isolated and there is an appropriate clinical abnormality. Recommendations about treatment are empirical since there have been no controlled trials of chemotherapy. When tested in the laboratory, the organisms are often resistant to antituberculous drugs, but there is considerable debate about the clinical relevance of this finding as patients appear to respond to treatment with drugs to which the organisms are resistant on in-vitro testing. There is general agreement that at least three drugs should be given for the entire treatment period, and that this period should be protracted, probably 2 years. Most regimens include rifampicin and isoniazid, regardless of the results of sensitivity testing, but the choice of the other two antituberculous drugs depends on the laboratory findings. The results of treatment have improved as the range of drugs available has widened, but even with intensive chemotherapy relapse is more common than in disease due to *M. tuberculosis*, and more patients die of progressive disease. Surgery was formerly advocated, particularly for infections with *M. kansasii*, but there were problems with postoperative recurrence when antibiotic cover for operation was inadequate. The results were not good unless the disease was sufficiently localised to permit resection well clear of the lesions with a wide margin of healthy lung. With the currently available drugs, surgery is not normally indicated. On in-vitro testing, the environmental mycobacteria may be sensitive to other antibiotics such as tetracyclines and erythromycin but it is not clear that these antibiotics have a useful place in treatment.

# Non-specific Measures

The introduction of effective chemotherapy requires reconsideration of former approaches. Rest is not necessary if drugs are taken. Hospital admission is not required unless the patient is acutely ill. While good nutrition is clearly important, chemotherapy is highly effective whatever the state of nutrition.

Corticosteroids have been used on a wide variety of indications and can be safely given if the patient is on effective antituberculous chemotherapy. The indications for their use are largely empirical. Many physicians give a short course of prednisolone to patients with pleural, pericardial or meningeal tuberculosis in the hope of preventing subsequent fibrosis (initial dose 30 mg/day tailing after 2 weeks to 10 mg/day for about 2 months). They may also be useful in the acutely ill non-reactive patient who is cachetic with little fever. Corticosteroids are useful in the management of severe sensitivity reactions and for desensitisation in drug hyper-sensitivity. Topical steroids are useful in the treatment of more severe reactions to tuberculin testing.

Surgery now has little place in the treatment of tuberculosis. The disadvantages of a surgical operation usually outweigh any benefit. Controlled trials in lymph node disease and bone tuberculosis show no benefit from surgery. Decompression is occasionally required for cord compression in spinal tuberculosis, but for the majority of patients chemotherapy and conservative management give better results. An abscess will usually reabsorb with chemotherapy. If drainage is required, aspiration, repeated if necessary, is preferred to surgical drainage. Surgery should only be undertaken under cover of effective antituberculous chemotherapy. Incisions should be carefully placed through healthy tissue and pri-mary closure should be attempted in order to minimise sinus formation and scar adherence.

## Infectivity and Segregation

Infectivity is confined to sputum-positive patients, and is maximal in the weeks preceding diagnosis when large numbers of bacilli are excreted. Within 2 weeks of starting chemotherapy with rifampicin, isoniazid and pyrazinamide, viable bac-terial counts in the sputum have fallen by 90%. For most purposes, infectivity can be assumed to have ended when effective chemotherapy starts. Isolation at the start of treatment has never been shown to be effective in the prevention of secon-dary cases, and should no longer be practised. If patients have to be admitted to hospital, they should be instructed in elementary hygiene in the disposal of sputum, and they should be nursed in a side-ward for the first 2 weeks. The prac-tice of continuing segregation until the sputum was direct and culture negative was never justified and should be abandoned. Infectivity for casual contacts at work and elsewhere is not high and segregation is not required unless the contacts are particularly susceptible, e.g. the immune suppressed or neonate when a 4-week period should elapse between start of chemotherapy and recommencing work.

Non-pulmonary tuberculosis is not infectious and segregation is not required.

## Contact Supervision

Examination of household contacts of cases of sputum-positive tuberculosis gives a worthwhile return of secondary cases (2%–5%) and should always be carried out. Initial examination comprising tuberculin test and chest X-ray should be carried out 3 months after the diagnosis of the source case unless the contact is symptomatic, when immediate investigation is required. A second examination at 6 months is probably worthwhile, but more protracted follow-up is not justified.

The yield from wider contact searching is generally low. Tuberculosis is infective, but its main infectivity is in relatively close contacts. Even with highly infectious cases, the return from examination of a large number of casual contacts is very low, and widespread examination is only justified if the contacts are particularly susceptible, e.g. young children or immune-suppressed patients. For highly infectious patients (sputum direct positive + + +), close contacts outside the home should be examined, and casual contacts in high risk groups such as children who have not received BCG should also be screened.

# Useful References

American Thoracic Society (1983) Statement on control of tuberculosis. Am Rev Resp Dis 128: 336–342

Banks J, Hunter JM, Campbell IA, Jenkins PA, Smith AP (1983) Pulmonary infection with *Mycobacterium kansasii* in Wales 1970–79: review of treatment and response. Thorax 38: 271–274

Bleiker MA, Styblo K (1978) The annual tuberculosis rate and its trend in developing countries. Bull IUAT 53: 295–303

Davies PD, Humphries MD, Byfield SP, Nunn AJ, Darbyshire JH, Citron KM, Fox W (1984) Bone and joint tuberculosis: a survey of notifications in England and Wales. J Bone Joint Surg 66B: 326–330

Essop AR, Posen JA, Hodkinson JH, Segal I (1984) Tuberculous hepatitis: a clinical review of 96 cases. Q J Med 53: 465–478

Glassroth J, Robins AG, Snider DE (1980) Tuberculosis in the 1980s. N Engl J Med 302: 1441–1450

Grange JM, Yates MD (1986) Infections caused by opportunist mycobacteria: a review. J R Soc Med 79: 226–229

Horne NW (1984) Control and prevention of tuberculosis: a code of practice Thorax 39: 321–325

Humphries MJ et al. (1984) Death occurring in newly notified patients with pulmonary tuberculosis in England and Wales. Br J Dis Chest 78: 149–158

ICMR/WHO Scientific Group (1980) Vaccination against tuberculosis. WHO, Geneva

Joint Tuberculosis Committee of the British Thoracic Association (1982) Notification of tuberculosis: a code of practice for England and Wales. Br Med J 284: 1454–1456

Joint Tuberculosis Committee of the British Thoracic Society (1983) Control and prevention of tuberculosis: a code of practice. Br Med J 287: 1118–1121

Katz I, Rosenthal T, Michaeli D (1985) Undiagnosed tuberculosis in hospitalised patients. Chest 87: 770–774

Kilmach OE, Ormerod LP (1983) Gastro-intestinal tuberculosis: a retrospective review of 109 cases in a district general hospital. Q J Med 56: 569–578

Leading article (1983) Tuberculosis in old age. Tubercle 64: 69–71

McKay AD, Cole RB (1984) The problems of tuberculosis in the elderly. Q J Med 53: 497–510

Medical Research Council Tuberculosis and Chest Disease Unit (1985) National survey of notifications of tuberculosis in England and Wales in 1983. Br Med J 291: 658–661

Medical Research Council Tuberculosis and Chest Disease Unit (1982) Tuberculosis in children in a national survey of notifications in England and Wales. Arch Dis Child 57: 734–741

Medical Research Council Tuberculosis and Chest Disease Unit (1982) The geographical distribution of tuberculosis notifications in a national survey of England and Wales (1978/9). Tubercle 63: 75–88

Miller EJW (1982) Tuberculosis in children. Churchill-Livingstone, Edinburgh

Mitchison DA (1985) The action of antituberculous drugs in short course chemotherapy. Tubercle 66: 219–225

Pagell WW, Symmonds FAH, McDonald N, Nassau E (1964) Pulmonary tuberculosis, 4th edn. Oxford University Press, London

Schraufnagel DE, Leech JA, Pollak B (1986) *Mycobacterium kansasii*: colonisation and disease. Br J Dis Chest 80: 131–137

Smith MJ, Citron KM (1983) Clinical review of disease caused by *Mycobacterium xenopi*. Thorax 38: 373–377

Sutherland I, Springett VH, Nunn AJ (1984) Changes in tuberculosis notification rates in ethnic groups in England and Wales between 1971 and 1978/9. Tubercle 65: 83–92

Traub M, Colchester ACF, Kingsley DPF, Swash M (1986) Tuberculosis of the central nervous system. Q J Med 53: 81–100

Yu YL, Chow WH, Humphries MJ, Wong RWS, Gabriel M (1986) Cryptic miliary tuberculosis. Q J Med 59: 421–428

# 9 Sarcoidosis

In 1889, Besnier described skin lesions due to the disease now known as sarcoidosis. In the following 60 years, lesions were described in various other systems, but it was not until the 1950s that the essentially generalised nature of sarcoidosis was recognised, and only in 1953 that the characteristic involvement of the mediastinal nodes was fully documented. The cause of sarcoidosis is still unknown and the natural history is unpredictable. There is no specific therapy.

## Pathology

Histologically the disease is characterised by tissue infiltration with non-caseating granulomas, and these may occur in any tissue. The cells of the granuloma are lymphocytes and macrophages, there is a marked tendency to giant cell formation, and inclusion bodies are often found in the giant cells. The granuloma is not unlike the granuloma of tuberculosis, but it does not caseate. Although the disease may be very widespread, the lesions are essentially focal rather than diffuse and they often do not disturb the normal tissue architecture. Granulomas may appear to be clinically or radiologically static, but they are characterised by a rapid cellular turnover. The presence of lesions implies activity, but the link between activity and the release of tissue-damaging mediators is unknown. When the disease becomes quiescent the granulomas regress, usually leaving no residual damage. Occasionally a fibrotic reaction is provoked with damage to tissue architecture and permanent scarring.

## Aetiology

The cause of the granuloma formation is obscure. Numerous hypotheses have been advanced, but none is satisfactory. The "infective" hypothesis is perhaps the best at present, but the transmissible agent has not been identified and the disease is certainly not infectious in the conventional sense. Given that mediastinal node involvement is almost universal, the portal of entry is probably the lung. The pattern of distribution of the lesions suggests subsequent haematogenous spread. Despite the resemblance of some of the features of the disease to tuberculosis and some other chronic infections, there is no convincing evidence that sarcoidosis is due to an atypical form of tuberculosis or any other bacterial infection, nor is there evidence to suggest that it is due to a toxic chemical.

Genetic factors play some part, as evidenced by the increased incidence within families and the effect of race on incidence. Associated immunological abnormalities are almost invariable but there is no evidence that the observed immunological abnormalities are causal. There is little change in the total number of lymphocytes in the peripheral blood but the number of T-lymphocytes is usually reduced. T-lymphocytes from the granuloma are activated. There is a polyclonal increase in immunoglobulins. Cell-mediated immunity is depressed and there is usually loss of hypersensitivity to tuberculin.

Bronchoalveolar lavage has provided some information about the nature of the lung lesion. Lymphocytes normally predominate in the lavage fluid, particularly in the early stages when their total numbers and their proportion relative to other cells are increased. There is some correlation between the numbers of lymphocytes obtained in lavage fluid and other indices of disease activity. Characterisation of the lymphocytes shows that the majority are T-lymphocytes, mainly T-helper cells. Macrophages are usually present and neutrophils may be found. Several mediators have been identified in the lavage fluid (monocyte chemotactic factor, helper factor, interleukin-1 and interleukin-2). It seems likely that these or other mediators from the granuloma induce tissue damage when it occurs. It has been suggested that bronchoalveolar lavage is a useful way to assess activity in sarcoidosis and that the findings may help to predict outcome, but there is considerable variability in the reported findings and its place in assessment and management remains uncertain. The granuloma in other tissues has not been intensively studied, but is presumed to be similar.

# Incidence

There are wide variations in incidence between different countries and races. The annual incidence of sarcoidosis in the United Kingdom is said to be about 4/ 100 000 per year. Sarcoidosis is more common in Ireland and the Scandinavian countries, and ten times more common in the negro races. The incidence of the disease is almost certainly underestimated. Many patients have no symptoms and underdiagnosis is known to be common, probably accounting for the apparent rarity of sarcoidosis in countries such as India.

# Clinical Picture

The onset of sarcoidosis is usually insidious with few symptoms. The diagnosis is most often made by the detection of an abnormality on a chest X-ray taken for some other purpose. Sarcoidosis may present acutely, most commonly as the combination of erythema nodosum and hilar adenopathy. Occasionally when the disease is very active general features of systemic illness with fever, malaise and weight loss occur, but symptoms are usually produced either by the local effects of a mass of sarcoid granuloma or by the tissue response which it elicits. In the majority of patients sarcoidosis is active for less than 3 years, but the disease can run a very protracted course. The acute forms tend to resolve relatively rapidly.

The manifestations of sarcoidosis are protean. Granulomas may be found at any site and are almost certainly present in many apparently uninvolved tissues. Estimates of site involvement are at best approximate, depending on the ease with which a site can be studied, and on the specialty of the reporting physician. Race is also important. Sarcoidosis is not only more common in those of negro race, but its manifestations are more florid and there is a greater tendency for extrathoracic sites to be involved. The frequency of site involvement may in general be summarised as follows:

1. Almost universal.
    a) Mediastinal nodes (histology if not on X-ray).
    b) Liver (histologically).
2. Common (50%–10% of cases).
    a) Lung and bronchi.
    b) Peripheral lymph nodes.
    c) Skin.
    d) Calcium metabolism.
    e) Eye.
3. Rare (<10% of cases).
    a) Bone.
    b) Heart.
    c) Parotid and lachrymal glands.
    d) CNS.
    e) Pleura.
    f) Synovium.
    g) ENT.

The commonest clinical presentations are asymptomatic hilar gland enlargement found on routine chest radiography, and erythema nodosum with hilar adenopathy, a form of the disease with a very good prognosis.

Mediastinal node and lung involvement are usually asymptomatic. Disproportion between the X-ray changes and the clinical picture may be striking. Mediastinal nodes, even if very large, virtually never produce symptoms, and extensive pulmonary infiltration may produce neither symptoms nor signs. The finding of a grossly abnormal chest X-ray in an asymptomatic individual with no abnormal physical signs is virtually pathognomonic of sarcoidosis. Extensive lung disease or bronchial involvement can cause cough, some mucus hypersecretion and shortness of breath. In extensive disease pulmonary function is impaired. The picture commonly is of a restrictive disorder; less commonly, there is an obstructive pattern as a result of extensive bronchial involvement. Pleural involvement is not often diagnosed on the chest X-ray but is frequently shown by special techniques such as CT scanning. It rarely produces an effusion.

Hepatic involvement is usually asymptomatic, but may be associated with general malaise or biochemical evidence of hepatocellular dysfunction; hepatomegaly is relatively rare and a frank "hepatitis-like" illness is most uncommon. Sarcoidosis in peripheral lymph nodes usually causes no specific symptoms, but may present a problem in differential diagnosis. Skin involvement is of several different types of which the most common is erythema nodosum, an allergic vasculitic lesion. Other skin manifestations include nodular infiltration, often in scars, and lupus pernio, a chilblain-like lesion affecting the face or digits. Hypercalciuria is common, but hypercalcaemia is rare, and neither is usually associated with symptoms. The abnormalities in calcium metabolism appear to be due to overproduction of $1,25\text{-}(OH)_2D_3$ by macrophages causing increased intestinal absorption of calcium. Eye involvement is characterised by keratoconjunctivitis or uveitis; both are commoner early in the disease and they may cause blindness.

Bone involvement is most often associated with periostitis and cystic lesions in the hands and feet which produce striking X-ray changes but rarely give rise to symptoms. Synovial sheath infiltration may produce an apparently severe "arthritis" in the hands but function is usually surprisingly well preserved. Cardiac involvement produces arrhythmias and cardiomyopathy. Sudden death due to arrhythmia is a well recorded complication, but the frequency and importance of cardiac involvement are uncertain. Sarcoid cardiomyopathy has a poor prognosis. Involvement of the central nervous system produces either a space-occupying effect from the mass of granuloma, or a meningitic picture. The outcome in CNS sarcoid is often poor, possibly as a result of ischaemic lesions produced by an associated granulomatous angiitis. Neuromyopathies are seen rarely. Involvement of salivary or lachrymal glands produces loss of secretion. Upper respiratory tract disease causes crusting, obstruction and bleeding and may be associated with destructive changes in the nose and sinuses. Splenic involvement is relatively rare. A wide variety of blood dyscrasias have been reported.

# Diagnosis

There are three parts to the diagnosis.

1.   To establish that sarcoidosis is the cause of the disease.
2.   To assess its extent.
3.   To assess its activity and likely outcome.

## Confirmation of Diagnosis

The diagnosis is easily missed. Sarcoidosis lacks specific clinical features and a high index of suspicion is required if it is to be diagnosed. As there is no specific therapy, caution is required in the pursuit of proof of diagnosis, unless it is necessary to exclude some other diseases such as lymphoma or tuberculosis. The extent to which the diagnosis is pursued depends on the clinical picture. The combination of a compatible clinical picture and a negative tuberculin test is often adequate and does not require histological confirmation. The pattern of disease progression is helpful in excluding alternative diagnoses, but if there is any doubt further support of the diagnosis is required, usually a Kveim test or tissue biopsy.

The Kveim test is a useful diagnostic method if a good antigen is available. The antigen, an extract of a sarcoid spleen, is injected intradermally, and the site of the injection biopsied 4–6 weeks later. In a positive reaction, classic sarcoid granulomas are seen at the site of injection. Problems arise as a result of variation in the potency of the antigen, and in the interpretation of the histology. Non-specific reactions occur and it can be difficult to discriminate between these and true positive reactions. With a good antigen and an experienced histopathologist, the results are generally comparable to those of biopsy of affected organs. Whenever possible the Kveim test should be undertaken before steroids are given as reactivity to the antigen tends to be depressed by steroids. The major drawback of the Kveim test is the delay in obtaining the result.

The alternative approach is to biopsy an affected tissue. The specialty of the physician tends to influence the site chosen. An accessible, obviously involved tissue should be selected. If there are superficial lymph nodes or skin lesions, this presents no problem. Failing these, most physicians would currently look to fibreoptic bronchoscopy. If there is any abnormality on the chest X-ray, either bronchial or transbronchial biopsy through the fibreoptic bronchoscope gives a high diagnostic yield, even when the bronchoscopic appearances are not grossly abnormal. If histological proof of diagnosis is essential, a Kveim test is not feasible, and no other site is apparent, there are three possible approaches: blind bronchial biopsy; biopsy of a mediastinal or scalene node; liver biopsy. They can all be expected to give positive histology in at least 80% of cases. Blind bronchial biopsy specimens usually but not invariably include an affected submucosal lymphatic. Problems occasionally arise in the interpretation of a granulomatous reaction from a lymph node draining an abnormal area of lung but an experienced histopathologist can usually distinguish these changes from sarcoidosis. The presence of a "granulomatous hepatitis" supports a diagnosis of sarcoidosis, but is less conclusive than the demonstration of the characteristic changes elsewhere.

If the clinical picture is compatible and the tuberculin test negative, there must be a very strong case to justify any investigation in pursuit of confirmation of diagnosis beyond a Kveim test, fibreoptic bronchoscopy, or biopsy of a superficial tissue under local anaesthesia.

## Assessment of Extent

The extent of involvement is assessed by evidence of clinical, radiological or biochemical abnormality. The more exhaustive the search, the more widespread is the disease likely to seem. Detailed search to determine the extent of involvement by sarcoidosis is not justified since disease involvement not producing symptoms is not generally an indication for treatment. Hypercalcaemia and, more debatably, extensive lung involvement are the main exceptions. All patients should have a chest X-ray and spirometry, and the serum calcium should be measured. Staging by chest X-ray is conventionally as follows: stage 1 — mediastinal node involvement, stage 2 — mediastinal nodes and lung, and stage 3 — lung involvement only. Further investigation should be undertaken only if there are definite symptoms.

### Assessment of Activity and Likely Outcome

Decisions about treatment of sarcoidosis are influenced by predictions of likely outcome. The basis of the predictions is imprecise. They depend on clinical assessment of activity and extent of involvement and are largely based on the progression of existing lesions or the development of new lesions. In the lung prognosis is related to extent of the disease. It is worse in patients with symptoms, and in those with a progressive fall in vital capacity or carbon monoxide transfer. Gallium scans and the cellular components of alveolar lavage fluid are sometimes used to assess activity though their role is less clear. Gallium is taken up by macrophages, and a positive gallium scan correlates quite well with radiological changes and other evidence of "active" lung disease but it is not clear how much additional information it provides. Alveolar lavage may be useful, but the reported findings thus far (1986) are too inconsistent for it to be established in routine clinical practice. Multiple site involvement and particularly extrathoracic site involvement carry a worse prognosis.

Activity of liver disease can be assessed by liver function tests, and abnormal calcium metabolism by repeated blood or urine calcium measurements. Sarcoid granulomas release angiotensin-converting enzyme (ACE), and activity in general can be assessed by changes in serum ACE levels. The changes are not specific, and they tend to parallel other obvious clinical, radiological and biochemical abnormalities.

It is probably true that while a number of methods give reasonable information about the extent and activity of the granulomas, none gives adequate information about prognosis. Decisions about treatment remain empirical.

# Treatment

There is no specific treatment. The granulomas at almost every site regress with corticosteroids, but the effect of steroids is suppressive, not curative. It is unlikely that they shorten the course of the disease. They should be given when sarcoidosis is producing severe symptoms, or is liable to produce tissue damage. Steroids must be continued as long as the disease remains active and threatens tissue damage, and moderately high doses (10+ mg prednisolone) may be required for a long time so that control of the disease may be bought at a fairly definite price in steroid side-effects. Except when given for control of symptoms, steroid therapy tends to be empirical. The indication is fear of irreversible tissue damage and, not surprisingly, there are considerable variations in the interpretation of this in clinical practice. The current trend is towards caution in the use of steroids.

When steroids are given, a clear objective of their use should be defined. The indications have varied widely between reported series, and there are no controlled trials on which judgement can be based. In general, there should be an initial high dose phase to attain control, followed by a gradual reduction to the lowest dose which maintains control. Maintenance therapy is usually required for several months, during which time it is hoped that the activity of the disease will subside. Treatment should be withdrawn slowly as rapid steroid withdrawal is liable to precipitate rebound reactivation. The optimum withdrawal rate is not known, but it is almost certainly longer than 3 months for the patient who has been treated for 6 months on a dose of 10 mg/day of prednisolone. Relapse will occur on steroid withdrawal if the disease has not "burned out", and a further treatment course will be required. There is no way of knowing when the disease has remitted other than by watching the effects of stopping treatment.

The response to steroids is affected by the site involved, and the role of steroid therapy is considered in relation to disease sites.

*Mediastinal Nodes.*    A benign condition on which steroids have little effect. Not indicated.

*Lung Involvement.*    Usually reserved for extensive lung disease with symptoms, or lung involvement thought by the physician to be likely to produce scarring. Currently there is less enthusiasm for steroids and a more conservative approach is adopted. Most physicians would reserve steroids for extensive persisting and deteriorating lung disease accompanied by symptoms, functional abnormality, particularly a reduced or falling vital capacity, or radiological changes suggesting the development of fibrosis in addition to infiltration. If symptoms are not severe, it is better to observe for evidence of deterioration rather than treat immediately. Initially prednisolone should be given in high dose (30–40 mg/day) for at least 1 month, monitoring change in symptoms, X-ray and vital capacity. High doses should be continued until the desired improvement has been produced. The dose should then be reduced to a maintenance level. This ideally would be less than 10 mg/day, but the dose will depend on its ability to maintain control of the disease. The initial high dose is usually required for at least 1 month and maintenance for at least 6 months. Slow withdrawal can then be tried. The treatment cycle should be repeated in the event of significant relapse. If steroid treatment is reserved for those with more severe abnormalities, it usually has to be prolonged, often for several years.

In general, treatment must be monitored by symptoms, changes on the chest X-ray and measurement of vital capacity. Repeated gallium scans or bronchoalveolar lavage have no place in routine follow-up. ACE measurements tend to parallel other indices such as the chest X-ray.

*Pleural Disease.*    If extensive or complicated by effusion treat with steroids. Usually requires shorter treatment course.

*Liver.*    The natural history of sarcoid involvement of the liver is not clear. Histologically the liver is almost invariably involved, and abnormalities in liver function are not infrequent. Although liver damage with portal hypertension has been reported, it is very uncommon and does not respond well to steroids. Steroids are usually given for a combination of non-specific systemic symptoms, and abnormalities in the liver function tests. Treat as for lung disease on clinical grounds with monitoring of enzyme abnormalities.

*Skin.*    Acute eruptive lesions often respond to steroids, but skin disease is rarely an indication for treatment unless extensive and disfiguring. More chronic lesions may respond to intralesional injection of steroids, but results are often poor.

*Erythema Nodosum ± arthralgia.*    Usually responds to analgesics or non-steroidal anti-inflammatory drugs. Response to a short course of steroids is usually dramatic. They should be given if local or general symptoms are severe and not responding to analgesics.

*Nose and Sinuses.*    There is usually some response to topical steroids — beclomethasone or budesonide. Systemic steroids have little effect.

*Salivary and Lachrymal Glands.*    Marginal response to steroid therapy only.

*Heart.*    Steroids are invariably given but there is little good evidence about their effect. While ST and T wave changes usually regress, and arrhythmias may be less frequent, it is not clear that steroids have any useful long-term effect. Treatment for arrhythmias or heart failure may be required.

*Hypercalcaemia and Bone Disease.*    Hypercalcaemia is not often associated with symptoms, but is liable to be persistent and may lead to stone formation or renal damage. It is suppressed by steroids, but treatment often has to be prolonged. Sunbathing and therapeutic use of vitamin D should be avoided and there may be a place for limiting dietary intake of calcium and vitamin D. Other bone changes are little affected, and bone disease is not usually an indication for steroids.

*Nervous System.*    There is usually some response where the granulomas produce a space-occupying effect as in cortical involvement or Bell's palsy from facial nerve involvement. The meningeal forms and the neuromyopathies respond relatively poorly.

*Eye.*    Topical steroids are usually effective in keratoconjunctivitis and anterior uveitis. Oral steroids should be given for posterior uveitis, and if there is any impairment of vision in anterior disease.

## Other Treatment

In patients with severe steroid-resistant disease, azathioprine has been shown to be of some benefit, and it may also be useful for a steroid-sparing effect. The benefits must be balanced against potentially more severe side-effects. As with steroids, there are no adequately controlled trials.

There are reports that a variety of other drugs such as chloroquine and some non-steroidal anti-inflammatory drugs have some therapeutic effect in sarcoidosis, but none has been shown to be of value clinically.

# Useful References

Cohen RD, Bunting PS, Meindok HO, Chamberlain DW, Rebuck AS (1985) Does serum angiotensin converting enzyme reflect intensity of alveolitis in sarcoidosis? Thorax 40: 497–500

Fleming HA (1986) Sarcoid heart disease. Br Med J 292: 1095–1096

Hillerdal G, Nou E, Osterman K, Schmekel B (1984) Sarcoidosis: epidemiology and prognosis. Am Rev Resp Dis 130: 29–32

Hunninghake GW, Garrett KC, Richerson HB, Fantone JC, Ward PA, Rennard SI, Bitterman PB, Crystal RG (1984) Pathogenesis of the granulomatous lung diseases. Am Rev Resp Dis 130: 476–496

James GD, Jones Williams W (1985) Sarcoidosis and other granulomatous disorders. WB Saunders, Philadelphia

Lin YH, Haslam PL, Turner-Warwick M (1985) Chronic pulmonary sarcoidosis: relationship between lung lavage cell counts, chest radiograph, and results of standard lung function tests. Thorax 40: 501–507

McNicol MW, Luce PJ (1985) Sarcoidosis in a racially mixed community. J R Coll Physicians Lond 19: 179–183

Neville E, Walker AN, James GD (1983) Prognostic factors predicting the outcome of sarcoidosis: an analysis of 818 patients. Q J Med 208: 525–533

Poole GW (1982) Editorial. The diagnosis of sarcoidosis. Br Med J 285: 321–322

Rizzato G (1986) Recent advances in sarcoidosis. Eur J Resp Dis 68: 1–6

Scadding JG, Mitchell DN (1985) Sarcoidosis, 2nd edn. Chapman and Hall, London

# 10  Alveolitis

## Definition

The term alveolitis was first used to describe the condition now called extrinsic allergic alveolitis. Its use was rapidly extended to include a number of other conditions such as "diffuse pulmonary fibrosis" and "interstitial pneumonia" for which the terms then in use were felt to be unsatisfactory. There were objections that the term "alveolitis" was not appropriate as some of these conditions involved the entire acinus including the small airways, but despite this the use of the term has persisted and seems to be widening to include other diseases with increased cellularity on bronchoalveolar lavage not due to bacterial infection. The use of the term alveolitis appears to convey a specific meaning, but this appearance is clearly not justified for the group of conditions it includes is a very heterogeneous one. However, they share to a variable extent a number of common features such as dyspnoea, diffuse shadowing on chest X-ray and a restrictive pattern of ventilatory impairment. At present, "alveolitis", rather like "pneumonia", appears to be a useful term to describe a group of diseases.

## Pathology

A variety of different histological classifications have been used, but none completely satisfactorily links tissue appearances to cause or prognosis. The presence of macrophages and pneumocytes in the alveoli, described as desquamative interstitial pneumonia (DIP), seems to represent an early stage in which response to treatment is more likely and prognosis more favourable. In the later stages the most prominent changes are thickening and fibrosis in the alveolar wall with distortion of alveolar structure and fewer cells in the lumen. The changes may be focal or diffuse, and they tend to be less easily reversed by treatment. The cell type in the infiltrate, such as the eosinophils in drug-induced alveolitis, may be characteristic of some types of alveolitis.

Alveolitis may be provoked by either inhaled or circulating agents, whose action may be either due to direct toxicity or may be immunologically mediated. With inhaled agents, the distribution of the changes tends to reflect the distribution of the inhaled material. The factors determining the distribution of changes due to circulating agents are not clear. Tissue damage in alveolitis is produced by liberation of mediators from the cells involved in the alveolitis — macrophages, neutrophils, eosinophils or lymphocytes. When fibrosis and scarring are produced a non-specific picture of permanent lung damage ensues.

The common conditions associated with alveolitis are as follows:

Cryptogenic fibrosing alveolitis.

Extrinsic allergic alveolitis.

Lung involvement by collagen disease:
    rheumatoid arthritis
    systemic lupus erythematosus (SLE)
    systemic sclerosis.

Exposure to chemical toxic agents:
    inhaled — asbestos, beryllium, oxygen
    circulating — cytotoxic agents, paraquat, amiodarone.

Radiation alveolitis.

Adult respiratory distress syndrome (ARDS).

Sarcoidosis.


## Bronchoalveolar Lavage and Alveolitis

Bronchoalveolar lavage (BAL) through the fibreoptic bronchoscope has made alveolitis much more accessible to study. The procedure involves wedging the bronchoscope in a third generation bronchus and instilling and gently sucking out buffered saline. It is well tolerated and can be repeated on several occasions. Total and differential white cell counts on the lavage fluid provide the basic information. Immunological and cytochemical studies can be carried out on the cells, and mediators can be identified, but these are not yet routine clinical techniques. The findings may eventually provide a more logical basis for classification, and more useful diagnostic, prognostic or therapeutic information. The technique clearly has great research potential, but its clinical role is not yet established.

There are differences in predominant cell types and mediators in the different diseases, but the findings are affected by factors such as the stage of the disease and they are not always consistent. Cryptogenic fibrosing alveolitis is characterised by a general increase in cell numbers, particularly neutrophils, and neutrophil collagenases and proteases are present in the fluid. The findings in the alveolitis of rheumatoid arthritis and systemic sclerosis resemble those of cryptogenic fibrosing alveolitis, while in extrinsic allergic alveolitis the cells tend to be lymphocytic, as they do in sarcoidosis (see Chap. 9).

The mechanism of progression from alveolitis to fibrosis depends on the nature of the alveolitis. The activated neutrophils of cryptogenic fibrosing alveolitis secrete collagenases and other enzymes which provoke fibrosis. They probably also secrete oxygen radicals which produce cellular damage. In extrinsic allergic alveolitis, lung damage appears to depend mainly on an immune complex vasculitis.

# Incidence

Alveolitis is almost certainly underdiagnosed. It is difficult to give figures for incidence other than for sarcoidosis (about 4/100 000 per year — see Chap. 9). Cryptogenic fibrosing alveolitis is much less common; exact figures are not available, but the incidence is probably about ten times less — around 4/million per year. There is no adequate information about the incidence of extrinsic allergic alveolitis though it has been suggested that there may be as many as 1000 new cases of farmer's lung each year in the United Kingdom. The presence of antibodies is not diagnostic of the disease, but they have been demonstrated in 54/1000 of the at-risk farming population. Estimates of the incidence of alveolitis in bird fanciers range between 0.5% and 7%. These figures suggest that the incidence of extrinsic allergic alveolitis is higher than that of fibrosing alveolitis.

Estimates of incidence of lung involvement in collagen disease suggest that about 1% of cases of rheumatoid arthritis will have alveolitis, almost invariably as part of an active general disorder. In SLE , about half of the patients with severe disease are said to have lung problems, though in some this is secondary to diaphragmatic weakness. Lung involvement appears to be relatively common in systemic sclerosis, affecting about half of the patients.

The incidence of alveolitis with asbestos exposure is related to the intensity and duration of exposure. Alveolitis with amiodarone appears to be dose related.

# The Clinical and Physiological Pattern

The clinical picture of established alveolitis is non-specific, with shortness of breath, diffuse shadowing on chest X-ray and a restrictive impairment of ventilatory function as the outstanding features. The differential diagnosis is from pulmonary oedema due to left ventricular failure or the diffuse infiltration of lymphangitic carcinoma. It is particularly important to establish the cause of the alveolitis. Both prevention and management depend on an accurate diagnosis of the underlying cause. When prevention is possible, it is far more effective than treatment. The diagnosis of the cause is often based on non-pulmonary features such as a history of exposure to a potentially damaging agent, evidence of disease at other sites, or abnormal immune responses.

The common presenting symptom is dyspnoea on exertion. There may be an irritating dry cough but sputum production is not a feature of the early stages of alveolitis. Extrinsic allergic alveolitis tends to be episodic in its early stages, and there is often a latent interval of 18–24 h between exposure and the development of symptoms, which may include systemic symptoms, particularly fever and general malaise. Finger clubbing is common in patients with fibrosing alveolitis and asbestosis but is rare in allergic alveolitis and sarcoidosis. Fine inspiratory crackles at the lung bases are common to most alveolitides, but are very rare in sarcoidosis. When the disease is severe central cyanosis may be present.

The characteristic physiological pattern is of small stiff lungs with impairment of gas exchange. The predominant abnormality is a loss of vital capacity from increased stiffness of the lung. Airway function is well preserved and the PEF and $FEV_1$ may even be increased in the early stages. Gas exchange is impaired, causing a fall in arterial $PO_2$ and an increased $A–aDO_2$. The $PCO_2$ is usually low. If these blood gas abnormalities are not very obvious at rest, they become striking on exercise. Carbon monoxide transfer is impaired. In the late stages, secondary polycythaemia, pulmonary hypertension and fluid retention may develop.

In most of the alveolitides there is a reasonably close relationship between radiological, clinical and physiological abnormality. The striking exception is sarcoidosis, where there may be extensive changes on the X-ray with little in the way of symptoms, physical signs or functional abnormality. This may relate to the essentially focal nature of the changes in sarcoidosis.

## The Natural History

The natural history depends primarily on the cause of the alveolitis. If there is an extrinsic cause, the pattern of evolution of the disease is determined by the pattern of exposure. Episodic exposure produces episodic symptoms, chronic exposure progressive disability. There is also great variability in the rate of evolution of the disease. There may be an acute fulminating illness like a rapidly progressive pulmonary oedema, an indolent scarcely progressive disorder or improvement, though this is rare unless an extrinsic cause is removed. Eventually, regardless of its cause, persisting alveolitis produces progressive irreversible pulmonary fibrosis. In the end stage there is a common picture of "honeycomb lung", with grossly fibrotic lung and intervening bronchiectatic bronchi. Persistent infection with cough and sputum is then added to the other problems.

## Diagnosis

Diagnosis of the presence of an alveolitis is not usually particularly difficult. The clinical, radiological and physiological patterns are fairly characteristic, and exclusion of pulmonary oedema and lymphangitic carcinoma rarely causes problems. In the immunosuppressed, an atypical response to infection may mimic alveolitis.

The main diagnostic problems lie in discriminating between the various causes of alveolitis. Investigation must often be primarily directed outside the lungs.

The history is of great importance. A detailed and specific occupational, recreational and drug history is essential; information should always be sought about exposure to birds. The history and general features normally indicate the presence of collagen disease. Serological tests for rheumatoid factor and antinuclear factor should be undertaken routinely. When there is any possibility of an extrinsic allergic alveolitis, attempts should be made to demonstrate circulating antibodies.

### Tissue Diagnosis

There is considerable uncertainty about the value of biopsy in management. Its use is restricted by the fact that there is no simple safe technique which reliably produces an adequate sample. Although lung biopsy is the only means of making an unequivocal diagnosis of alveolitis, histology rarely indicates the cause of the alveolitis and it does not at present give unequivocal information about prognosis. In most patients, biopsy proof of diagnosis is not required, but it is necessary if there is real uncertainty about the diagnosis and other causes of diffuse infiltration cannot be excluded. Histology also contributes to understanding of the primary disease process and may in time permit better classification, as renal biopsy has for nephritis.

Bronchoscopy and transbronchial biopsy can be relatively readily carried out through the fibreoptic bronchoscope but the tissue specimen obtained is small. It is usually adequate to diagnose sarcoidosis and to exclude malignancy, but it is less useful for other alveolitides. The samples obtained may not be representative as relatively normal lung is biopsied more readily than fibrotic tissue, and histological examination of such small specimens is not easy. Percutaneous biopsy provides a rather larger sample, but has similar problems. Both techniques have a risk of haemorrhage or pneumothorax. When histological proof of the diagnosis is needed, open biopsy from an affected area provides an adequate and more representative sample and seems to be the most satisfactory procedure, but even minithoracotomy techniques require an anaesthetic and a surgical procedure in patients who are often not particularly fit. The procedure should only be undertaken if there are strong grounds for requiring histological proof of diagnosis.

# Specific Alveolitides

*Cryptogenic Fibrosing Alveolitis.*    This presents the "classic" clinical picture. The spectrum ranges from a very chronic, scarcely progressive disease to a rapidly evolving disorder which is fatal within a few months. Radiological involvement is usually maximal in the lower zones. Symptoms are not specific. Diagnosis can be made on the presence of the combination of clubbing, fine crackles at the lung bases, the appropriate changes on the chest X-ray and in lung function, together with exclusion on clinical grounds of other causes of alveolitis. Immunological abnormalities, such as a positive antinuclear factor or rheumatoid factor at low titre occur in 25%–50% of patients, but none seems to be specifically causal. Histological confirmation of diagnosis is not usually required, but may given some prognostic information. When the pattern is that of a cellular desquamative interstitial pneumonia, response to steroids is more likely. Bronchoalveolar lavage may support the diagnosis.

*Extrinsic Allergic Alveolitis.*    The diagnosis depends on a history of exposure to a potential allergen, either at work or leisure, and the demonstration of the presence of circulating antibodies to the allergen. The pattern of association between symptoms and work and of remission during holidays is strongly suggestive of the diagnosis, although it may be masked by a latent period between exposure and the development of symptoms. Specific questioning is required to identify the increasing number of potential occupational causes (mouldy hay, mushroom spores, humidifiers, cork or sugar-cane dust etc) or recognise leisure hazards such as exposure to birds. Patients may be aware of a risk not recognised by the doctor.

The disease tends to progress in episodes following exposure, although the delay of up to 24 h between exposure and the development of symptoms is sufficiently long that the importance of exposure may not be realised, and with continuous low grade exposure an apparently progressive pattern may mask the diagnosis. Systemic features such as fever and gastrointestinal upset may also be found. Clubbing is rare. On the chest X-ray the abnormalities tend to be in the midzones. In the early stages the infiltrate has an inconspicuous "ground glass" appearance which is easily missed if the X-ray is of poor quality. Once the diagnosis is suspected, serological tests for circulating antibodies should be carried out. These can be positive in exposed subjects in the absence of evidence of disease, but the combination of an appropriate clinical picture and circulating antibodies to the relevant antigen is considered virtually diagnostic.

The significance of the presence of antibodies in the absence of symptoms, radiological or functional abnormalities, is difficult to assess. Surveys of populations at risk have shown that antibodies are present in many more people than are affected by disease. They presumably define an at-risk population in whom further antigen exposure should be avoided, either completely by change in activity (e.g. disposing of pet birds) or by modification of working pattern if change in occupation is not feasible (e.g. in farming).

*Collagen Disease* (see Chap. 12).    Lung involvement is common in collagen disease, but it is usually only one aspect of a generalised disorder; it is rarely the primary problem or an indication for treatment.

Fibrosing alveolitis is one of several pulmonary manifestations of rheumatoid arthritis. Although lung disease can predate arthritis, the presence of other features of rheumatoid disease usually make the diagnosis of the cause of the alveolitis relatively easy. The presence of high titres of rheumatoid factor in the blood (>1:80) is helpful. Lower titres are not specific as they are found in many patients with cryptogenic fibrosing alveolitis.

In the more severely affected patients with SLE, lung involvement is common and includes diffuse alveolitis. The clinical picture is complicated by other manifestations of the disease, including muscle involvement with respiratory muscle weakness leading to the picture described as the "shrinking lung". In systemic sclerosis, pulmonary involvement produces a picture similar to that of fibrosing alveolitis; the diagnosis must be made on the presence of other features.

*Chemical Agents.*    Heavy exposure to asbestos can produce asbestosis, an alveolitis similar to that of cryptogenic fibrosing alveolitis. It is rare with less than 3 years' unprotected exposure to a dusty environment, and usually develops more than 10 years after the main exposure. A history of asbestos exposure and the presence of other features compatible with asbestosis exposure, such as pleural plaques on the chest X-ray, help to confirm the diagnosis. Asbestos exposure and asbestosis increase the incidence of lung cancer; in some series as many as half of the patients with asbestosis died from carcinoma of the lung. The risk is greatly increased in cigarette smokers.

Much more rarely, other chemical agents such as beryllium produce an acute pneumonic picture or a diffuse pulmonary fibrosis. Diagnosis depends on a history of exposure, but may require biopsy and histochemical examination for confirmation. Cobalt exposure produces a similar chronic change — "hard metal disease".

In experiments on animals high oxygen concentrations have been shown to produce an alveolitis. In patients with the adult respiratory distress syndrome who require prolonged ventilation with very high inspired oxygen concentrations (50% +), oxygen "toxicity" may be an important factor in the development of fibrosis (see Chaps. 6 and 23).

*Drugs and Alveolitis.*    See Chap. 12.

*Radiation.*    External radiation in sufficiently high dose produces a localised alveolitis with subsequent fibrosis. Problems were particularly severe with early supervoltage treatment of carcinoma of the breast and bronchus when the radiation dose to normal tissues was high. With improved equipment and dose planning, this complication is now becoming rare.

# Treatment

## Cryptogenic Fibrosing Alveolitis

The natural history of cryptogenic fibrosing alveolitis is unpredictable, as is the response to treatment. There is no specific therapy, but some patients respond to steroids. Although a good response is more likely in the early stages, when the alveolar reaction is more cellular, prediction of response from histology is not reliable. Unless there are contraindications, all patients with significant or increasing symptoms should have a trial of steroids. Treatment should generally be tried early, before there is irreversible fibrotic damage. Prednisolone should be given initially in high dose (30–40 mg/day), and response monitored by change in symptoms, chest X-ray and vital capacity. Monitoring of change in carbon monoxide gas transfer, although frequently carried out, probably does not provide useful additional information. When the optimum response has been obtained the dose should be tailed down to a maintenance level, which generally has to be continued indefinitely. Azathioprine should be tried in patients who do not respond to steroids or who require a high maintenance dose of prednisolone which produces significant side-effects (e.g. >15 mg/day). Neither steroids nor azathioprine benefit the patient with advanced disease and fibrotic lungs.

The prognosis in fibrosing alveolitis is poor. The response to treatment is variable, unpredictable and often disappointing. Most series report good responses in 20%–30% of patients. In the more favourable "cellular" group, a mean survival of 12 years has been reported, but mortality as great as 66% at 2 years has been reported in those not responding to steroids.

### Extrinsic Allergic Alveolitis

Prevention is more important than treatment. Early diagnosis and antigen avoidance are essential. When the antigen involved is not associated with the patient's work complete avoidance may be feasible, but this is much more difficult when the antigen is associated with the patient's occupation. The ideal solution, change of occupation, is often not possible and the emphasis must then be on measures to reduce antigen load. Working methods should be reviewed with the aim of reducing antigen production. Many antigens are associated with contamination by moulds, and this can be reduced by improved working practices, the use of fungicides and better ventilation. Care in cleaning and sterilisation of humidifier systems prevents mould growth as well as Legionella infection. When exposure to atmospheric contamination is unavoidable, the use of filters and respirators may prevent antigen inhalation, but those that are effective are difficult to wear in a working environment. Ordinary "breathing masks" offer no protection.

Acute episodes often regress spontaneously, but if severe, treatment with corticosteroids is usually effective. Up to 40 mg prednisolone/day may be required, the dose depending on the severity of the episode. Progress is monitored by disappearance of fever and signs of systemic illness, by resolution of radiological abnormalities and improvement in vital capacity. Treatment may have to be given for 6–8 weeks. When chronic changes are established, a formal steroid trial is worthwhile, but the response is usually poor. The medicolegal implications of the diagnosis should be borne in mind, and in the more disabled the possibility of compensation should be considered.

### Diffuse Lung Involvement in Collagen Disease

Lung involvement is rarely an indication for treatment, and response to treatment is usually poor (see Chap. 12). There is a rather greater chance of response in rheumatoid disease and SLE, and virtually no chance of a response in systemic sclerosis. A formal steroid trial should be undertaken in rheumatoid disease and SLE when there is severe or increasing lung involvement. Great care should be taken with dose reduction as relapse of the underlying condition may be precipitated, even in non-responders. Azathioprine should be tried in non-responders with rheumatoid lung or SLE, but appears to be of no value in systemic sclerosis, in which condition there are some reports of benefit with penicillamine.

### Chemical Agents

There is no treatment for asbestosis, but removal from asbestos exposure may delay progression. Beryllium lung disease in its acute form tends to respond to steroids, and there may also be some response in the more chronic progressive disease. Steroids should always be tried if there are major lung problems. With these agents, environmental control to prevent exposure is essential.

As with extrinsic allergic alveolitis, the possibility of compensation should be borne in mind.

### Treatment of End-stage Pulmonary Fibrosis

There is no specific therapy. With the development of honeycomb lung and bronchiectasis, the treatment of secondary infection becomes important. Pulmonary hypertension and cor pulmonale occur in the later stages of the more chronic diseases and diuretics may then be required for fluid retention. Long-term oxygen therapy may be helpful in relieving breathlessness.

# Useful References

Banham SW, McSharry C, Lynch PP, Boyd G (1986) Relationship between avian exposure, humoral immune response, and pigeon breeders' disease among Scottish pigeon fanciers. Thorax 41: 274–278

Becklake MR (1976) Asbestos-related diseases of the lung and other organs: their epidemiology and implications for clinical practice. Am Rev Resp Dis 114: 187–227

British Thoracic Society Research Committee Report (1984) A national survey of bird fanciers' lung: including its possible association with jejunal villous atropy. Br J Dis Chest 78: 75–86

Cormier Y, Belanger J, Laviolette M (1986) Persistent broncho-alveolar lymphocytosis in asymptomatic farmers. Am Rev Resp Dis 133: 843–847

Crystal RG, Bitterman PB, Rennard SI, Hance AJ, Keogh BA (1984) Interstitial lung diseases of unknown cause (part 1). N Engl J Med 310: 154–164

Crystal RG, Bitterman PB, Rennard SI, Hance AJ, Keogh BA (1984) Interstitial lung diseases of unknown cause (part 2). N Engl J Med 310: 235–244

Crystal RG, Reynolds HY, Kalica AR (1986) Bronchoalveolar lavage. Chest 90: 122–131

Editorial (1975) Farmer's lung. Br Med J: 189–190

Hendrick DJ, Marshall R, Faux JA, Krall JM (1981) Protective value of dust respirators in extrinsic allergic alveolitis: clinical assessment using inhalation provocation tests. Thorax 36: 917–921

Hunninghake GW, Garrett KC, Richerson HB, Fantone JC, Ward PA, Rennard SI, Bitterman PB, Crystal RG (1984) Pathogenesis of the granulomatous lung diseases. Am Rev Resp Dis 130: 476–496

Morgan WKC, Seaton A (1984) (eds) Occupational lung diseases, 2nd edn. WB Saunders, Philadelphia

Tukiainen P, Taskinen E, Holsti P, Korhola O, Valle M (1983) Prognosis of cryptogenic fibrosing alveolitis. Thorax 38: 349–355

Turner-Warwick M, Burrows B, Johnson A (1980) Cryptogenic fibrosing alveolitis: clinical features and their influence on survival. Thorax 35: 171–180

Turner-Warwick M, Lebowitz M, Burrows B, Johnson A (1980) Cryptogenic fibrosing alveolitis and lung cancer. Thorax 35: 496–499

# 11 Lung Tumours

This chapter is mainly concerned with primary lung tumours, most of which are carcinomas arising in the bronchial epithelium. Primary lung cancer is an epidemic disease of this century. In the past it was almost certainly underdiagnosed, but there is little doubt that it was a relatively rare condition until the 1940s. In most western countries it is now the commonest cancer in men, and the second commonest in women. This dramatic increase in incidence is clearly related to the emergence of cigarette smoking as a common habit in the course of this century.

## Bronchial Carcinoma

### Histological Classification

Bronchial carcinomas show a diversity of histological type. Their natural history depends both on histological type and the degree of differentiation. There is often considerable variability in the histological appearance of lung tumours and in interpretation by the histopathologist. Caution is therefore required in the interpretation of the histology. Classifications are less clear cut than might be expected. In particular, the relatively small samples obtained by bronchoscopic biopsy may be unrepresentative of the tumour as a whole, either in type or degree of differentiation. A variety of different classifications has been used, including a fairly elaborate one adopted by the World Health Organisation. None is entirely satisfactory or universally adopted. The simplest classification is:

Squamous cell carcinoma — comprising about 50%
Small cell carcinoma — comprising about 35%
Adenocarcinoma — comprising about 15%
Alveolar cell carcinoma — comprising about 1%

Several classifications, including that of the WHO, incorporate a "large cell" group which probably comprises a variety of poorly differentiated carcinomas.

Squamous cell and small cell carcinoma arise in the bronchial epithelium, and the incidence of both is closely related to smoking habits. Adenocarcinoma arises in the mucous glands and its incidence shows no relation to smoking habits. It was previously the commonest type of lung cancer in women, but is now becoming relatively less common as the incidence of smoking-related tumours rises. Most squamous cell carcinomas and adenocarcinomas are differentiated and have a relatively good prognosis. Small cell carcinoma, which is essentially undifferentiated, grows rapidly and is usually widely disseminated at the time of diagnosis. It has a very poor prognosis.

## Aetiological Factors

The vast majority of primary lung cancers (squamous cell and small cell carcinomas comprising 85%–90% of all tumours) are due to malignant change in the bronchial epithelium induced by exogenous carcinogens in cigarette smoke. There is a consistent increase in incidence with increasing numbers of cigarettes smoked, with a 20-fold increase in those smoking more than 20 cigarettes/day. International differences in incidence can be accounted for by differences in the numbers of cigarettes smoked and in the smoking pattern. The lower incidence of carcinoma in smokers in the United States despite a high cigarette consumption is almost certainly related to the habit of leaving a large stump. In those who stop smoking, the increase in risk declines rapidly, halving within 5 years, and falling to about twice that of life-long non-smokers after 10 years. The incidence of lung cancer in pipe and cigar smokers is increased to a lesser extent (about five times that of non-smokers).

It is probable that atmospheric pollution also contributes to the development of lung cancer, and that this accounts for the increased incidence in urban as opposed to rural areas. This effect is relatively weak compared with that of cigarette smoking, urban rates being less than twice rural rates. The change in incidence in men in the United Kingdom is probably due to the combined effects of smoking and atmospheric pollution. The generations born in the first 20 years of this century have had a very high risk of developing lung cancer and this has persisted as the group has aged. Subsequent generations of men show a lower incidence. A similar cohort effect is occurring much later in women, reflecting changes in smoking habits starting during the 1939–45 war.

Specific occupational factors are important in groups at risk, but make a relatively small contribution (2%–3%) to the overall incidence. The increase in incidence of lung cancer in asbestos workers and those exposed to radon is well known. Other chemicals (chromate, nickel, arsenic, haematite and aromatic polycyclic hydrocarbons) also increase the risk of developing lung cancer. They have a weaker effect than cigarette smoking, but they probably all potentiate the risk from smoking.

The cause of adenocarcinoma in the lung, as at other sites, is not known. Pulmonary fibrosis predisposes to the development of alveolar cell carcinoma.

## Incidence

In most westernised countries where smoking is common, lung cancer is by far the most common form of malignant tumour. In 1983 in England and Wales there were 27 600 deaths from lung cancer in men and 9400 in women. In that year there were 12 600 deaths from carcinoma of the breast, 10 300 from carcinoma of the colon, and 9400 from carcinoma of the stomach.

The international variations in incidence are striking, with a low incidence in many Third World countries (Table 11.1). The large part of this variation is explicable on the basis of different national "smoking histories". The incidence of bronchial carcinoma is already rising in Third World countries as cigarette smoking becomes more common.

**Table 11.1.** Death rates from carcinoma of the lung (males, 1977, WHO figures)

|                    | Deaths/100 000 population |
| ------------------ | ------------------------- |
| England and Wales  | 310                       |
| USA                | 194                       |
| France             | 135                       |
| Japan              | 75                        |
| Egypt              | 7                         |
| Sri Lanka          | 4                         |

## Natural History

Bronchial carcinoma tends to present relatively late. It is possible to make some estimate of tumour growth rates by measuring the increase in size of lesions on the chest X-ray. Extrapolation from these figures suggests that most lung carcinomas have been present for several years before diagnosis. There are few structures in the lung to produce symptoms and small lesions (<1 cm in diameter) are not detected easily by radiological screening. The natural history and prognosis of bronchial carcinoma depend mainly on histological type. As a group, squamous cell carcinomas have the least aggressive behaviour pattern. The total 5-year survival from diagnosis is around 5%, the 5-year survival following surgery is 20% to 30%, and the 5-year survival when the disease is sufficiently localised to permit curative resection is as high as 50%. The figures for adenocarcinoma are similar, with a rather poorer survival rate in those whose disease is less well localised at the time of diagnosis. At the time of diagnosis, small cell carcinoma is almost invariably widely disseminated and the prognosis is very poor, with a median survival from diagnosis of approximately 3 months in the untreated patient. Even with aggressive treatment in cases of apparently limited disease, median survival is still less than 1 year.

Squamous cell and adenocarcinoma often spread locally, producing pleural, pericardial, mediastinal or chest wall involvement. They spread by the lymphatics and haematogenously to distant organs. Virtually any tissue may be involved, but the commonest sites for metastases are the hilar, mediastinal and cervical nodes, and liver, bone and brain. In small cell carcinoma haematogenous spread with multiple organ involvement is almost invariable at the time of diagnosis, hence the very poor prognosis. Local spread is less striking. Paraneoplastic syndromes are relatively common in bronchial carcinoma, with neuropathy and myopathy occurring in 10%–15%, particularly in the more advanced stages of the disease. Ectopic hormone production is usually associated with small cell carcinoma — ACTH with biochemical changes of Cushing's syndrome, and antidiuretic hormone (ADH) with hyponatraemia. Hypercalcaemia due to circulating tumour products causing abnormal calcium metabolism is associated with squamous cell carcinoma. A wide variety of other endocrine disturbances are described, but these are less frequent.

**Clinical Presentation**

Symptoms are not specific. Central tumours involving the major bronchi tend to cause cough, haemoptysis if they ulcerate, or distal infection if they obstruct secretion drainage. In general, central tumours present earlier than peripheral lesions which can become quite large before they cause symptoms. Chest pain and increasing shortness of breath tend to be associated with more widespread disease. Pain results from extension to involve pleura, chest wall or mediastinum. Breathlessness usually results from collapse due to major bronchial obstruction, infection or pleural effusion. A few patients present with superior mediastinal obstruction, a distressing condition due to tracheal and superior vena caval compression by enlarged mediastinal nodes. Many patients present with symptoms due to metastases; it is unwise to diagnose a primary cerebral tumour in a smoker if the chest has not been X-rayed. Some patients, particularly those with small cell tumours, present with non-specific symptoms, or paraneoplastic syndromes. As chest X-rays are often taken as a more or less routine part of medical examination, the diagnosis may be made in this way in an asymptomatic individual, or in one with no respiratory symptoms.

In smokers and those with preceding chronic chest disease, many of the symptoms associated with lung cancer may already be present. Change in the pattern of symptoms or the development of new or unexpected respiratory symptoms is then important in suggesting the diagnosis of carcinoma — change in cough, increasing shortness of breath, haemoptysis, new chest pain, a slowly resolving chest infection, etc. The incidence of bronchial carcinoma is so great in heavy smokers, and the clinical features potentially so protean, that a very high index of suspicion is essential. In a heavy smoker (20+/day) it is a reasonable working hypothesis that any unexplained respiratory symptom or unusual opacity on the chest X-ray is due to carcinoma until proved otherwise.

**Prevention**

Despite apparent advances in treatment, there has been little change in overall survival from lung cancer. Prevention is the only way in which significant inroads can be made into mortality. Cigarette smoking is the overwhelming risk factor — 80%–90% of lung cancer would disappear if cigarette smoking ceased. In the United Kingdom there has been a reduction in the prevalence of cigarette smoking in the last decade (in men from 52% to 38% and in women from 41% to 33%), but total tobacco consumption remains high and cigarette smoking in teenagers who will be the next generation of lung cancer patients has not shown the same fall. Further action is urgently required, and this must be in the "political" sphere. The success of anti-smoking clinics is limited and substitutes such as synthetic smoking material or nicotine chewing gum have not had the success that would be required to effect significant change, nor is their long-term safety certain.

Control of other carcinogens — of which industrial exposure to asbestos and chromates appear to be the most important — must also be rigorous.

## Early Detection

It has been suggested that high risk groups should be screened by regular chest radiographs and sputum cytology or bronchoscopy, and there is some evidence that such programmes increase the rate of detection of treatable lesions. These programmes thus far have been selective, they need large resources, and the return is small. Overall they do not make a useful contribution to the problems of lung cancer.

## Investigation

The objective of investigation is to confirm the diagnosis and establish the possibility of treatment. It is necessary to know both the extent and histological type of the tumour if appropriate treatment is to be given.

A chest X-ray is mandatory and fibreoptic bronchoscopy is usually indicated. It often provides histological confirmation of the diagnosis, and gives information about the extent of central tumour spread. Sputum cytology may be helpful in patients who are clearly unfit for bronchoscopy. If it is necessary to establish histological type and these methods fail, other techniques such as direct needle biopsy of the tumour or lymph node biopsy should be considered (see Chap. 1).

The subsequent approach is very much influenced by the type and stage of disease. For patients with squamous cell and adenocarcinoma, the optimum treatment is surgical resection if the disease is sufficiently localised and the patient's general health and respiratory function are adequate to make useful postoperative survival likely. Investigation of these patients is therefore orientated towards assessment of operability, and involves some form of staging. For patients with small cell lung carcinoma, chemotherapy appears to be the optimum treatment, and a different investigative approach is indicated. In patients with manifestly inoperable disease, treatment is directed to symptom control. It may be helpful to confirm the diagnosis and investigation may be required to assess and treat complications, but there is usually no justification for intensive investigation.

## *Approach to the Potentially "Surgical" Patient*

Surgery is absolutely contraindicated if local spread prevents closure of the bronchial stump after resection; the signs are abnormal rigidity or mucosal infiltration of the proximal bronchial tree and these are assessed at bronchoscopy. Local spread to involve the chest wall or mediastinum, or the known presence of lymph node metastases or distant spread, are also near-absolute contraindications to operation. It is also essential to take into account lung function, age and general fitness. Apart from tumour recurrence, respiratory insufficiency is the commonest cause of death after surgery. Adequate lung function is required to permit reasonable survival. There is on average a 15% loss of vital capacity and 1-s forced expiratory volume after lobectomy and a 30% loss after pneumonectomy. Lobectomy is feasible if the preoperative $FEV_1$ is greater than 1.5 l, and pneumonectomy if greater than 1.8 l. The mortality of surgery rises sharply in patients over the age of 70 years, and resection would rarely be considered in a patient aged more than 75 years. Poor general fitness and intercurrent illness also increase operative morbidity and mortality.

There are considerable variations in the pattern of preoperative assessment. Staging such as "TNM" staging provides a basis for assessment of operability of the tumour. It attempts to assess local spread of the tumour (T), the presence of lymph node spread (N) or distant metastases (M).

T — local assessment of tumour.
1. Bronchoscopic evidence of tumour extent and bronchial wall involvement. Fibreoptic or rigid bronchoscopy will usually provide this evidence, as well as giving histological typing.
2. Clinical or radiological evidence of local spread to involve pleura, mediastinum or chest wall. The presence of a pleural effusion is always ominous. A serous effusion does not necessarily indicate pleural involvement, but a blood-stained effusion almost always does.

N — lymph node involvement either in the mediastinum or cervical region. There is controversy about assessment of mediastinal nodes. It is generally accepted that obvious involvement of mediastinal nodes is a contraindication to surgery, but it is not clear that the more elaborate techniques of preoperative assessment improve the results of resection, although they do reduce the number of cases found to be inoperable at thoracotomy. Some surgeons accept the findings of the plain chest X-ray, others require preoperative CT scanning of the mediastinum, and some carry out a routine preoperative mediastinoscopy. While a detailed assessment of resectability before thoracotomy seems to be highly desirable, survival does not appear to have been improved by mediastinoscopy. Approach to routine assessment of mediastinal lymph nodes remains a matter of individual custom.

Other evidence of intrathoracic spread usually secondary to lymph node involvement includes phrenic or recurrent laryngeal paralysis and oesophageal involvement either by compression or invasion. These would all be regarded as contraindications to surgical resection, as would involvement of the scalene node, often the first extrathoracic node to be involved.

M — evidence of distant metastases.

For most sites, clinical evidence is adequate, but liver function tests should be part of routine assessment as liver involvement is often not clinically apparent. If they are abnormal, a liver scan or ultrasound examination should be carried out to exclude metastases. Distant metastases whatever their site are a contraindication to surgery.

## Approach to the Patient with Small Cell Carcinoma

Once the histological type is established a simple staging into localised (restricted to one hemithorax) or generalised disease is used, and has prognostic significance. Patients are often subjected to very detailed investigation as part of clinical trials of chemotherapy in an attempt to define optimum regimes of treatment. Such investigation is not required under other circumstances.

## Approach to the Patient with Inoperable or Disseminated Disease

In patients whose disease is already widespread it may be helpful to establish histological type. A wide variety of techniques, such as cytological examination of sputum, bronchial aspirates or effusions, direct needle biopsy of lung lesions, or biopsy of other superficial metastases, may be useful. However, if potentially curative treatment is not being given, investigation should be restricted to tests which are likely to identify treatable complications and to provide help in management. The necessity for any investigation, particularly an invasive investigation, should be carefully considered.

## Treatment

The available treatments are as follows:

1. Surgical resection — for squamous cell or adenocarcinomas of limited extent when age and lung function do not contraindicate surgery.
2. Chemotherapy — for small cell carcinoma.
3. Radiotherapy — may have a place in radical treatment of squamous cell carcinoma and is useful in palliation, e.g. of superior mediastinal obstruction, localised painful metastases, cerebral secondaries etc.
4. Palliation — for many patients (approximately 55% of the total) for whom curative surgery is not possible and aggressive chemotherapy or radiotherapy is not indicated.

## Surgery

The requirements for successful surgery have been defined. The operation rate for squamous cell and adenocarcinoma is usually 20%–25% with an operative mortality of 5%–10%. The overall 5-year survival of surgically treated patients is about 25%. As is common in surgery for neoplastic disease at any site, better results are obtained with disease amenable to a more limited procedure (segmental resection or lobectomy). Patients requiring pneumonectomy usually have more advanced disease and the results are less satisfactory.

## Chemotherapy

The main indication is small cell carcinoma where there is good evidence that chemotherapy prolongs survival and gives a reasonable quality of life. A wide variety of drugs have been tried (nitrogen mustard, cyclophosphamide, vincristine, adriamycin, CCNU, etc.) in varying combinations and dosage cycles with and without supplemental radiotherapy. There is thus far little evidence of "cure". Five-year survivals are still very rare, but there is undoubted evidence of prolongation of survival. Median survival ranges between 6 and 16 months, depending on the extent of disease at the time of diagnosis, and there is a 7% survival at 2 years. The more energetic chemotherapeutic regimens have a high incidence of side-effects, both the disagreeable such as vomiting and hair loss, and the serious such as bone marrow failure and infection. Although these regimens may prolong survival, this is often at the cost of an unacceptably low quality of life. Slightly less energetic regimens can achieve both prolongation of survival and symptom control so that the quality of life is actually improved. Priority in chemotherapy must be to obtain the greatest possible prolongation of survival together with a reasonable quality of life. The optimum compromises have not yet been defined.

Chemotherapy can be used for palliation in squamous cell carcinoma. Symptom control is usually achieved, and there may be considerable regression of metastases on the chest X-ray, but useful prolongation of survival is not achieved. Adenocarcinoma in the lung, as elsewhere, is relatively resistant to chemotherapy.

## Radiotherapy

Squamous cell and small cell carcinomas respond to radiotherapy, whereas adenocarcinoma is relatively refractory. However, radiotherapy tends to be a second choice in treatment. Surgery is preferred for squamous cell carcinoma. In small cell carcinoma radiotherapy is used to supplement chemotherapy. Radiotherapy is potentially curative, but early attempts at radical radiotherapy produced severe radiation side-effects, particularly postradiation fibrosis in the lung. With high energy radiation it is possible to give large tumour doses without these side-effects. In trials of radical radiotherapy in localised disease, 1-year survival was rather better than for surgery, largely because of absence of operative mortality. Five-year survival was less good — around 6% as opposed to 20% for surgery. Radical radiotherapy may have a place in patients with localised disease in whom surgery is contraindicated. With improved techniques, survival times are increasing and side-effects are fewer. There is some constitutional upset, but radiation "pneumonitis" and postirradiation fibrosis are usually localised. Oesophagitis is common, but usually transient. Skin reactions are rarely severe. Treatment appears to be well tolerated, even by older patients.

Palliative radiotherapy is useful in the control of symptoms and treatment of complications. Control of symptoms is usually very good in bone pain, persistent haemoptysis and superior mediastinal obstruction. When radical radiotherapy is given for superior mediastinal obstruction, there may also be some improvement in overall survival despite the widespread nature of the disease. Dyspnoea due to major bronchial obstruction by tumour can often be relieved. Radiotherapy is useful in patients with symptoms from cerebral metastases which are not adequately controlled by steroids and anticonvulsants. In general, the smaller doses of radiation used in palliative radiotherapy produce few side-effects. However, as with any treatment, there should be a specific indication for radiotherapy; it should not be offered routinely to the patient with an inoperable lesion.

## Palliative Treatment

For more than half of the patients with bronchial carcinoma there is no specific treatment. Overall mortality is high, about 90% at 1 year, and management is largely symptomatic. This large group of patients requires emotional support as well as symptom control. Complications should be treated when they cause symptoms. Persistent cough should be suppressed and infection treated. Radiotherapy is helpful in the control of pain from bony metastases and of haemoptysis. It is usually worthwhile to treat dyspnoea due to major bronchial obstruction either by radiotherapy or by laser diathermy. Pleural effusions producing breathlessness should be aspirated. If they recur, topical chemotherapy with mepacrine or bleomycin often obliterates the pleural space, preventing further recurrence and improving symptom control. When cerebral metastases produce headaches or paralysis, high dose dexamethasone (12 mg/day) should be given; anticonvulsants should be given for fits. Radiotherapy may also be useful for solitary cerebral secondaries.

Endocrine disturbances other than hypercalcaemia do not usually produce symptoms. Hypercalcaemia is common in the late stages of the disease, and not uncommon at an earlier stage in squamous cell carcinoma, even in the absence of metastases. It appears to be due to circulating parathormone-like substances and abnormal prostaglandin activity in bone. Adequate fluid intake is essential; prednisolone 30 mg/day is often also given, although evidence of its efficacy is lacking. Non-steroidal anti-inflammatory drugs are useful for bone pain. Other endocrine disturbances tend to occur in the late stages of the disease and may not produce symptoms. The need for treatment should always be questioned. Hyponatraemia due to excess ADH activity usually responds to fluid restriction, and symptoms from excess cortisol secretion to metyrapone. These complications also respond to reduction of tumour bulk by chemotherapy or radiotherapy.

In the terminal stages of the disease pain is common, and its cause should be identified. Patients dying of lung cancer may have pain for other reasons and appropriate treatment should be given. If the pain is due to spread of lung cancer, it should always be possible to control it. Analgesics should be given regularly, starting with simple agents such as aspirin or paracetamol, but, if the pain is not controlled, working rapidly up to the use of opiates. Morphine is an invaluable agent, controlling pain and cough and often contributing to a state of mild euphoria. The principles of its use have been clearly laid down in many publications from hospices. Regular dosage is required to build up and maintain analgesic levels. There is no place for intermittent or on-demand ("prn") therapy. The dose should be increased in the course of a few days until pain control is attained. Initially, morphine or diamorphine should be given 4-hourly and the dose increased until the pain is controlled. High total doses may be required and drowsiness may be a problem initially, but this usually wears off in a few days. Nausea responds to antiemetics. The major continuing problem with opiates is constipation, and great care is required to maintain bowel function. It is easiest to use morphine in solution as the hydrochloride during the initial stage of establishing an effective analgesic dose. It can be continued or, when the daily requirement is known, a sustained release tablet (MST$^r$) can be substituted. There is no good evidence that diamorphine is more effective than morphine or that combined preparations containing alcohol, phenothiazines, cocaine etc. offer any additional benefit. In the late stages of the disease there is no substitute for morphine, and there need be no concern about addiction. Other methods of pain control may also be required. Non-steroidal anti-inflammatory drugs such as indomethacin and salicylates are helpful in the control of bone pain, and radiotherapy may be useful for localised lesions. Other methods of pain control such as nerve blocks may occasionally be required.

The general management of the patient is important. Emotional support of both patient and family is essential. Attention to apparently minor physical problems is of great importance. Much of the discomfort of dying is due to them, and the prevention or treatment of problems such as a painful skin or mouth is an essential part of care. Care can be given in hospital, in a hospice or at home. The attitudes of the staff are of more importance than the place.

### The Solitary Peripheral Lesion

A number of patients present with an apparently solitary peripheral lesion on X-ray, often an incidental finding in an asymptomatic individual. All such lesions should be assumed to be carcinomas unless there is convincing evidence in support of an alternative diagnosis. The investigative approach often requires different techniques. Tomography or CT scanning may be helpful in showing calcification, as in a tuberculoma, or an abnormal vascular pattern in an angioma, or they may reveal other unsuspected lesions suggesting secondary rather than primary carcinoma. Bronchoscopy should be carried out, although the lesion may appear to be peripheral and likely to be beyond the range of vision. X-ray control is required so that the affected segment can be entered. Brushing or washing provides material for cytological examination, and biopsy is worthwhile. The lesion may be accessible for direct transcutaneous biopsy or aspiration for cytology. The techniques used in assessment depend on the locally available skills. If the diagnosis cannot be made by other means, solitary peripheral lesions should be regarded as carcinomas and should be resected after normal routine preoperative investigation.

# Other Intrathoracic Tumours

## Alveolar Cell Carcinoma

This tumour probably arises in alveolar epithelium. It is relatively rare (about 1%–2% of all lung tumours). It tends to spread widely through alveolar walls and may be multicentric. Its aetiology is unknown. There is no association with cigarette smoking, but there is an association with diseases such as fibrosing alveolitis. The symptoms are similar to those of bronchial carcinoma but are more variable and the radiological appearances are non-specific. Diagnosis is difficult in the presence of pre-existing abnormality and tends to be delayed. In later stages diffuse involvement of both lungs produces severe dyspnoea, the picture resembling that of carcinomatous lymphangitis. The diagnosis is sometimes made after resection of an otherwise undiagnosed lung lesion. Bronchoscopy is not particularly helpful. Transbronchial biopsy is useful if the diagnosis is suspected. For solitary lesions treated by resection, the prognosis is rather better than that of bronchial carcinoma (40% 5-year survival). Resection should be attempted whenever it is technically feasible. The prognosis for the diffuse form is very poor. The disease does not respond to radiotherapy or chemotherapy.

## Pleural Tumours

Primary pleural tumours are rare. Mesothelioma, the commonest, is nearly always the result of asbestos exposure. The exposure may have been trivial and will almost invariably have occurred many years previously. Mesothelioma tends to be locally invasive, infiltrating both chest wall and lung, and producing a particularly unpleasant local pain. Diagnosis is difficult and there is a risk of needle track involvement if percutaneous biopsy techniques are used. Surgical resection is rarely possible. Mesotheliomas do not respond to radiotherapy or chemotherapy. Median survival is around a year. Pain relief is the most important aspect of treatment, but can be difficult. In the United Kingdom mesothelioma is recognised as an industrial disease, compensation is available (information can be obtained through a DHSS office), and all deaths should be notified to the Coroner.

## Bronchial Adenoma

Bronchial adenomas are benign tumours of the bronchial wall which may be locally invasive, extending both into the bronchial lumen and outside the bronchial wall into the peribronchial tissues. Histologically they are a mixed group, the majority being carcinoid tumours. They cause symptoms from irritation of cough-sensitive areas by pedunculated lesions, by ulceration causing recurrent haemoptysis, by bronchial obstruction, or, more rarely, with features of the carcinoid syndrome from ectopic hormone secretion. Adenomas are rare (<1% of tumours in surgical centres). They are often readily visible through the bronchoscope, but require formal excision because of their tendency to extension through the bronchial wall. Most are locally invasive, but distant metastases are rare. They should be resected.

## Metastatic Lesions

Secondary tumours frequently present in lung and pleura. The diagnosis may be readily apparent, but is sometimes made only after thoracotomy. Once diagnosed, management is normally symptomatic. Occasionally resection of a solitary metastasis from a primary site such as a hypernephroma may be worthwhile. Metastases normally produce few symptoms. They may cause pleural effusion which should be managed by aspiration, and possibly local chemotherapy when reaccumulation is rapid and symptoms troublesome. Chemical agents such as tetracycline or mepacrine or antimitotic agents such as bleomycin are injected into the pleura after most of the fluid has been removed. The pleura is then aspirated again as thoroughly as possible so that the resulting reaction causes adherence of the parietal and visceral layers. If significant quantities of fluid are left in the pleura, the results are usually poor.

Lymphangitic carcinoma is a particularly distressing form of metastatic disease. The common primary sources are the lung itself, the upper gastrointestinal tract, and the breast. Diffuse lymph node involvement with lymphatic permeation and obstruction produce a stiff oedematous lung and a radiological picture of diffuse infiltration. Lymphangitic carcinoma is commonly associated with pleural effusion; its presence may be suspected if dyspnoea is not relieved or increases on aspiration of the fluid. Severe dyspnoea is eventually invariable, and responds very poorly to treatment. If the primary lesion is in the breast, chemotherapy or hormonal therapy should be tried, although results are usually poor. Generous use of opiates is normally indicated.

# Useful References

Bailar JC (1984) Screening for lung cancer — where are we now? Am Rev Resp Dis 130: 541–542

Belcher JR (1983) Thirty years of surgery for carcinoma of the bronchus. Thorax 38: 428–432

Coggon D, Acheson DE (1983) Trends in lung cancer mortality. Thorax 38: 721–723

Doll R, Peto R (1981) Causes of cancer. Quantitative estimate of avoidable risks in US today. Oxford University Press, London

Edwards CW (1984) Alvolar cell carcinoma: a review. Thorax 39: 166–171

Geddes DM (1979) The natural history of lung cancer: a review based on rates of tumour growth. Br J Dis Chest 73: 1–17

Gregor A (1984) Radiotherapy for inoperable non-small cell carcinoma of the bronchus. In: Smyth JF (ed) The management of lung cancer, Arnold, London

Hetzel MR, Nixon C, Edmondstone W, Mitchell CM, Millard FJC, Nansen EM, Woodcock AA, Bridges CE, Humberstone AM (1985) Laser therapy in 100 tracheobronchial tumours. Thorax 40: 341–345

Hillerdahl G (1983) Malignant mesothelioma 1982: a review of 4710 published cases. Br J Dis Chest 77: 321–327

Horn JW, Kessler LG (1986) Falling rates of lung cancer in men in the United States. Lancet I: 425–426

Lamb D (1984) Histological classification of lung cancer. Thorax 39: 161–165

Le Roux BT (1984) The surgical management of bronchial carcinoma. In: Smyth JF (ed) The management of lung cancer. Arnold, London

Lung cancer study group (1984) Prognostic factors in patients with resected stage I non-small cell lung cancer. Cancer 54: 1802–1813

Matsuda M, Horai T, Nakamura S, Nishio H, Sakuma T, Ikegami H, Tateishi R (1986) Bronchial brushing and bronchial biopsy: comparison of diagnostic accuracy and cell typing reliability in lung cancer. Thorax 41: 475–478

Melamed MR, Flehinger BJ, Zaman MB, Heelan RT, Perchick SA, Martini N (1984) Screening for early lung cancer. Chest 86: 44–53

Morgan WKC (1979) Industrial carcinogens: the extent of the risk. Thorax 34: 431–433

Ogilvie C (1980) Physician among surgeons: thoughts on pre-operative assessment. Thorax 35: 881–883

Rossing TH, Rossing RG (1982) Survival in lung cancer. Am Rev Resp Dis 126: 771–777

Souhami RL (1985) Chemotherapy in non-small cell bronchial carcinoma. Thorax 40: 641–645

Spiro SG (1985) Chemotherapy for small cell lung cancer. Br Med J 290: 413–441

Spiro SG, Goldstraw P (1984) The staging of lung cancer. Thorax 39: 401–407

Stevenson JC (1985) Malignant hypercalcaemia. Br Med J 291: 421–422

Stolley PD (1983) Lung cancer in women — five years later, situation worse. N Engl J Med 309: 428–429

Vogelsang GB, Abeloff MD, Ettinger DS, Booker SV (1985) Long term survivors of small cell carcinoma of the lung. Am J Med 79: 49–56

# 12 The Lungs in Systemic Disease, Pulmonary Eosinophilia and Drug Reactions

## The Lungs in Systemic Disease

### Connective Tissue Disorders

Pleural and pulmonary complications are common in the connective tissue disorders. Estimates of incidence depend on the methods used to detect them and, in patients with rheumatoid arthritis for example, have ranged from 2% when chest radiographs alone were used to 45% when pulmonary function tests were included. The main management decisions centre on the use of corticosteroids. These are very effective in suppressing some of the pleural and pulmonary complications but completely ineffective in others. The decision to use corticosteroids for specific respiratory problems must consider the effect of steroids on other aspects of these multisystem diseases. Steroid trials need care since, if steroid withdrawal is too abrupt, the underlying disease may flare up.

#### Rheumatoid Arthritis

Rheumatoid arthritis is associated with a wide variety of pleural and pulmonary complications (Table 12.1). Pleural effusions, usually unilateral, affect men more than women and often last for months and sometimes years before resolving spontaneously. Fluid may be serous or turbid and it contains mainly lymphocytes and neutrophils. It characteristically has a low glucose content (<1.6 mmol/l) and high levels of lactic dehydrogenase, cholesterol and rheumatoid factor. The surface of the parietal pleura at thoracoscopy has a granular appearance. Empyema is a rare cause of pleural effusion in these patients.

    Fibrosing alveolitis (rheumatoid lung) is discussed in Chapter 10. In one in five patients it precedes the development of arthritis. Diagnostic difficulties can occur because treatment with both gold and penicillamine can cause a similar clinical and radiological picture, and although eosinophilia is more likely with drug-induced alveolitis, it is not invariable. The radiological features of generalised bronchiectasis can also cause confusion, though a good history and pulmonary function tests should separate this from alveolitis.

**Table 12.1.** Complications of rheumatoid arthritis and their treatment

| Complication | Treatment |
| --- | --- |
| Pleural thickening and pleural effusions | Usually remits after several months; repeat aspirations if causing symptoms |
| Fibrosing alveolitis (rheumatoid lung) | Steroid trial if symptoms and function deteriorate |
| Rheumatoid nodules | Mainly a diagnostic problem, can be single or multiple, usually asymptomatic, treatment not usually indicated |
| Bronchiectasis | As for other forms of bronchiectasis |
| Pulmonary hypertension due to intimal hypertrophy in the pulmonary artery | Difficult |
| Drug-induced lung disease (gold, penicillamine) | Stop drugs, give steroids if severe |
| Infections | Prompt treatment with antibiotics |
| Rheumatoid pneumoconiosis | Variable static or downhill course (?more common in patients on penicillamine — should be discontinued) |
| Obliterative bronchiolitis | Steroids disappointing but worth a try |

Obliterative bronchiolitis is a rare cause of breathlessness in patients with rheumatoid arthritis with a poor prognosis. The diagnosis should be suspected in a breathless patient when the chest X-ray is normal or shows hyperinflation only, and pulmonary function tests show a combination of irreversible airways obstruction, large lung volumes with gas trapping and well preserved transfer factor for carbon monoxide.

The management of the specific pleural and pulmonary complications of rheumatoid arthritis is outlined in Table 12.1. Infection and bronchiectasis are treated conventionally. On the whole, corticosteroids are disappointing in the more progressive and symptomatic problems such as fibrosing alveolitis and obliterative bronchiolitis. Pleural effusions may respond to corticosteroids though this does not normally justify their use. Repeat aspiration of pleural fluid should be carried out when symptoms necessitate.

## Other Collagen Diseases

Collagen diseases may have direct effects on the pleura, lung, respiratory muscles or pulmonary vascular bed, or they may predispose to secondary problems such as aspiration pneumonia and infection. Some of the well recognised complications are listed in Table 12.2. The complications of systemic lupus erythematosus and dermatomyositis can develop fairly rapidly, but on the whole respond well to steroids. The changes in systemic sclerosis develop more insidiously but are unresponsive to treatment.

### Wegener's Granulomatosis

In Wegener's granulomatosis, necrotising vasculitis and glomerulonephritis are associated with granulomata of the upper respiratory tract and lungs. The granulomata can lead to ulceration and bone destruction in and around the nose,

Table 12.2. Some complications of collagen diseases

| | | | |
|---|---|---|---|
| SLE | Pleurisy, pleural effusion<br>Basal lung collapse ⎫<br>Diaphragmatic weakness ⎬ shrinking lung<br>Fibrosing alveolitis<br>Obliterative pulmonary vascular disease | | Overall good response to steroids ± azathioprine |
| Systemic sclerosis | Fibrosing alveolitis (scleroderma lung)<br>Aspiration pneumonia<br>Obliterative pulmonary vascular disease | | Steroids not helpful<br>Treat infections promptly |
| Dermatomyositis | Muscle weakness — ⎫<br>    intercostals/diaphragm, ⎬<br>    larynx/pharynx ⎭<br>Cancer, including lung cancer | Ventilatory failure<br>aspiration | Good response to steroids usually |
| Ankylosing spondylitis | Bilateral apical fibrosis | | No treatment |
| Sjögren's syndrome | Bronchiolitis obliterans | | No treatment shown to be effective |

pharynx and larynx. Lung involvement usually consists of single or multiple irregular nodules of varying size and characteristically cavitated, or, more rarely, of diffuse lung infiltration. These may be asymptomatic or may cause cough, dyspnoea or pleurisy. Pulmonary vasculitis can lead to pulmonary hypertension. Systemic features mainly involve the kidneys, skin and joints. Biopsy of nasal lesions is helpful for diagnosis.

The prognosis without treatment is poor, with median survival counted in months. Steroids alone are unhelpful. Treatment with azathioprine or cyclophosphamide is extremely effective. When granulomata are limited to the thorax the prognosis is much better.

## Pulmonary Haemosiderosis and Goodpasture's Syndrome

Idiopathic pulmonary haemosiderosis is a rare disease affecting children predominantly and occasionally young adults. It presents with recurrent episodes of haemoptysis, iron deficiency anaemia out of proportion to the degree of haemoptysis, pyrexia and breathlessness. The transfer factor for carbon monoxide (TLCO) is increased with lung haemorrhage and may be helpful in distinguishing recent pulmonary haemorrhage from other causes of pulmonary shadowing. Occult bleeding is confirmed by finding haemosiderin-laden macrophages in sputum or lavage fluid. Intrapulmonary haemorrhage can cause fatal haemoptysis or may lead to pulmonary hypertension, respiratory failure and cor pulmonale. Prognosis is poor, with a mean survival of around 2 years. Symptomatic treatment includes blood transfusion for anaemia, and oxygen as necessary. Steroids may be helpful for acute lung haemorrhage but do not appear to alter the underlying course of the disease; immunosuppressive drugs may do so, but experience is limited. High doses of inhaled steroids are reported to have contained lung haemorrhage in one patient.

In Goodpasture's syndrome, pulmonary haemosiderosis is associated with a proliferative glomerulonephritis and the presence of antiglomerular basement membrane (anti-GBM) antibodies in blood, kidneys and on pulmonary alveolar basement membrane. The disease, which affects both sexes and all ages, presents with haemoptysis, dyspnoea and fatigue. The nephritis is usually rapidly progressive though some patients have survived for a long time without treatment. The overall prognosis in untreated patients however is only 4 months. Diagnosis is confirmed by finding anti-GBM antibody in the serum or by finding linear IgG deposition on the glomerular capillary basement membrane on renal biopsy.

Patients with Goodpasture's syndrome have responded to a combination of plasmapheresis and immunosuppressive drugs, usually high dose steroids and cyclophosphamide, with dialysis if necessary. Cigarette smoking should be discontinued and any infection treated promptly since both can precipitate lung haemorrhage. Bilateral nephrectomy was tried in an attempt to reduce the renal antigen load but no clear effect has been shown, and with more effective treatment it is not justified.

## Amyloid

The lung is often involved in both primary and secondary amyloid though it is usually asymptomatic. Primary amyloid may cause diffuse lung shadowing, pulmonary nodules or deposits in the airways and larynx. It is often mistaken for carcinoma. Secondary amyloid is more likely to involve the pulmonary blood vessels, again rarely causing symptoms. Bronchial amyloid has been treated successfully with laser therapy. High dose oral steroids may slow progress in diffuse disease and their use is worth a trial if symptoms are troublesome.

## Eosinophilic Granuloma (Histiocytosis X)

Pulmonary involvement in children or young adults usually causes progressively increasing breathlessness, often complicated by recurrent episodes of spontaneous pneumothorax and occasionally by other manifestations of the disease such as diabetes insipidus or osteolytic skeletal lesions. There may be no abnormal signs in the chest or crepitations may be present. The chest X-ray shows diffuse bilateral mottling initially, followed by the changes of "honeycomb lung". The course of the disease is variable, usually being slowly progressive but occasionally remitting. Progression is often associated with the development of irreversible airways obstruction, hyperinflation and recurrent pneumothoraces. Diagnosis may not require confirmation if other manifestations of the disease are present, but otherwise will usually require lung biopsy or bronchoalveolar lavage to identify the characteristic histiocytes and foam cells. An open lung biopsy provides a good opportunity to carry out a pre-emptive pleurodesis to prevent pneumothorax.

Corticosteroids are difficult to assess in a rare disease such as this with a variable course. They have been reported to help some patients but not others. Immunosuppressive drugs and radiotherapy have been unhelpful. Penicillamine appears to have caused improvement in patients deteriorating rapidly despite high doses of corticosteroids and should be tried in this situation. Recurrent pneumothoraces require pleurodesis.

# Alveolar Proteinosis

This is a rare condition in which pulmonary alveoli are filled with a PAS (periodic acid–Schiff) lipid-rich proteinaceous material, probably as a consequence of impaired clearing of alveolar surfactant. The patient is usually male, aged between 30 and 50, with rather non-specific symptoms of dyspnoea, cough and sometimes fever. Some patients have no symptoms, whereas others deteriorate rapidly. Chest signs are often absent, though crepitations and finger clubbing may occur. The chest X-ray in contrast is often rather dramatic, with patchy bilateral fluffy perihilar shadowing which can resemble pulmonary oedema. The diagnosis is made by demonstrating characteristic lamellar bodies on electron microscopic examination of sputum, lung washings or lung biopsy specimens. Without treatment, approximately one-third of patients improve, one-third stay the same and one-third deteriorate. Treatment with bronchoalveolar lavage is effective so it is important to consider the diagnosis and ask for electron microscope studies on available specimens.

Bronchoalveolar lavage has superseded treatment with inhaled trypsin which carried the theoretical risk at least of producing emphysema. One lung is lavaged with up to 20 l of warm isotonic buffered saline containing heparin and acetylcysteine under general anaesthesia. The procedure is carried out on the opposite lung a few days later. Symptomatic improvement occurs within 24 h; radiological clearing is rather slower. Repeat lavage is usually necessary after varying periods of time, though rarely less than 6 months. In some, improvement has been maintained for several years.

# Pulmonary Eosinophilia

Pulmonary eosinophilia is characterised by transient pulmonary infiltrates in association with a blood eosinophil count in excess of $0.5 \times 10^9/l$. The pulmonary infiltrate consists of large numbers of eosinophils with some mononuclear cells in alveolar walls and exudate. Replacement by fibrous tissue occurs in severe and progressive disease. Other pathological features may be present, depending on the underlying cause, such as airway changes in allergic bronchopulmonary aspergillosis.

Classification of the various forms of pulmonary eosinophilia has been exceptionally confusing. A classification based on the underlying cause is most logical (Table 12.3), though occasional patients defy neat categorisation.

**Table 12.3.** Features of pulmonary eosinophilia

| | Blood eosinophils | IgE | Airways | Treatment | Other |
|---|---|---|---|---|---|
| Helminth infestation | $2–4 \times 10^9/l$ | | | | CXR — multiple nodular or ill-defined opacity |
| *Ascaris lumbricoides* | ++ | ++++ | No | Anti-helminthic drugs | |
| *Toxocara canis* | ++ | +++ | | | Hepatosplenomegaly and hyperglobulinaemia |
| Schistosoma | ++ | +++ | | | |
| Filaria | ++ | +++ | Cough and wheeze | Diethyl-carbamazine | |
| ABPA | ++ | ++ | Asthma | Prednisolone | |
| Systemic vasculitis | +++ | | Asthma | Prednisolone | Shades into Wegener's, weight loss, malaise |
| Cryptogenic pulmonary eosinophilia | +++ | Normal | About 50% no evidence of bronchiectasis | Prednisolone causes rapid improvement | Systemic symptoms; occasionally liver, spleen, lymph nodes enlarged |

## Helminth Infestations

The helminths most frequently associated with pulmonary eosinophilia are shown in Table 12.3. Symptoms vary with the parasite in question and are most prominent in tropical pulmonary eosinophilia due to filariasis. Blood eosinophil levels are usually very high ($2 - 4 \times 10^9/l$), as are IgE levels. Treatment consists of eradicating the helminth. Diethylcarbamazine produces dramatic improvement in patients with filariasis and a therapeutic trial is a useful diagnostic test.

## Allergic Bronchopulmonary Aspergillosis (ABPA)

ABPA is characterised by recurrent episodes of pulmonary eosinophilia in a patient who is usually both atopic and asthmatic. It accounts for about 80% of pulmonary eosinophilia in the United Kingdom and is diagnosed on the history, radiological findings and an immediate positive skin test to *Aspergillus fumigatus*. However, a positive skin test response to *A. fumigatus* is seen in some atopic individuals who do not have clinical features of ABPA, so appropriate clinical features are also needed to make the diagnosis. Serum precipitins to *A. fumigatus* can be obtained in up to 90% of patients with ABPA, depending on the technique and the concentration of serum used. The pulmonary infiltrate is thought to result from the combination of an immediate IgE and an IgG–complement-mediated response to *A. fumigatus* in medium-sized bronchi. The bronchi become obstructed with mucin-containing fungal hyphae, eosinophils and leucocytes and these may be expectorated as casts. However, they may also become adherent to the mucosa, causing damage to the bronchial wall and proximal bronchiectasis.

Patients with ABPA usually present with deteriorating asthma, transient pulmonary shadows and sometimes with constitutional upset. An occasional patient does not have asthma. The pulmonary infiltrate and bronchoconstriction respond to oral steroids in the early stages, but if the infiltrates are not treated promptly, bronchial damage and fibrosis can lead to cor pulmonale in a small number of patients. The majority of patients presenting with this clinical picture have a positive skin test to *A. fumigatus*, but about 20% with an identical clinical picture do not. An immunological response to other moulds has been found on rare occasions, but in the majority of patients with a negative skin test the cause is unknown.

Treatment for ABPA is aimed at suppressing acute episodes of pulmonary eosinophilia promptly with corticosteroids to try to prevent the development of irreversible airways obstruction. Pulmonary infiltrates should be treated promptly with 30 mg prednisolone for 3 weeks, with a repeat chest X-ray and spirometry at that time. The dose of steroids should be reduced gradually when the infiltrate has cleared. Patients who are developing progressively severe airways obstruction usually require long-term oral steroids. Young patients with discrete episodes and good reversibility of their airways obstruction are better managed by treating their asthma conventionally with inhaled drugs and reserving oral steroids for episodes of pulmonary infiltration. Patients should be encouraged to keep steroids at home with instructions to start them promptly if they develop pleurisy, chest tightness or a fall in peak flow rate. Inhaled steroids do not appear to prevent the episodes of infiltration, though higher doses of inhaled steroids have not been studied. There is no place for antifungal agents since *Aspergillus* is ubiquitous.

### Systemic Vasculitis

Pulmonary eosinophilia is a rare, though well known, complication of polyarteritis nodosa. It also occurs in related vascular disorders where classification is again confusing. The Churg–Strauss syndrome refers to patients who are usually young, female and atopic with moderately severe asthma and a very high blood eosinophil count who present with systemic vasculitis and pulmonary infiltrates. Renal involvement is less frequent than with classic polyarteritis nodosa and the overall prognosis and response to steroids rather better.

The pulmonary manifestations of systemic vasculitis usually respond well to corticosteroids. Prognosis is mainly influenced by the severity of renal involvement which often dictates whether additional treatment such as cytotoxic drugs should be added.

### Drug-induced Pulmonary Eosinophilia

See Drug-induced Lung Disease (below).

### Cryptogenic Pulmonary Eosinophilia

Of patients presenting with non-drug-induced pulmonary eosinophilia, no cause can be found in about 20% in the United Kingdom. This group appears to include two main clinical pictures. The first consists of patients with clinical and radiological features identical to those of ABPA but in whom there is no evidence of hypersensitivity to *A. fumigatus*. Management is similar to that for ABPA. The other pattern is dominated by systemic symptoms, predominantly fever, malaise and weight loss, associated in some patients with an enlarged liver, spleen or lymphadenopathy. About half will have asthma, usually starting in adult life. The radiological features vary but may show a generalised peripheral pattern of lung shadowing sometimes described as the photographic negative of pulmonary oedema. Serum IgE levels are usually normal, in contrast to pulmonary eosinophilia due to helminths or ABPA. Oral corticosteroids produce a dramatic improvement in both symptoms and radiological abnormalities within a few days. It may be possible to discontinue steroids after a few months without relapse, but some patients require continuous treatment for many years.

## Respiratory Problems due to Drugs and Paraquat

Drugs may interfere with respiratory function in a predictable way, as with opiates or β-adrenoceptor antagonists, by hypersensitivity reactions or by direct toxic effects on the lung. Several drugs and chemicals are taken up preferentially by the lung and this may explain the predisposition for lung involvement of some compounds, such as paraquat. A simple classification of adverse drug effects on respiratory function is shown in Table 12.4. Drug effects which would be anticipated are not discussed here, nor are drugs which might affect lungs indirectly by causing muscle weakness or by predisposing to infection. Drugs causing bron-

**Table 12.4.** Classification of drug-induced lung disease

1. Depression of respiratory control — opiates, sedatives, anaesthetics, etc.
2. Asthma
   a) Pharmacological ⎫  see Chapter 4
   b) Idiosyncratic   ⎭
3. Alveolar
   a) Pulmonary eosinophilia
   b) Diffuse alveolar damage ± fibrosis
   c) Systemic lupus erythematosus-like syndrome (overlaps with pleural)
   d) Allergic alveolitis — pituitary snuff
   e) ?Goodpasture's syndrome
4. Pulmonary vascular disease
   a) Pulmonary thromboembolism
   b) Pulmonary hypertension
5. Pleural

choconstriction and respiratory depression are mentioned in Chapters 4 and 6 respectively.

## Drug-induced Lung Disease

Many drugs cause pulmonary shadowing on the chest X-ray, dyspnoea and crepitations, though there are considerable differences in presentation and prognosis. Current attempts to classify drug-induced lung disease are crude, for several reasons. Much of the information on individual drugs has come from reports of one or two cases only, and these are often in patients with conditions, such as rheumatoid arthritis, which may themselves affect the lungs. In addition, some drugs appear to be capable of causing different presentations in different patients. It is probably more appropriate at present to describe the main clinical patterns of presentation, recognising that some drugs may cause more than one pattern of response.

### Pulmonary Eosinophilia

Patchy or diffuse lung infiltration is seen in association with lung crepitations and a somewhat variable blood eosinophilia. Symptoms usually develop a few days after starting the drug, in contrast to lung problems due to cytotoxic drugs, for example. Symptoms are likely to recur if the drug is reinstituted, but tend to be less severe. The condition usually resolves when the drug is withdrawn but will respond more rapidly if steroids are given. Some of the drugs involved are listed in Table 12.5.

### Diffuse Alveolar Damage

Several drugs cause diffuse lung shadowing, without blood eosinophilia. This may in part be due to oxidant damage since for some of the cytotoxic drugs there is evidence that oxygen therapy will increase lung damage further. Patients may present acutely or insidiously with breathlessness, a dry cough and crepitations. Pulmonary function tests show a restrictive disorder with a low TLCO. Lung histology shows thickened alveolar walls containing fibrous tissue and intra-alveolar

**Table 12.5.** Drugs causing eosinophilic pneumonia

Antibiotics
   Sulphonamides, nitrofurantoin, penicillin tetracycline,
   sulphasalazine, para-amino salicylic acid
Imipramine
Chlorpropramide
Chlorpromazine
Aspirin, ?phenylbutazone
Carbamazepine
Gold salts, ?penicillamine
Procarbazine
Methotrexate

desquamative cells. This picture is seen with several cytotoxic and immunosuppressive drugs (busulphan, bleomycin and methotrexate most frequently) and more recently with the antiarrhythmic drug amiodarone. Nitrofurantoin can probably cause this pattern as well as acute pulmonary eosinophilia.

It is not clear yet whether these changes are due to a hypersensitivity reaction or to a direct toxic effect of the drug. Some of the evidence favours a hypersensitivity reaction in that the condition will often reverse if detected early, is said to respond to steroids and a mild eosinophilia is seen in an occasional patient with amiodarone lung disease, for example. However, with some drugs such as bleomycin the effect is clearly related to dose and renal function. Lung problems are rare with cumulative doses of less than 150 mg but occur in up to 10% of patients receiving more than 500 mg. With amiodarone the effect is probably dose related, most patients having received more than 600 mg daily, though problems can occur with doses below 400 mg daily. The relationship with dose is less clear with other drugs. The lung lesions will usually improve if the drug is stopped at an early stage but otherwise can be progressive and fatal. Approximately one-third of patients with amiodarone lung disease have died, the remainder have usually improved, apparently helped by steroids in some instances.

Attempts to detect early disease using pulmonary function tests such as the TLCO have given conflicting results so far. Regular chest X-rays and alerting the patient to early symptoms are important.

### A Systemic Lupus Erythematosus-like Syndrome

Patients usually present with systemic symptoms of fever, weight loss and arthralgia. When the lungs are involved, pleurisy and pleural effusions tend to dominate the picture but more diffuse lung shadowing can occur. The drugs concerned include hydralazine, procainamide, isoniazid and sulphonamides. The response appears to be dose related for some drugs such as hydralazine and procainamide, but not for others. Antinuclear factor is positive but DNA antibodies are usually low or absent, in contrast to SLE. The syndrome usually regresses once the drug is withdrawn.

Less common presentations include an allergic alveolitis (from porcine and bovine preparations of nasal snuff) and Goodpasture's syndrome from penicillamine.

### Drug-induced Pleural and Pulmonary Vascular Disease

Methysergide can cause pleural fibrosis. This was also seen with oral practolol before it was taken off the market, but has not been associated consistently with any other β-adrenoceptor antagonist.

The association between the contraceptive pill and pulmonary thromboembolism is well known. The incidence has decreased since the oestrogen content of the pill has been reduced. Pulmonary hypertension resembling primary pulmonary hypertension was seen in patients using an appetite-suppressant drug (aminorex) in Europe and has occurred very rarely in patients taking amphetamine-like agents, fenfluramine and phenformin.

## Oxygen Toxicity

The dangers of uncontrolled oxygen therapy for patients with carbon dioxide retention are discussed in Chapters 6 and 23. High concentrations of inspired oxygen can cause absorption atelectasis even in normal subjects, but they also have a direct toxic effect on the lung, causing an adult respiratory distress syndrome picture (see Chap. 23).

## Paraquat Poisoning

There have been many fatalities from the widely used herbicide paraquat. These usually follow accidental and non-accidental ingestion, though percutaneous absorption from paraquat sprays and even intravenous administration have been responsible. Paraquat accumulates in the lung where it produces oxygen radicals which damage alveolar pneumocytes in a similar way to high concentrations of oxygen (see Chap. 23). Paraquat also causes hepatic and renal failure and ingestion causes oral and pharyngeal ulceration, but these are usually reversible. It is the pulmonary complications which normally determine the outcome.

The signs and symptoms of pulmonary involvement may be delayed for several days after ingestion. They consist of breathlessness and lung crepitations with impaired TLCO and hypoxaemia. With lesser degrees of poisoning, the pulmonary changes will resolve on supportive measures alone. With severe poisoning, symptoms can progress rapidly with death occurring within a week. A small number of patients have a more protracted downhill course, with increasing respiratory failure causing death up to 1 month after ingestion. However, the majority of patients who survive the first week will recover. A fatal outcome occurs in about 50% of patients ingesting the liquid concentrate of paraquat, but is very rare in patients ingesting the granular form available for domestic use.

Since there is no treatment for lung damage due to free radicals, the initial treatment, orientated towards reducing absorption of paraquat from the gut, is crucially important. Gastric aspiration and lavage should be followed with oral Fuller's Earth (20% w/v) and magnesium sulphate (5% w/v) in doses of 250 ml 4-hourly for 48 h. Large volumes of intravenous fluids are needed to replace the fluid lost from the bowel and to ensure a urine output of at least 3 l a day. Plasma paraquat levels are a guide to prognosis. Peritoneal dialysis is ineffective and haemodialysis and forced osmotic diuresis disappointing. Charcoal haemoperfusion is under assessment and plasmapheresis has been tried. Lung irradiation appears to have helped one patient with severe pulmonary damage.

# Useful References

*Lungs in Systemic Disease*

Basset F, Soler P, Jaurand MC, Bignon J (1977) Ultrastructural examination of broncho-alveolar lavage for diagnosis of pulmonary histiocytosis X: preliminary report on 4 cases. Thorax 32: 303–306
Editorial (1985) Alveolar haemorrhage. Lancet II: 853–854

Fauci AS, Haynes BF, Katz P, Wolff SM (1983) Wegener's granulomatosis: prospective clinical and therapeutic experience with 85 patients for 21 years. Ann Intern Med 98: 76–85

Lacronique J, Roth C, Battesti J-P, Basset F, Chretien J (1982) Chest radiological features of pulmonary histiocytosis X: a report based on 50 adult cases. Thorax 37: 104–109

Macfarlane JD, Dieppe PA, Rigden BG, Clark TJH (1978) Pulmonary and pleural lesions in rheumatoid disease. Br J Dis Chest 72: 288–300

Morgan PGM, Turner-Warwick M (1981) Pulmonary haemosiderosis and pulmonary haemorrhage. Br J Dis Chest 75: 225–242

## Alveolar Proteinosis

Costello JF, Moriarty DC, Branthwaite MA, Turner-Warwick M, Corrin B (1975) Diagnosis and management of alveolar proteinosis: the role of electron microscopy. Thorax 30: 121–132

Du Bois RM, McAllister WAC, Branthwaite MA (1983) Alveolar proteinosis: diagnosis and treatment over a 10-year period. Thorax 38: 360–363

## Pulmonary Eosinophilia

Geddes DM (1986) Pulmonary eosinophilia. J R Coll Phys Lond 20: 139–145

## Lung Problems due to Drugs

Cooper JAD, White DA, Matthay RA (1986) Drug-induced pulmonary disease, Part 1: Cytotoxic drugs. Am Rev Resp Dis 133: 321–340

Cooper JAD, White DA, Matthay RA (1986) Drug-induced pulmonary disease, Part 2: Noncytotoxic drugs. Am Rev Resp Dis 133: 488–505

Darmanata JI, van Zandwijk N, Duren DR, van Royen EA, Mooi WJ, Plomp TA, Jansen HM, Durrer D (1984) Amiodarone pneumonitis; three further cases with a review of published reports. Thorax 39: 57–64

Gibson GJ (1983) Drug induced pulmonary disease. In: Weatherall DJ, Ledingham JGG, Warrell DA (eds) Oxford textbook of medicine. Oxford University Press, Oxford, pp 101–103

Higenbottam T, Crome P, Parkinson C, Nunn J (1979) Further clinical observations on the pulmonary effects of paraquat ingestion. Thorax 34: 161–165

Holmberg L, Boman G (1981) Pulmonary reactions for nitrofurantoin. Eur J Resp Dis 62: 180–189

Lok-Wan Liu F, Cohen RD, Downar E, Butany JW, Edelson JD, Rebuck AS (1986) Amiodarone pulmonary toxicity: functional and ultrastructural evaluation. Thorax 41: 100–105

Penn RG, Griffin JP (1982) Adverse reactions to nitrofurantoin in the United Kingdom, Sweden, and Holland. Br Med J 284: 1440–1442

Proudfoot AT, Stewart MS, Levitt T, Widdop B (1979) Paraquat poisoning: significance of plasma-paraquat concentrations. Lancet II: 330–332

Van Barneveld PWC, Van der Mark ThW, Sleijfer DTh, Mulder NH, Schraffordt Koops H, Sluiter HJ, Peset R (1984) Predictive factors for bleomycin-induced pneumonitis. Am Rev Resp Dis 130: 1078–1081

# 13 Pneumothorax and Pleural Effusions

## Pneumothorax

Spontaneous pneumothorax occurs most often in fit young patients, characteristically tall, thin and male, where it is usually due to rupture of a small subpleural bleb at the apex of the lung. Pneumothorax can also occur as a result of trauma, investigative procedures or underlying disease — staphylococcal pneumonia, asthma, emphysema, tuberculosis and carcinoma or, rarely, in patients with Marfan's syndrome or in association with menstruation (catamenial pneumothorax). Management is usually straightforward in the young and fit but it can be very difficult in those with other chest problems. A pneumothorax is described as open or closed depending on whether the leak is sealed or not.

A tension pneumothorax requires emergency decompression. Insertion of any hollow needle into the pleural space will suffice. Otherwise the decision to treat or not in fit patients depends on symptoms and the size of the pneumothorax. If left alone, a pneumothorax will resolve at the rate of about 1.25% per day once the leak is sealed. Breathing high concentrations of oxygen will increase the rate of reabsorption fourfold but this is not practicable for active young people. A partial pneumothorax of less than about a third of the lung volume in a relatively asymptomatic patient can be left safely as long as the patient is warned to seek help if symptoms increase. In patients with a larger pneumothorax or significant symptoms, air should be removed by simple aspiration or by intercostal tube drainage. Simple aspiration can be carried out by inserting a Teflon cannula into the pleural space and gently aspirating air with a 60-ml syringe via a plastic three-way tap with the exit tubing sealed underwater. Aspiration should be continued until resistance against the catheter is felt or 4 l has been removed. In the former case, a repeat chest X-ray should be taken 3–4 h later and, if the lung remains expanded, the patient can be allowed home, with instructions to return if symptoms recur. If 4 l of air are removed without resistance being felt, the pneumothorax is probably open, and a chest X-ray will confirm that no expansion has occurred. Simple aspiration is more likely to be effective in patients with smaller pneumothoraces, where the leak is likely to have sealed, and in those without underlying lung problems.

Intercostal tube drainage attached to an underwater seal is indicated when simple aspiration fails, when the patient is distressed and where there are underlying lung problems. With a closed pneumothorax the lung will expand rapidly over a few hours and additional suction is not required. If expansion does not occur with an underwater seal alone, it can usually be achieved by continuous suction from a vacuum pump with a pressure of 2–4 kPa (15–30 mmHg). It is important that the lung should be fully expanded even if it is bubbling vigorously, since the pleura is then more likely to seal around the leak. Suction should not be removed during nursing procedures or visits to the X-ray department and should be continued for 24 h after full expansion. Continuing failure to re-expand despite suction for 48 h is unusual. Bronchoscopy with suction of retained secretions will occasionally allow a collapsed lung to expand more fully. Otherwise surgical help is needed, in the form of a thoracoscopy to release adhesions, or pleurectomy.

A small pneumothorax will usually cause marked symptoms in patients with underlying lung disease and these should be treated promptly, irrespective of size. In patients with emphysema, care is needed to distinguish pneumothoraces with adhesions from emphysematous bullae.

Pneumothoraces recur in about 10% of patients. Surgical pleurectomy will prevent further recurrence and should be considered on the second recurrence if the pneumothorax is unilateral but at an earlier stage in subjects with a previous contralateral pneumothorax. Pleurectomy is the procedure of choice for young subjects since it has a very low recurrence rate and has the attraction of not leaving irritant chemicals in the body. For patients with underlying pulmonary problems, chemical pleurodesis with talc, dextrose or another irritant may be safer.

# Pleural Effusions

Management of pleural effusion depends on the underlying cause, so establishing the diagnosis is essential. The main causes of pleural effusions are heart failure, malignant disease, tuberculosis, other infections and pulmonary embolism. The underlying cause may be suspected from the history and clinical examination, but since patients with a condition such as rheumatoid arthritis may have a pleural effusion for other reasons, all effusions should be aspirated if there is any diagnostic doubt. The exceptions are those due to heart failure where diuretic treatment should be given, and occasionally in other situations where the clinical picture leaves no doubt about the cause of the effusion.

Examination of the pleural fluid will determine whether it is a transudate, exudate or empyema and which cells and possibly which organisms are present. It will detect malignant cells in approximately half the patients with a malignant pleural disease and allow tubercle bacilli to be cultured in a quarter of patients with tuberculous pleural disease. Multiple pleural biopsies will increase the diagnostic yield for tuberculosis to almost 100% in addition to giving a rapid answer and should therefore be taken routinely at the time of diagnostic aspiration.

Large pleural effusion of whatever cause should be aspirated if the patient is breathless or uncomfortable. Removing 1 litre on alternate days will prevent the development of pulmonary oedema which occasionally complicates over-rapid aspiration.

# Useful References

Archer GJ, Hamilton AAD, Upadhyay R, Finlay M, Grace PM (1985) Results of simple aspiration of pneumothoraces. Br J Dis Chest 79: 177–182

Hirsch A, Ruffie P, Nebut M, Bignon J, Chretien J (1979) Pleural effusion: laboratory tests in 300 cases. Thorax 34: 106–112

Riordan JF (1984) Management of spontaneous pneumothorax. Br Med J 289: 71

Spencer Jones J (1985) A place for aspiration in the treatment of spontaneous pneumothorax. Thorax 40: 66–67

# 14 Methods of Drug Administration

Many drugs which act on the airways are effective topically. Increasing use of the inhaled route to deliver drugs has been an important development because it allows maximum effect on the airways to be achieved with smaller doses of drugs and fewer side-effects. This chapter considers the principles involved and the devices available and discusses the advantages and disadvantages of the different routes of administration for patients with respiratory disorders.

## Inhaled Route

Inhalation is used predominantly for drugs with a direct effect on the airways, particularly drugs for asthma and bronchitis. It is the preferred route of administration for β-agonists and corticosteroids and is the only route used for antimuscarinic drugs and sodium cromoglycate. Antibiotics are occasionally given by inhalation to achieve higher local concentrations or reduce systemic side-effects. Theophylline is too insoluble to be effective when given by inhalation.

### Particle Size

Drugs for inhalation are given as an aerosol consisting of liquid or solid particles in a gas. The fate of the particles on inhalation is very dependent on their size. The optimum size for particles designed to settle in the airways is 2–5 μm. Larger particles are filtered out in the upper airways, while smaller particles remain suspended and leave the lung in the expired air. Ideally, therapeutic aerosol particles should all be the same size (monodisperse) but this is technically difficult to achieve. The more heterodisperse the aerosol, the less drug deposits in the airways.

Particle size is best expressed as mass median aerodynamic diameter — the particle size containing the median mass. The emphasis on mass is important since it is the size of the particles containing most of the drug which determines how much drug enters the airways. With a wide particle size distribution, terms such as mean diameter are meaningless; 90% of particles could be in the 2–5 µm range while 90% of the drug was contained in particles >10 µm.

## Delivery Methods

Several methods are used to deliver drugs by inhalation.

1. *Metered dose inhalers.* These usually contain 100–400 doses of drug in powdered form combined with a chlorofluorocarbon propellant. The inhalers are robust, fit conveniently into a pocket or handbag and are actuated relatively easily by pressure on the cannister, though some power and co-ordination are required. It is very important to ensure that patients are taught to use them correctly. This requires explanation and demonstration supervised by a doctor, nurse or technician. The patient should be told:
a)  to shake the cannister thoroughly to disperse the drug particles throughout the propellant,
b)  to breathe out ("empty your lungs" is easier to follow),
c)  to breathe in slowly, activating the aerosol during early inspiration,
d)  to hold their breath at full inspiration for about 10 s.

Many patients fail to use their inhalers correctly, usually due to incorrect time of activation, breathing in too rapidly, or failure to hold the breath on inspiration. Explanation and demonstration must be routine when an aerosol is first prescribed. Occasional spot checks should also be carried out and can easily be done at the time of pulmonary function tests. Placebo-containing cannisters can be obtained from the manufacturers for demonstration purposes. Adaptors are available to help patients with arthritis.

Particles leave the metered dose inhaler at 70 mph. Around 80% of the dose impacts in the mouth and oropharynx and is subsequently swallowed. A further 10% sticks in the apparatus or is exhaled so that only 10% enters the lung (Fig. 14.1). It is the 10% which is inhaled which produces nearly all the bronchodilatation. With drugs such as the non-catecholamine β-agonists, the ingested fraction is absorbed but the amount is very small when compared with the oral dose necessary to achieve the same bronchodilator effect — for salbutamol one inhalation of 100 µg (approximately 80 µg absorbed) causes a similar amount of bronchodilatation as a 4 mg oral dose. For other inhaled drugs the ingested fraction has little pharmacological activity, either because it is poorly absorbed (antimuscarinic drugs and sodium cromoglycate) or because of first pass metabolism (topical steroids, catecholamines).

The safety of the propellants has been questioned. High concentrations of fluorocarbons sensitise the myocardium to catecholamine or hypoxia-induced arrhythmias in animals, and young, previously fit, people have died after inhaling large amounts of freon from polythene bags. However, studies of deliberate overdosage from a metered dose inhaler in man suggest that the risk from propellant alone is minimal unless the inhaler is grossly overused or misused.

2. *Dry powder inhalers.* A capsule containing the powdered drug with a bulking agent is inserted into a turbo inhaler and perforated within the inhaler. The

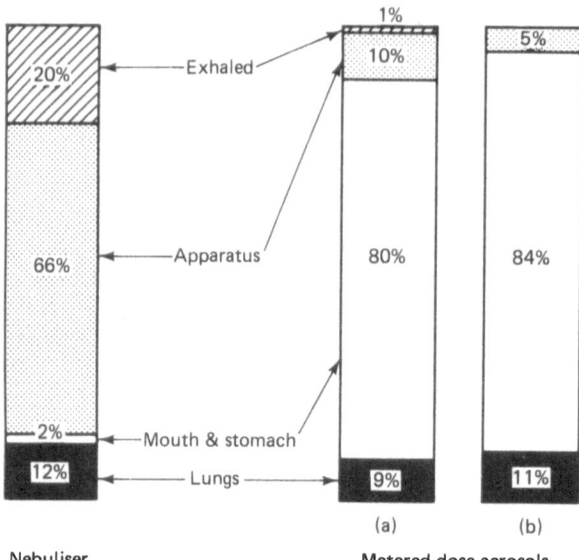

**Fig. 14.1.** Fractional distribution of radiolabelled marker following inhalation from an "Inspiron mini-Neb" jet nebuliser (Lewis et al. 1985) compared with two studies of fractional distribution from a metered dose inhaler (Newman et al. 1981, Spiro et al. 1984). (Reproduced with permission.)

drug is sucked in with the airstream as the patient inspires through the inhaler. The technique was introduced for sodium cromoglycate (Spinhaler R) and has been used more recently for salbutamol and beclomethasone dipropionate (Rotahaler R). Roughly the same proportion of drug enters the lungs as with the metered dose inhaler — around 10%. The dry powder is irritant for some patients but in general the inhalers are effective. Because they only deliver drug during inspiration, they are particularly useful for young children and for patients unable to co-ordinate a metered dose inhaler properly.

3. *Metered dose inhaler plus spacer*. Spacing devices between the metered dose inhaler and the patient reduce the velocity of the particles entering the mouth and also reduce particle size by allowing time for evaporation of propellant. Drug impaction in the mouth and oropharynx is decreased and the percentage of the dose entering the airways is increased. Dependence on timing and inhaler technique is less critical. Spacing devices reduce the incidence of oral candidiasis with inhaled steroids considerably by reducing drug impaction in the oropharynx.

The effectiveness of a spacing device depends on its size and shape. The larger spacing devices now available (around 750 ml) are more effective than the small extension tubes, though more cumbersome. They are unnecessary for most patients who get near maximum benefit from one or two puffs from a metered dose inhaler alone, but they are helpful for certain groups of patients. For most of these patients the spacer is only needed at night, or night and morning, and it can then be left at home where size is less of a problem. The spacing device has a one-way valve which should close on expiration, but occasionally this fails to occur because the patient is unable to generate an adequate flow.

The main indications for spacing devices are:
a)  patients with persistently poor inhaler technique, despite adequate teaching,
b)  patients who get candidiasis with inhaled steroids,
c)  patients with nocturnal asthma who require a higher dose of inhaled β-agonist and steroid at night,
d)  patients with severe asthma who require higher doses of drugs; spacing devices can be a reasonable alternative to a nebuliser in these patients.

4. *Nebulisers.* Nebulisation involves the fragmentation of a solution into small particles. Nebulisers can be used with IPPB but this does not appear to confer any advantage and they are usually used during spontaneous breathing. A mouthpiece or face mask is equally effective, though the face mask may be better for young children.

Nebulisers are of two main types, jet nebulisers and ultrasonic nebulisers. Jet nebulisers are driven by a stream of compressed air which, when forced through a narrow orifice, creates a negative pressure by the Venturi principle (Fig. 14.2). Fluid is drawn up by the negative pressure in such a way that it collides with the gas

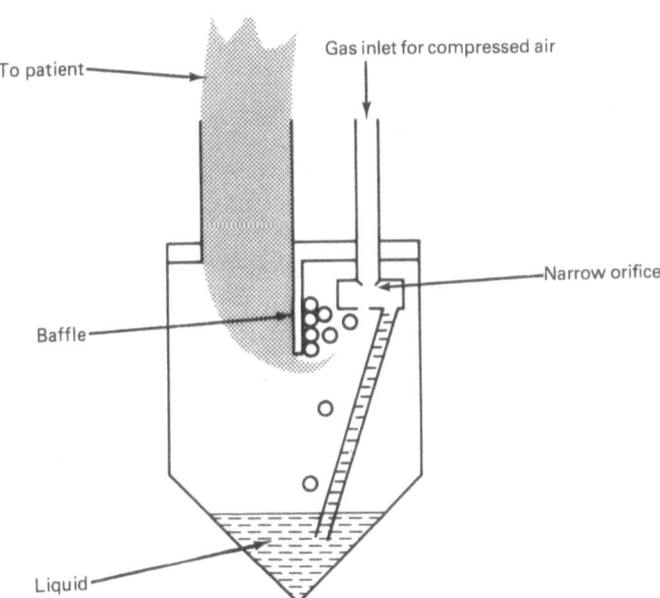

**Fig. 14.2.** A jet nebuliser. The compressed air creates a negative pressure when it expands and this sucks fluid up the feeder tube, the fluid fragmenting when it hits the jet of air.

jet and is fragmented. Baffles surrounding the nebuliser outlet return large particles to the reservoir while allowing smaller particles to leave the nebuliser in the airstream. The compressed gas is normally obtained from a compressor unit or gas cylinder. Particle size is inversely related to flow rate and for most nebulisers a driving flow rate of about 8 l/min will produce optimum particle size and a reasonably short nebulisation time. Higher flow rates tend to disconnect the tubing. The reducing valves on most compressed gas cylinders and pipelines in hospitals provide a similar flow rate but the valve provided for domiciliary use in the United Kingdom gives a maximum flow rate of 4 l/min. Although this is less than ideal, it has not been shown to make a difference in practice, though the longer nebulisation time might encourage patients at home to discontinue nebulisation before the nebuliser is empty.

In the ultrasonic nebuliser the vibration of a piezo-electric crystal fragments the surface of the nebuliser solution overlying it. Particle size depends on the vibrating frequency of the crystal. Larger particles are returned to the reservoir by a baffle, and the smaller particles are removed in the airstream. Nebulised solution only leaves the nebuliser chamber during inhalation. Ultrasonic nebulisers are quieter than jet nebulisers and may be more robust, but experience of their use is more limited.

## Factors Affecting the Dose of Drug Delivered by Nebuliser

The effective dose of a drug which a patient inhales from a nebuliser depends on:

1. The type of nebuliser, and in particular its residual volume and the particle size it produces
2. The flow rate
3. The duration of nebulisation.

Because nebulisers can differ considerably in these respects, results from studies with one nebuliser should not be extrapolated uncritically to nebulisers in general. Studies with the "Inspiron Mini-Neb" jet nebuliser, driven by air at 8 l/min, showed that 86% of the drug leaving the nebuliser was either exhaled or remained in the apparatus. Only 2% impacted in the upper airway and 12% entered the lungs (see Fig. 14.1). The proportion of the nebulised dose entering the lungs is thus very similar to that from a metered dose inhaler. Dose-response studies show that the amount of bronchodilatation produced by a β-agonist is similar dose for dose, whether given from a metered dose inhaler or from an Inspiron nebuliser. Plasma drug levels and side-effects are higher, however, with the metered dose inhaler, probably because its use involves breath holding at full inspiration where a large alveolar surface is available for drug absorption.

## Precautions for Use of Nebulisers

1. *Driving gas.* Compressed air should always be used for patients with chronic bronchitis and carbon dioxide retention since oxygen can cause carbon dioxide

narcosis. In some asthmatic patients nebulised β-agonists might potentiate hypoxaemia, and although this has not been shown to be a significant problem it would seem sensible to use oxygen when possible.

2. *Infection.* Swabs from nebulisers will often grow bacteria, though infection has not been recognised as a problem in practice. Nebulisers should be washed in clear water after use and dried thoroughly. More stringent precautions are required in intensive care units.

3. *Servicing.* Nebulisers should be serviced regularly to ensure that they are working properly and, in the domiciliary setting, to ensure they are being used correctly.

4. *Contamination of the atmosphere.* If antibiotics are being given, expired air should be diverted to reduce the chance of antibiotic resistance. Some antibiotic solutions discolour furniture and need to be vented externally.

## Indications for Use of Nebulisers

The indications for nebulisers have not yet been fully established. They are mainly used for patients unable to use other forms of inhaler or when a high dose of drug by inhalation is indicated. They are used to administer the following drugs.

1. *Beta agonists.* Nebulisers are usually used to administer higher doses of β-agonists. Metered dose inhalers would not be suitable for high doses of β-agonists, even if this were technically possible, because although the degree of bronchodilatation is similar, side-effects are increased for the same drug dose when compared with the nebulised route.

Nebulised β-agonists are used mainly in two situations:

a) In acute asthma higher doses of β-agonists can be given quickly and conveniently by nebuliser. They are now used widely, by patients at home, by general practitioners and in hospitals.

b) In chronic severe airways obstruction nebulisers may be used to give high doses of β-agonists on a regular basis. It is probable that some of these patients could be managed equally well with a spacing device and metered dose inhaler. The indications for nebulised therapy in this group are not yet clear.

2. *Ipratropium.* Nebulised ipratropium has been used to treat severe asthma in hospital (see Chap. 16).

3. *Sodium cromoglycate and corticosteroids.* Young children who cannot use an inhaler can be given sodium cromoglycate or occasionally topical steroids by nebuliser.

4. *Antibiotics.* Inhaled antibiotics provide an additional method of control of respiratory infection, though the indications for this form of treatment are uncertain. They can only be given by nebulisation (see Chap. 7).

Further details on the indications in particular situations are given in the relevant chapters.

# Oral Route

Most non-catecholamine β-agonists are available as tablets and elixirs. The oral dose is much higher than that given by metered dose inhaler so that despite some conjugation, blood levels are higher and side-effects increased for a given amount of bronchodilatation. Oral preparations should be reserved for patients unable to use the inhaled route, for example adults with physical problems such as arthritis or small children, for whom elixirs of β-agonists can be useful.

Methylxanthines are relatively insoluble and can only be given orally or intravenously. Steroids are given orally for most respiratory disorders, apart from chronic asthma, when inhaled steroids will often remove the need for oral steroids.

# Parenteral Therapy

In the acutely ill patient the intravenous route can be used to administer β-agonists, theophyllines, steroids and antibiotics. Effective doses can be given, but the higher blood levels produced are liable to give rise to more severe side-effects. However, intravenous medication is normally required for a short time only and the possibility of side-effects must be weighed against vagaries of absorption and any uncertainty about the efficacy of inhaled drugs. The use of the intravenous route is discussed in more detail in relation to both specific diseases and individual drugs.

# Useful References

Clarke SW, Newman SP (1984) Therapeutic aerosols 2 — Drugs available by the inhaled route. Thorax 39: 1–7

Clay MM, Pavia D, Newman SP, Clarke SW (1983) Factors influencing the size distribution of aerosols from jet nebulisers. Thorax 38: 755–759

Cushley MJ, Lewis RA, Tattersfield AE (1983) Comparison of three techniques of inhalation on the airway response to terbutaline. Thorax 38: 908–913

Draffan GH, Dollery CT, Williams FM, Clare RA (1974) Alveolar gas concentrations of fluorocarbons -11 and -12 in man after use of pressurised aerosols. Thorax 29: 95–98

Gunawardena KA, Patel B, Campbell IA, Macdonald JB, Smith AP (1984) Oxygen as a driving gas for nebulisers: safe or dangerous? Br Med J 288: 272–274

Hadfield JW, Windebank WJ, Bateman JRM (1986) Is driving gas flow rate clinically important for nebuliser therapy? Br J Dis Chest 80: 50–54

Hartley JPR, Nogrady SG, Seaton A (1979) Long-term comparison of salbutamol powder with salbutamol aerosol in asthmatic out-patients. Br J Dis Chest 73: 271–276

Lewis RA, Fleming JS (1985) Fractional deposition from a jet nebuliser: how it differs from a metered dose inhaler. Br J Dis Chest 79: 361–367

Newman SP, Clarke SW (1983) Therapeutic aerosols 1 — Physical and practical considerations. Thorax 38: 881–886

Newman SP, Pavia D, Moren F, Sheahan NF, Clarke SW (1981) Deposition of pressurised aerosols in the human respiratory tract. Thorax 36: 52–55

Newman SP, Millar AB, Lennard-Jones TR, Moren F, Clarke SW (1984) Improvement of pressurised aerosol deposition with Nebuhaler spacer device. Thorax 39: 935–941

Spiro SG, Singh CA, Tolfree SEJ, Partridge M, Short MD (1984) Direct labelling of ipratropium bromide aerosol and its deposition pattern in normal subjects and patients with chronic bronchitis. Thorax 39: 432–435

# 15 Sympathomimetic Amines

Sympathomimetic therapy started serendipitously in 1900 when desiccated adrenal gland was given to patients with asthma "to reduce oedema of the bronchial mucosa" and was found to be effective. Within 2 years the active substance had been isolated and purified, and variously named adrenaline, suprarenin and epinephrine. Synthetic compounds were subsequently produced, ephedrine in the 1920s and isoprenaline in 1940. The various sympathomimetic amines available in the 1940s were known to have different and sometimes opposite effects on different tissues. The reason for these anomalies became apparent in 1948 when Ahlquist identified two receptors subserving different functions, which he named $\alpha$- and $\beta$-adrenoceptors. Subsequently, Lands et al. in 1967 were able to subdivide $\beta$-receptors into $\beta_1$- and $\beta_2$-adrenoceptors and to show that $\beta_2$-receptor stimulation was responsible for bronchodilatation. This paved the way for the introduction of more $\beta_2$-selective sympathomimetic amines in the 1960s.

## Chemistry

The basic structure of the sympathomimetic amines is a benzene ring attached to two carbon atoms and an amine group (Fig. 15.1). The distinctive features of each sympathomimetic amine depend on the substitutions on this basic structure. In general, $\beta$-agonist activity increases and $\alpha$-agonist activity decreases as the size of the substituent on the amine group increases.

Most substitutions also reduce potency (biological activity per unit weight of drug) for $\beta$-adrenoceptors with respect to isoprenaline, but since loss of potency is more marked for $\beta_1$ than $\beta_2$ effects, some degree of $\beta_2$-selectivity is introduced. $\beta_2$-adrenoceptor agonists vary in their selectivity but none is $\beta_2$-specific, i.e. they all stimulate $\beta_1$-receptors to a lesser, but dose-dependent, extent.

Certain general points can be made about the structure–activity relationships of sympathomimetic amines.

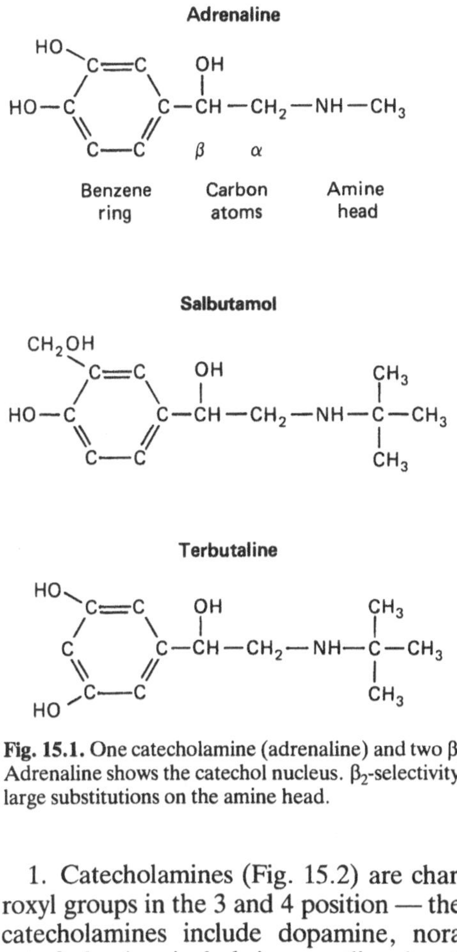

**Adrenaline**

| Benzene ring | Carbon atoms | Amine head |

**Salbutamol**

**Terbutaline**

**Fig. 15.1.** One catecholamine (adrenaline) and two $\beta_2$-selective agonists (salbutamol and terbutaline). Adrenaline shows the catechol nucleus. $\beta_2$-selectivity with salbutamol and terbutaline is related to the large substitutions on the amine head.

1. Catecholamines (Fig. 15.2) are characterised by a benzene ring with hydroxyl groups in the 3 and 4 position — the catechol nucleus. Naturally occurring catecholamines include dopamine, noradrenaline and adrenaline; synthetic catecholamines include isoprenaline, isoetharine and rimiterol.

2. Non-catecholamines have other substitutions or a repositioning of the hydroxyl groups on the benzene ring (see Fig. 15.1). These modifications make the drug less potent than isoprenaline but resistant to breakdown by catechol-O-methyltransferase (COMT). Non-catecholamines include salbutamol, terbutaline, orciprenaline and fenoterol.

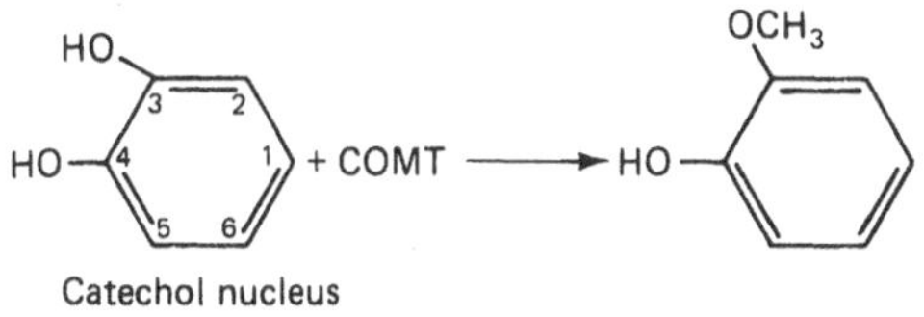

Catechol nucleus

**Fig. 15.2.** 3-O-Methylation of the catechol nucleus by catechol-O-methyltransferase (COMT).

3. Large substitutions on the amine head increase $\beta_2$-selectivity.

4. Substitutions on the $\alpha$-carbon atom and large substitutions on the amine head (e.g. salbutamol, terbutaline) block oxidation by monoamine oxidase (MAO).

5. Drugs with a lone benzene ring, such as amphetamine and ephedrine, show increased penetration of the central nervous system.

# Formulation

Both catecholamines and non-catecholamines are available for inhalation by metered dose inhaler, and some of the more $\beta_2$-selective agonists are available for inhalation by other methods (dry powder inhaler, nebuliser solution, etc). Only the non-catecholamines are effective when given orally and these are available as tablets and in some instances as an elixir. A slow-release formulation of salbutamol is available. Several of the $\beta_2$-selective agonists are available for intramuscular and intravenous use.

# Mode of Action

Bronchial muscle tone is due to calcium-dependent coupling of actin and myosin. This is reduced when the myosin light chain is phosphorylated, a reaction promoted by intracellular cyclic 3,5-adenosine monophosphate (cyclic 3,5-AMP) through activation of specific proteinkinases (Fig. 15.3). The concentration of cyclic 3,5-AMP is determined by the relative activity of adenylate cyclase and the phosphodiesterase enzymes which metabolise cyclic 3,5-AMP to adenosine monophosphate. $\beta$-Agonists increase cyclic 3,5 AMP through adenylate cyclase activation.

All the $\beta$-agonists in use as bronchodilators act directly on $\beta$-adrenoceptors. Recent work with radiolabelled adrenoceptor ligands has helped to clarify their mode of action. $\beta$-Agonists combine with adrenoceptors on the cell membrane to initiate a chain of events which in bronchial smooth muscle leads to bronchodilatation. The membrane–receptor complex consists of three components, all of which exist in an active and an inactive form: the $\beta$-adrenoceptor, the transducer (diguanine nucleotide regulatory protein) and the catalyst (adenylate cyclase) (Fig. 15.3). Stimulation of the $\beta$-adrenoceptor by an agonist causes a transient sequential change of each from the inactive to the active form, the agonist–adrenoceptor complex stimulating the transducer which when activated stimulates adenylate cyclase. Activation of adenylate cyclase catalyses the intracellular conversion of adenosine triphosphate (ATP) to cyclic 3,5-AMP.

$\beta_2$-Receptors have a mass of around 60 000 daltons and a half-life of 20–30 h in cultured cells. In the presence of high concentrations of agonist, they may be removed from the cell surface (down regulation) or the receptor may be phos-

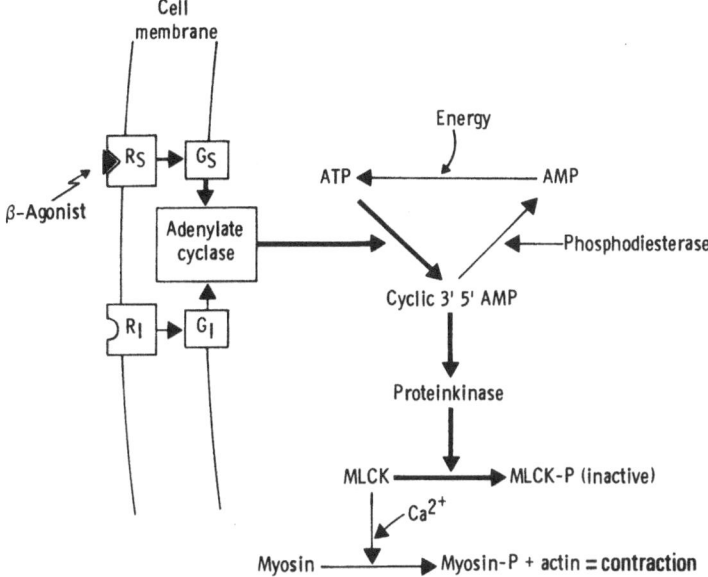

**Fig. 15.3.** Events following binding of the β-agonist to the β-adrenoceptor (Rs). This stimulates the regulatory protein (Gs), which in turn stimulates adenylate cyclase. Adenylate cyclase is also controlled by an inhibitory regulatory system (Ri and Gi). Other abbreviations include adenosine triphosphate (ATP), cyclic 3,5-adenosine monophosphate (cyclic 3,5-AMP) and myosin light chain kinase (MLCK).

phorylated and inactivated. The reverse occurs with low agonist concentrations so that β-adrenoceptor numbers are then increased. This feedback control mechanism helps to protect the cell against excessive agonist stimulation and provides increased sensitivity when agonist concentrations are low. This could reduce the effectiveness of β-agonist drugs but it does not appear to do so in practice, possibly because there are "spare" receptors in the lung so that the maximum tissue response is not necessarily altered by a reduction in receptor numbers. Other hormones such as cortisone also alter receptor numbers.

Some sympathomimetic agents, such as amphetamine and tyramine and to a lesser extent ephedrine, act indirectly by displacing noradrenaline from sympathetic nerve terminals. Consequently they show a reduced response with increasing dosage as noradrenaline stores are depleted.

# Pharmacokinetics

### Catecholamines

Catecholamines are well absorbed from the buccal mucosa and the lung but when administered orally they are almost completely conjugated and inactivated. Once absorbed, exogenous catecholamines, like endogenous adrenaline and nor-adrenaline, are subject to removal by two active uptake mechanisms and to metabolism by two widely distributed enzymes, COMT and MAO. Hence catecholamines have a relatively short half-life.

Uptake 1, in which catecholamines are taken up into the sympathetic nerve ter-minal to be stored in granules, is an important method for terminating the action of adrenaline and noradrenaline. It is inhibited by certain drugs including amphetamine, cocaine and imipramine. Uptake 2 involves the uptake of catecholamines, including isoprenaline, into non-neuronal tissue such as smooth muscle cells where metabolic degradation occurs. It is inhibited by steroids.

The main metabolic pathways for catecholamines is 3-O-methylation of the catechol nucleus by COMT and cleavage of the sympathomimetic amine between the α carbon atom and the amine group by MAO (see Fig. 15.2). In general, 3-O methylation by COMT is the more important, but MAO is also necessary. This is illustrated by the dangerous hypertension which can occur in patients on MAO inhibitors following ingestion of food containing tyramine or drugs such as ephedrine which cause the rapid release of noradrenaline from sympathetic nerve endings. The metabolic products of catecholamines following inactivation by COMT and MAO are excreted in the urine. There is little conjugation of endogenous or intra-venously administered sympathomimetic amines.

### Non-catecholamines

Non-catecholamines are well absorbed from the buccal mucosa and the lung. When given orally they are partially conjugated, but enough active drug is absorbed to allow the oral route to be effective. They are not taken up by either uptake mechanism nor are they subjected to degradation by COMT. $\beta_2$-selective amines with large substitutions on the amino group also tend to be resistant to deamination by MAO. Non-catecholamines therefore have a longer half-life than catecholamines. The drugs are excreted partly unchanged in the urine and partly as inactive conjugates.

# Pharmacological Actions

The main actions effected through $\beta_1$- and $\beta_2$-receptors are shown in Table 15.1. Drugs with a greater affinity for $\beta_2$-adrenoceptors ($\beta_2$-selective) provide less cardiac stimulation for a given degree of bronchodilatation in asthma.

### Airways

$\beta_2$-Agonists have several pharmacological actions which could contribute to bron-chodilatation. Their direct relaxant effect on bronchial smooth muscle is almost

**Table 15.1.** Adrenoceptors responsible for the main actions and side-effects of sympathomimetic amines in clinical practice

| Tissue | Receptor | Response |
|---|---|---|
| Airways | $\beta_2$ | Bronchodilatation, reduction in mediator release from mast cells, increased mucus production, increased ciliary activity |
|  | $\alpha_1$ | ?Bronchoconstriction, ?increased mediator release from mast cells |
| Heart | $\beta_1$ | Tachycardia, inotropic action |
| Blood vessels | $\beta_2$ | Dilatation, fall in blood pressure, compensatory reflex increase in heart rate |
|  | $\alpha_1$ | Constriction |
| Uterus | $\beta_2$ | Relaxation |
| Muscle | $\beta_2$ | Tremor |
| "Metabolic" | $\beta_2$ | Increased glucose, insulin, lactate, pyruvate, NEFA, glycerol and ketone bodies; decreased potassium, phosphase, calcium and magnesium |

certainly the most important. They are in addition, however, potent inhibitors of mast cell degranulation, much more so than sodium cromoglycate, and they may inhibit mediator release from other secretory cells. They decrease mucosal oedema, increase mucus secretion and enhance ciliary function, and these additional effects may contribute to the response to $\beta$-agonists with chronic therapy. The relative importance of these different actions is difficult to determine and is not distinguished by measurements such as the $FEV_1$.

Some bronchodilatation occurs in all subjects, both normal subjects and those with asthma and chronic bronchitis. The increase in $FEV_1$ is usually greatest in patients with asthma, though there is usually some response in patients with other chronic disorders associated with airways obstruction. Normal subjects usually show a 30%–100% increase in measurements which do not involve a maximum inspiration such as specific airway conductance or flow rates from partial flow–volume curves. They show little change in $FEV_1$ because the preceding maximum inspiration removes resting vagal bronchoconstriction.

It was anticipated that $\beta$-agonists and theophylline might produce a synergistic effect on the airways since theophylline caused phosphodiesterase inhibition in vitro. However, the majority of clinical studies have failed to confirm this (see Chaps. 4 and 17).

## Metabolic Actions

Intravenous $\beta_2$-agonists have been shown to produce several metabolic changes in both normal and asthmatic subjects. These include an increase in glucose, insulin, non-esterified fatty acids (NEFA), glycerol, lactate, pyruvate, ketone bodies and a fall in serum potassium, phosphate, calcium and magnesium. Although this list sounds impressive, the only metabolic changes which appear to cause clinical problems are the fall in potassium and, very rarely, the increase in glucose and lactate in diabetic patients. Metabolic changes can also occur after oral $\beta$-agonists, including an increase in high density lipoprotein cholesterol levels. Nebulised β-agonists are much less likely to cause metabolic changes though a small fall in serum potassium has been documented. Patients with severe asthma show similar metabolic abnormalities, presumably due to release of endogenous catecholamines, and these may be accentuated by intravenous β-agonists.

## Cardiac Effects

The change in heart rate following a β-agonist depends on the dose, route of administration, severity of asthma, and other drugs being administered, in addition to the $\beta_2$-selectivity of the drug. Patients with severe asthma and a tachycardia prior to treatment usually show a fall in heart rate with intravenous therapy as their asthma improves, whereas patients with less severe asthma are more likely to show an increase in heart rate.

Tachycardia and palpitations can be caused by both $\beta_1$- and $\beta_2$-adrenoceptor stimulation. The $\beta_1$ effect is due to direct stimulation of cardiac $\beta_1$-receptors. The $\beta_2$ effect is, in part at least, indirect, due to stimulation of peripheral vascular $\beta_2$-receptors causing a fall in systemic vascular resistance and a reflex tachycardia through vagal withdrawal. $\beta_2$-Selective drugs cause less tachycardia for a given degree of bronchodilatation than drugs such as isoprenaline or adrenaline. Tachycardia occurs more often with systemic therapy. With the inhaled route, heart rate is only likely to increase with the higher doses given by nebuliser.

Arrhythmias can also be induced by sympathomimetic agents, though how frequently they occur and how important they are is not known. Serious arrhythmias may occur as a result of $\beta_2$-agonist therapy, though if they do they are clearly rare. It is almost impossible to establish whether patients who die from asthma have had an arrhythmia since they usually die at home and there have been few ECG records of cardiac rhythm at the time of death. The finding of widespread mucous plugging in patients with asthma at autopsy does not exclude an arrhythmia as the final event.

$\beta_2$-Agonists have been used in cardiogenic shock and low cardiac output states to increase cardiac output and reduce systemic vascular resistance.

## Arterial Oxygen Tension

Patients with airways obstruction show a small decrease in arterial oxygen tension following inhalation of both selective and non-selective β-agonists. The fall is usually small (0.5 kPa, 3–4 mmHg) but larger changes up to 1.5 kPa (10 mmHg) can occur and could be important in hypoxaemic patients. Conversely, arterial $PO_2$ has sometimes increased in patients receiving higher doses of $\beta_2$-agonists intravenously or by nebuliser. These conflicting findings are probably due to two separate actions of β-agonists. Arterial $PO_2$ will tend to fall as β-agonists increase ventilation–perfusion mismatching by overriding vasoconstriction due to hypoxaemia, and will tend to rise as β-agonists increase cardiac output and mixed venous $PO_2$.

## Tremor

An exaggeration of normal physiological tremor is a common side-effect of $\beta_2$-agonists. Stimulation of $\beta_2$-adrenoceptors on skeletal muscle fibres and muscle spindles increases the gain on the normal servomechanism associated with the stretch reflex.

## Development of Tolerance to the Effects of $\beta$-Agonists

The terms tolerance and tachyphylaxis are used to describe the progressive impairment of the response to a drug with increasing doses of the drug. The reduction in $\beta$-adrenoceptor numbers and the impaired receptor function which follow increasing $\beta$-agonist stimulation ($\beta$-receptor desensitisation) are one possible mechanism for this effect. However, other mechanisms could be involved, such as impaired drug access due to increased mucus production, altered drug pharmacokinetics or intracellular adaptation to increased receptor stimulation.

It was suggested, following the epidemic of asthma deaths in the 1960s, that patients tending to overuse their isoprenaline inhalers might have become tolerant to the bronchodilator effect of isoprenaline. As a consequence, their airways would fail to bronchodilate normally, not only in response to an inhaled $\beta$-agonist but also in response to endogenous catecholamines released during an acute attack of asthma.

Tolerance to increasing doses of $\beta$-agonists in man is known to occur for some actions such as tremor and cyclic AMP production from lymphocytes, but there are large differences in the susceptibility of different tissues. Fortunately, the airways of asthmatic patients seem to be very resistant to the development of tolerance. Change in airway responsiveness is easily determined by repeat measurements of the response to a $\beta$-agonist using either PEF or $FEV_1$, and measurements in patients taking regular $\beta$-agonist therapy over many years suggest that tolerance is very uncommon. There is some uncertainty about whether it occurs in some patients with higher doses of $\beta$-agonists but tolerance has not been demonstrated in the majority of studies using recommended doses. The possibility that it might occur with higher doses is one reason to limit the dose given by nebuliser to the minimum which will achieve the maximum effect.

# Side-effects

$\beta$-Agonists have a very wide safety margin, particularly the $\beta_2$-selective agonists. This accounts for the very wide range of doses administered. The main side-effects are as follows.

1.  *Tremor*. Tremor is rarely a problem with low dose inhaled therapy. It is more likely to be a nuisance with oral treatment or with high doses by nebuliser. It

tends to decrease if the patient persists with treatment, due to the development of tolerance.

2.  *Muscle cramp*.
3.  *Palpitations*. These are unusual with inhaled $\beta_2$-selective drugs. They can be a problem with non-selective drugs, when $\beta$-agonists are given by routes other than inhalation and with higher doses given by nebuliser.
4.  *Hypokalaemia*. This only appears to cause clinical problems with parenteral administration or when patients are on other potassium-lowering drugs such as steroids.
5.  *Arrhythmias*. These are very rare but might account for some deaths.
6.  *Development of tolerance*. This is also very rare but may occur with very high doses.

# Which β-Agonist?

In clinical practice the main points to consider when selecting a $\beta_2$-agonist are $\beta_2$-selectivity, duration of action and whether the drug is available in the formulation required (Table 15.2). Only drugs with a direct action on $\beta_2$-adrenoceptors should be used. The more selective the agent used the greater the margin of safety.

## $\beta_2$-Selectivity

When the $\beta_2$-selectivity of $\beta$-agonists is assessed in man it is always considerably less than would be expected from studies on isolated tissues. This is because the fall in peripheral vascular resistance following $\beta_2$-stimulation causes a vagally mediated reflex increase in heart rate so that the tachycardia is greater than would be expected from in-vitro studies. The studies in man are the relevant ones for clinical practice. They show roughly seven- to tenfold $\beta_2$-selectivity for salbutamol compared to isoprenaline. Salbutamol and terbutaline appear to be similar in terms of $\beta_2$-selectivity, with fenoterol and orciprenaline being slightly less $\beta_2$-selective.

## Duration of Action

The duration of action of any bronchodilator depends on the dose given: the higher the dose the longer the half-life. For sympathomimetic amines it also depends on whether the drug is a catecholamine or not. Catecholamines have a fairly rapid onset of action, producing near-maximum bronchodilatation within 5 min of inhalation. They also have a relatively short duration of action, varying from 30 min to 2 h depending on dose. The onset of bronchodilatation following

**Table 15.2.** Clinical and pharmacological features of sympathomimetic amines

| British name | American name | $\beta_2$-selectivity | Approximate time to peak effect after inhalation (min) | Half-life for inhaled drug* | Do acti of i ($\mu$g |
|---|---|---|---|---|---|
| Catecholamines | | | | | |
| Adrenaline | Epinephrine | No | ? | ? | — |
| Isoprenaline | Isoproterenol | No | 5 | 30–90 min | 80 |
| Rimiterol | | Yes | 5 | 30–90 min | 200 |
| Isoetharine | Isoetharine | Yes | 5 | 30–90 min | 350 |
| Non-catecholamines | | | | | |
| Salbutamol | Albuterol | Yes | 15 | 3–8 h | 100 |
| Fenoterol | | Yes | 15 | 3–8 h | 180 |
| Terbutaline | Terbutaline | Yes | 15–30 | 3–8 h | 250 |
| Orciprenaline | Metaproterenol | Partial | 15 | 4+ h | 670 |
| Ephedrine | Ephedrine | No | — | — | — |

*These figures are very dependent on dose (see text).
†Relative to isoprenaline.
‡Not available in UK.

inhalation of the non-catecholamines is slightly slower but 80% of peak effect is seen by 5 min and values close to maximum by 15 min. Bronchodilatation lasts for 3–6 h with recommended doses. Salbutamol, terbutaline and fenoterol have a slightly longer duration of action than orciprenaline.

## Other Factors

Differences in potency (e.g. orciprenaline 20 mg = salbutamol 4 mg), are un-important since lower potency is easily compensated for by giving a larger dose of drug. There is no evidence that any one $\beta$-agonist causes a greater maximal effect than any other drug. Some patients claim to respond better to one $\beta$-agonist than another but these preferences are inconsistent and in general are probably due to other factors pertaining at the time that the drug was taken.

# Drugs

### $\beta_2$-Selective Non-catecholamines

These are the drugs of choice for bronchodilatation since they combine the better safety profile associated with $\beta_2$-selectivity with a reasonably long duration of action. Salbutamol, terbutaline, fenoterol and orciprenaline are used most widely.

### $\beta_2$-Selective Catecholamines

These include rimiterol, which is similar in its metabolism and time profile to iso-prenaline, and isoetherine, which is similar except that it is conjugated to a lesser extent in the gut wall.

### Isoprenaline

Isoprenaline, the first relatively pure $\beta$-agonist to be used widely, is a non-selective $\beta$-agonist with little $\alpha$-adrenoceptor activity. It causes more tachycardia for a given degree of bronchodilatation than the newer, more selective $\beta_2$-agonists and as a catecholamine its action is relatively shortlived. It is conjugated in the gut wall to an inert sulphate so is ineffective when given orally. Although it has been the yardstick for the assessment of newer drugs, it has been superseded in clinical practice by the $\beta_2$-selective agonists.

### Ephedrine

Ephedrine, a non-catecholamine, has no place in the modern treatment of respiratory disorders. Side-effects such as insomnia and retention of urine are fairly common due to penetration of the central nervous system and lack of $\beta_2$-selectivity. Since it acts in part by release of noradrenaline from sympathetic nerve terminals, it is dangerous in the presence of MAO inhibitors.

### Adrenaline

Adrenaline is used for severe asthma in some countries, though rarely in the United Kingdom. It appears to cause more adverse cardiac effects than $\beta_2$-agonists, as would be expected from its $\alpha$-adrenoceptor agonist activity and lack of $\beta_2$-selectivity.

# Indications for $\beta$-Agonists

$\beta_2$-Agonists are one of the most widely prescribed groups of drugs in the clinical pharmacopoeia; estimates suggest that 3 million puffs are inhaled from metered dose inhalers each day in the United Kingdom. Their wide safety margin and maintained therapeutic effectiveness over many years have caused them to be the usual drug of first choice for any patient with airways obstruction in whom there is some reversibility.

### Asthma

$\beta_2$-Agonists are usually the first drug to be tried in patients with asthma. The dose and means of administration will vary with the severity and form of asthma (see Chap. 4).

### Chronic Bronchitis

Although patients with chronic bronchitis show much less reversibility, a small response may cause a useful improvement in symptoms. There appears to be little to choose between an inhaled $\beta_2$-agonist and ipratropium bromide as initial treatment (see Chap. 5).

### Other Conditions

Patients with other conditions in which airways obstruction occurs, such as cystic fibrosis and bronchiectasis, often benefit from $\beta_2$-agonists. A therapeutic trial of $\beta_2$-agonists is indicated in any patient with airways obstruction.

# Route of Administration

Whenever possible, $\beta_2$-agonists should be given by inhalation since this allows bronchodilatation to be achieved with less drug absorption and fewer side-effects than either the oral or intravenous route.

### Inhaled Route

The metered dose inhaler is the most widely used means of delivering $\beta_2$-agonists by inhalation and it is usually convenient and effective. Care is needed to make sure that it is used correctly (see Chap. 14). Although only 10% of the drug enters the lungs, this is adequate to achieve maximal or near-maximal bronchodilatation in most patients. For patients unable to use a metered dose inhaler, other means of inhalation should be tried. These include a dry powder inhaler, a metered dose inhaler attached to a spacing device, or a nebuliser. The indications for these are discussed in Chapter 14.

### Oral Route

Only non-catecholamines are effective when given orally. This route usually produces more side-effects than the inhaled route for a given degree of bronchodilatation and it should only be used when there are problems in using any form of inhaler. It has been suggested that the oral route might provide better access to small airways than the inhaled route in patients with severe airways obstruction, but the majority of patients have shown less rather than more bronchodilatation with the oral route.

When given orally, $\beta_2$-agonists reduce pulmonary vascular resistance. It has been argued that this might be useful for patients with chronic bronchitis and pulmonary hypertension, but evidence that it is of long-term benefit is needed before oral treatment can be recommended in view of its increased side-effects.

### Parenteral Route

Certain $\beta_2$-agonists are available for intramuscular or intravenous administration. The intramuscular route is used very rarely for self-administration of terbutaline or adrenaline by patients with very brittle asthma. For intravenous administration, the selective $\beta_2$-agonists can be given as a bolus or, more commonly, by infusion, and this route is sometimes necessary for patients with acute asthma. It is also used in non-respiratory conditions such as threatened abortion and cardiogenic shock.

# Useful References

Ahlquist RP (1948) A study of adrenotropic receptors. Am J Physiol 153: 586–600

Conolly ME, Davies DS, Dollery CT, George CF (1971) Resistance to beta-adrenoceptor stimulants, a possible explanation of the rise in asthma deaths. Br J Pharmacol 43: 389–402

Handslip PDJ, Dart AM, Davies BH (1981) Intravenous salbutamol and aminophylline in asthma: a search for synergy. Thorax 36: 741–744

Harvey JE, Tattersfield AE (1982) Airway response to salbutamol: effect of regular salbutamol inhalations in normal, atopic and asthmatic subjects. Thorax 37: 280–287

Lands AM, Arnold A, McAuliff JP, Luduena FP, Brown TG (1967) Differentiation of receptor-systems activated by sympathomimetic amines. Nature 214: 597–598

Larsson S, Svedmyr N (1977) Bronchodilating effect and side-effects of beta$_2$-adrenoceptor stimulants by different modes of administration (tablets, metered aerosol and combinations thereof). Am Rev Resp Dis 116: 861–869

Larsson S, Svedmyr N, Thiringer G (1977) Lack of bronchial beta-adrenoceptor resistance in asthmatics during long-term treatment with terbutaline. J Allergy Clin Immunol 59: 93–100

Lefkowitz RJ, Caron MG, Stiles GL (1984) Mechanisms of membrane-receptor regulation. Biochemical, physiological, and clinical insights derived from studies of the adrenergic receptors. N Engl J Med 310: 1570–1579

Leslie D, Coats PM (1977) Salbutamol-induced diabetic ketoacidosis. Br Med J 3: 768

O'Brien IAD, Fitzgerald-Fraser J, Lewis IG, Corrall RJM (1981) Hypokalaemia due to salbutamol overdosage. Br Med J 282: 1515–1516

Prior JG, Cochrane GM, Raper SM, Ali C, Volans GN (1981) Self-poisoning with oral salbutamol. Br Med J 282: 1932

Swillens S, Dumont JE (1980) A unifying model of current concepts and data on adenylate cyclase activation by beta-adrenergic agonists. Life Sci 27: 1013–1028

Tattersfield AE (1983) Autonomic bronchodilators. In: Clark TJH, Godfrey S (eds) Asthma. Chapman and Hall, London, pp 301–335

Tattersfield AE (1985) Tolerance to beta-agonists. Clin Resp Physiol 21: 1s–5s

# 16 Antimuscarinic Drugs

Atropine and ipratropium bromide are anticholinergic drugs which act by competitive inhibition of acetylcholine at parasympathetic muscarinic receptors. Antagonism at nicotinic receptors is only seen with very high doses.

Plants of the *Datura* genus, containing atropine and related alkaloids, are known to have been used for asthma 300 years ago. Their intoxicating effects on the central nervous system had been made use of much earlier, by Mark Antony's troops in Asia Minor, for example. Inhaled *Datura* was introduced into Britain from India in 1802, and by the 1850s belladonna and stramonium were being recommended for asthma. Stramonium was regarded as being the most specific for asthma and was inhaled via cigarettes, cigars and assorted inhaler devices. The popularity of antimuscarinic drugs waned earlier this century with the introduction of theophyllines and sympathomimetic amines but the introduction of more selective antimuscarinic drugs has caused some reappraisal of their use.

## Chemistry

Atropine and hyoscine are the most important naturally occurring antimuscarinic alkaloids (Table 16.1). They consist of esters of the aromatic acid tropic acid attached to an organic base, tropine or scopine.

The main synthetic antimuscarinic drugs are:

Tertiary ammonium compounds
    atropine sulphate
    hyoscine
Quaternary ammonium compounds
    atropine methonitrate
    ipratropium bromide

The tertiary compounds are incompletely ionised at physiological pH. The small non-ionised portion (less than 1%) is able to cross the blood–brain barrier and cause central nervous system effects. Quaternary ammonium derivatives,

**Table 16.1.** Source of some natural alkaloids with antimuscarinic activity

| Source | Popular name | Alkaloids |
|---|---|---|
| *Atropa belladonna* | Deadly nightshade, belladonna | Atropine = 1 hyoscyamine |
| *Datura stramonium* | Stinkwood, thornapple, devil's apple | Atropine = 1 hyoscyamine |
| *Hyoscyamus niger* | Henbane, hogbean | Hyoscine = scopalamine (USA) |

such as atropine methonitrate and ipratropium bromide (Fig. 16.1), are highly polar and lipid insoluble, and consequently much less well absorbed across biological membranes such as the lung and gastrointestinal tract. They are more potent than the tertiary compounds, have a longer duration of action, and being fully ionised at physiological pH, do not cross the blood–brain barrier. Ipratropium may have an additional advantage over atropine methonitrate in that it appears to demonstrate some pharmacological selectivity for the airways.

# Formulation

When used as bronchodilators, the drugs are only given by the inhaled route. Side-effects following systemic absorption of tertiary compounds are unacceptable and the quaternary derivatives are not absorbed after oral administration. With

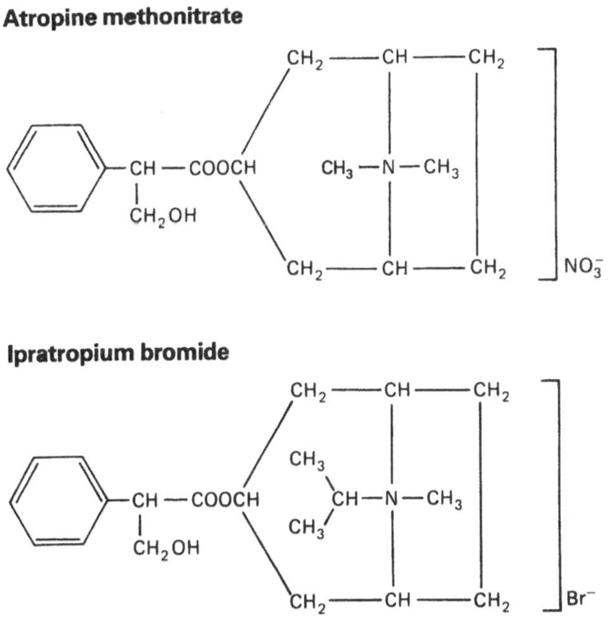

**Atropine methonitrate**

**Ipratropium bromide**

**Fig. 16.1.** Atropine methonitrate and ipratropium bromide.

lation, bronchodilatation is achieved with doses which produce undetectable blood levels. The intravenous dose of ipratropium needed to produce the same degree of bronchodilatation as conventional inhaled doses produces plasma levels a thousand times higher, with associated systemic symptoms from parasympathetic blockade.

Inhaled atropine is only available in combination with other compounds such as adrenaline. Ipratropium bromide is available as a metered dose inhaler and nebuliser solution.

# Mode of Action

The antimuscarinic drugs are competitive antagonists of acetylcholine at muscarinic receptors. Their intracellular mechanism of action has not been fully clarified. Occupancy of the muscarinic receptor by agonists such as acetylcholine appears to be associated with inhibition of adenylate cyclase, intracellular formation of cyclic 3,5-GMP and opening up of ion channels in the cell membrane. The relative importance of each of these in causing bronchoconstriction has not been established.

# Pharmacokinetics

Following absorption, atropine is partly hydrolysed in the liver and partly excreted unchanged in the urine. The quaternary derivatives are poorly metabolised and excreted largely unchanged in urine and faeces. The small proportion of ipratropium which is absorbed has a half-life in serum of 3–4 h and is slowly converted to metabolites which are inactive or have weak anticholinergic activity and which, with ipratropium itself, are excreted in urine.

# Pharmacological Effects

Bronchodilatation following the administration of antimuscarinic drugs is usually attributed to inhibition of vagal bronchoconstrictor activity by competitive antagonism at muscarinic receptors on bronchial smooth muscle. Reduction in mast cell mediator release or subtle changes in mucus production, mucociliary clearance or in the inflammatory response may contribute to the bronchodilatation but, as with other drugs, the importance of these mechanisms in patients is difficult to determine.

The bronchodilator response to atropine and ipratropium is slower than the response to β-agonists, being about 75% maximum at 15 min and taking about 1 h to achieve a maximal or near-maximal effect. The reason for the relatively slow onset of action is not clear, but it occurs with all antimuscarinic drugs irrespective of route of administration. The duration of bronchodilator action of atropine sulphate (half-life 2–3 h) is less than that of atropine methonitrate and ipratropium, which are similar, with a half-life of 3–6 h, depending on dose.

The dose–response data available for the antimuscarinic drugs suggest that near-maximal response will occur with 1–2 mg for atropine sulphate, 0.5–1 mg for atropine methonitrate, and between 80 μg and 120 μg for ipratropium. Peak bronchodilatation is almost as great for 40 μg ipratropium but the response is less well sustained. The paucity of dose–response data may account for the initial marketing of a relatively low dose of ipratropium (18 μg/metered dose) and the large variation in the dose of atropine in proprietary preparations (50–500 μg/metered dose).

## Studies of Bronchial Reactivity

Antimuscarinic drugs are often used to probe the role of vagally mediated bronchoconstriction in the airway response to bronchial provocation. It is difficult, however, to determine how much of the inhibition seen with an antimuscarinic drug is due to inhibition of reflex effects and how much to bronchodilatation alone. Any drug which causes bronchodilatation would be expected to alter the response to a provocation challenge for several reasons — redistribution of inhaled stimulus towards or away from relevant receptors, geometric factors affecting the relationship between change in radius and change in flow, and a redistribution of the balance of peripheral and central components to total resistance. Care is needed before assuming that small changes following an antimuscarinic drug are necessarily reflecting a vagally mediated reflex contribution to bronchoconstriction.

Overall, high doses of atropine and ipratropium have had relatively small effects on bronchial responsiveness to stimuli such as histamine and exercise in asthmatic patients, in contrast to β₂-agonists where the increased bronchodilatation seen with increasing doses has been associated with a progressive reduction in bronchial reactivity. They have usually had no effect on antigen-induced bronchoconstriction.

## Effect on Sputum Volume, Viscosity and Mucociliary Clearance

The effect of atropine on mucociliary clearance is disputed but in some studies it has caused a reduction in sputum production, ciliary beat frequency and mucociliary transport. In contrast, ipratropium by metered dose inhaler, in doses up to 200 μg t.d.s. regularly for 1 month, has not been shown to cause a change in the volume and viscosity of saliva or sputum, nor a reduction in mucociliary clearance. In some studies mucociliary clearance has increased following ipratropium.

However, no direct comparison of atropine and ipratropium by the same route in the same patients has been reported and there are no data, as yet, on the effect of higher doses of nebulised ipratropium on mucociliary clearance. The reason for the apparent difference between atropine and ipratropium is unclear.

# Side-effects

When given by inhalation in recommended doses, both atropine methonitrate and ipratropium bromide cause very few side-effects. This is due to the introduction of bronchial selectivity by using the inhaled route and to lack of penetration of the central nervous system. Ipratropium may cause a dry mouth and some patients dislike the taste and the relatively slow onset of action. Problems with sputum viscosity have not been seen. Paradoxical bronchoconstriction has occurred very rarely when the drug is given by metered dose inhaler. It was seen more often with nebulised ipratropium when the nebuliser solution was hypotonic. With the current isotonic nebuliser solution, it is less common but can still occur in very hyperreactive patients. Systemic side-effects such as tachycardia are not a problem with ipratropium, though it is not recommended for patients with narrow angle glaucoma. When the drug is given by nebuliser local atmospheric contamination can cause topical absorption by the eye and glaucoma.

When antimuscarinic drugs are absorbed systemically, side-effects are common and due almost entirely to predictable pharmacological effects (Table 16.2). Severe side-effects including hallucinations and convulsions are seen with accidental or deliberate overdosage of oral drugs. They are also seen with the abuse of drugs, plants of the *Datura* species or asthma cigarettes (Potter's Asthma Remedy = *D. stramonium*) which are still available in chemist shops. Treatment consists of gastric lavage, sedation by drugs without anticholinergic activity, oxygen and assisted ventilation if necessary. The anticholinesterase drug physostigmine penetrates the central nervous system but carries the risk of inducing bronchoconstriction in asthmatic patients.

**Table 16.2.** Side-effects of antimuscarinic drugs

| | |
|---|---|
| 1. Seen with inhaled drug | Dry mouth |
| 2. Very uncommon with any inhaled drug | Tachycardia |
| | Blurred vision |
| | Glaucoma |
| | Hesitancy in passing urine, urinary retention |
| 3. Usually associated with overdose of oral drug or drug abuse | Difficulty in speaking and swallowing |
| | Visual hallucinations |
| | Flushed skin |
| | Disorientation |
| | Delirium and convulsions |

# Clinical Studies

The findings of a large number of clinical studies in patients with chronic bronchitis and asthma using different drugs, dosages and routes of administration can be summarised as follows.

1. In single dose studies, patients with chronic bronchitis have shown a similar degree of bronchodilatation with conventional doses of atropine and isoprenaline, and a similar response to inhaled ipratropium 40 µg and salbutamol 200 µg. The few longer term studies have shown similar findings to the single-dose studies. One study found a similar increase in $FEV_1$ with these doses of ipratropium and salbutamol, but a greater increase in exercise tolerance with salbutamol.

2. When recommended doses of an antimuscarinic drug and $\beta_2$-agonist are compared in patients with asthma, the majority have a greater response to the β-agonist. This is less true in the older patient with late onset asthma.

3. Two recent studies found that large doses of nebulised ipratropium (500 µg) were as effective as nebulised salbutamol (10 mg) in patients with acute asthma. Ipratropium was free from side-effects in these studies.

4. The combination of recommended doses of ipratropium and a β-agonist has usually shown a small additive effect — of the order of 10%–20% further improvement in $FEV_1$ over that seen with either drug alone. The same was true when high dose nebulised β-agonist and ipratropium were combined. Whether this small additional effect is worthwhile will depend on clinical circumstances.

# Clinical Indications

1. Antimuscarinic drugs can be used as an alternative to a β-agonist as first line treatment in patients with chronic bronchitis. They might be preferable for patients with cardiac arrhythmias.

2. They may be helpful for patients with asthma who do not respond to or cannot use a β-agonist, particularly in the older late onset asthmatic patient.

3. They can be useful as additional therapy in patients with chronic bronchitis or asthma who continue to be symptomatic despite appropriate doses of a β-agonist and, in the case of asthma, a prophylactic drug. Pulmonary function tests should be used to help to assess whether this addition is worthwhile.

4. They may have a role in acute asthma. In view of the occasional report of bronchoconstriction with nebulised ipratropium, it would seem sensible to try a nebulised β-agonist first in severely ill patients. The two drugs can be combined in the nebuliser.

# Useful References

Conolly CK (1982) Adverse reaction to ipratropium bromide. Br Med J 285: 934–935

Gandevia B (1975) Historical review of the use of parasympatholytic agents in the treatment of respiratory disorders. Postgrad Med J 51 (Suppl 7): 13–20

Gomm SA, Keaney NP, Hunt LP, Allen SC, Stretton TB (1983) Dose response comparison of ipratropium bromide from a metered dose inhaler and by jet-nebulisation. Thorax 38: 297–301

Gross NJ, Skorodin MS (1984) Anticholinergic, antimuscarinic bronchodilators. Am Rev Resp Dis 129: 856–870

Mann JS, George CF (1985) Anticholinergic drugs in the treatment of airways disease. Br J Dis Chest 79: 209–228

Mann JS, Howarth PH, Holgate ST (1984) Bronchoconstriction induced by ipratropium bromide in asthma: relation to hypotonicity. Br Med J 289: 469

Pavia D (1984) Lung mucociliary clearance. In: Clarke SW, Pavia D (eds) Aerosols and the lung. Butterworths, London, pp 127–155

Tattersfield AE (1981) Measurement of bronchial reactivity: a question of interpretation. Thorax 36: 561–565

Tattersfield AE (1982) Bronchodilator drugs. Pharmac Ther 17: 299–313

Ward MJ, Fentem PH, Roderick Smith WH, Davies D (1981) Ipratropium bromide in acute asthma. Br Med J 282: 598–600

# 17 Theophylline and Related Xanthines

The name theophylline ("divine leaf") refers to the leaves of the tea plant which contain a small amount of theophylline. Naturally occurring methylxanthines also include theobromine found in cocoa and caffeine found in coffee beans, cocoa and cola nuts. Methylxanthines cause central nervous system stimulation, an observation traditionally attributed to an Arabian shepherd who noticed that goats played all night after eating berries of the coffee plant. Theophylline was extracted from tea leaves in 1888, its formula identified in 1895 and its bronchodilator action in animals established early this century. Although its potential value as a bronchodilator for asthma was noted in 1921, it was not evaluated systematically until the late 1930s when it came into more general use.

Theophylline, like other methylxanthines, is difficult to administer in doses which are both safe and effective, due to the combination of large intersubject differences in metabolism and a relatively small therapeutic window. This has stimulated investigations into its mode of action and a search for preparations and related compounds with a greater margin of safety.

## Chemistry

Theophylline is a methylated xanthine, like most xanthines with bronchodilating activity studied so far (Fig. 17.1). The formulae of theophylline, xanthine (dioxypurine) and the purine uric acid, to which they are closely related, are shown in Fig. 17.2. Substitutions in different positions of the xanthine molecule cause predictable changes in function (Fig. 17.3). Derivatives of theophylline with substitutions in the N-7 position, e.g. diprophylline, are less potent than theophylline, and show more erratic absorption and a shorter half-life. They have no advantage over theophylline and are not considered further. A non-methylated alkylxanthine, enprofylline, is currently being investigated as part of a search for xanthine drugs with fewer side-effects.

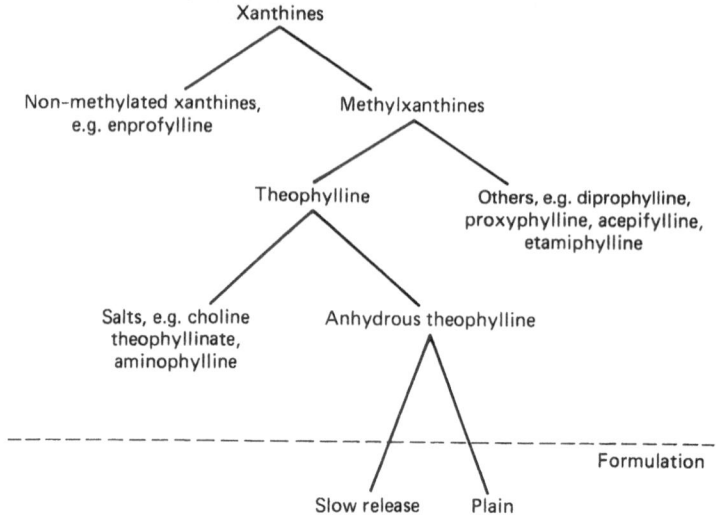

**Fig. 17.1.** Clinical classification of xanthine drugs.

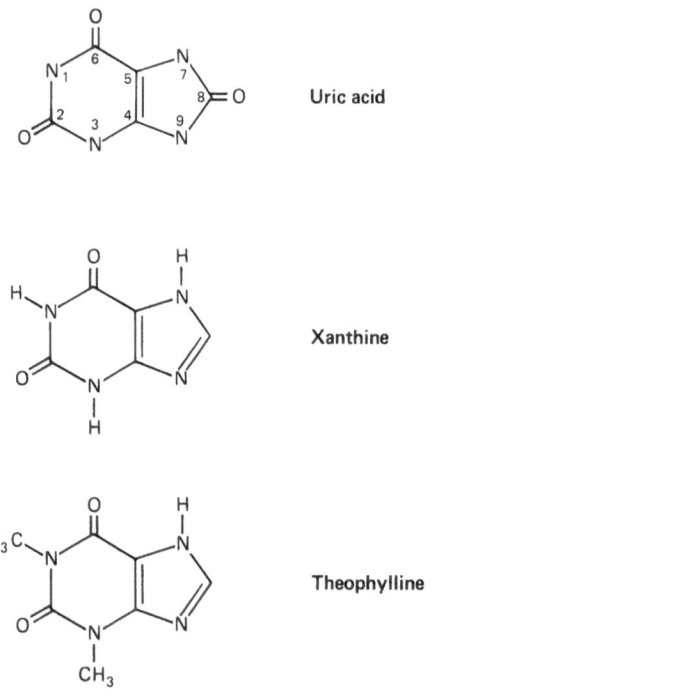

**Fig. 17.2.** Formulae of uric acid, xanthine and theophylline.

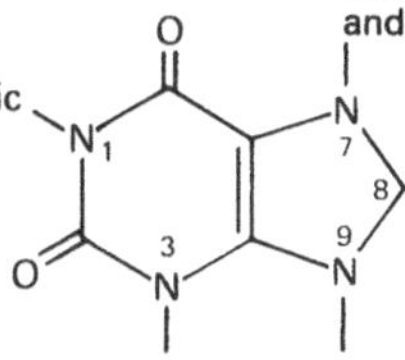

Essential for adenosine
antagonism
Bronchodilator and toxic
potency may increase

Decreased bronchodilator
and toxic potency

Unchanged bronchodilator
potency

Toxic potency and
adenosine antagonism may
increase

Essential for increased
bronchodilator potency
Toxicity may increase

General loss of
potency

**Fig. 17.3.** Effect of different substitutions on the xanthine molecule (Persson 1983, reproduced with permission).

# Formulation

Theophylline is available for oral administration as anhydrous theophylline or as salts such as choline theophyllinate. The salts are more soluble than theophylline itself, but this confers no particular advantage since uncoated anhydrous theophylline is completely absorbed. None of the salts of theophylline has any proven advantage over anhydrous theophylline for oral use. Recently emphasis has concentrated on improving the predictability and rate of absorption of oral theophylline and several new slow-release formulations of theophylline have been designed. These decrease the rate of drug dissolution, so that theophylline is absorbed slowly from the gastrointestinal tract over several hours.

The ethylenediamine salt aminophylline is 20 times more soluble than theophylline and this is an important advantage for intravenous use. Ethylenediamine constitutes 15% by weight and dissociates from theophylline in the body. It is normally inert but can cause allergic reactions. Intramuscular aminophylline is absorbed slowly but its administration is too painful to recommend.

Theophylline is absorbed from the rectum and suppositories and retention enemas are available. However, they can cause proctitis and absorption is often erratic. Their use has diminished as better slow-release oral formulations have become available. Inhaled theophylline has an unpleasant taste and because of its poor solubility causes negligible bronchodilatation even when inhaled for 20 min.

# Mode of Action

In-vitro studies of bronchial smooth muscle show that theophylline, like β-agonists, causes functional antagonism of any bronchoconstrictor stimulus. Bronchial smooth muscle relaxation with β-agonists is associated with increased levels of intracellular cyclic AMP following adrenoceptor stimulation of adenylate cyclase (see Chap. 15), and the increase in cyclic 3,5-AMP is thought to mediate bronchodilatation through phosphorylation of myosin light chain kinase. When theophylline was shown to increase intracellular cyclic 3,5-AMP levels by phosphodiesterase inhibition (Fig. 17.4), it was assumed that bronchodilatation following treatment with theophylline was also due to an increase in cyclic 3,5-AMP levels, in this case following phosphodiesterase inhibition (PDI). More recently however, several lines of evidence suggest that this mechanism is unlikely.

1. The dose of theophylline causing PDI ($5-10 \times 10^{-4}$ mol/l) is much higher than the plasma levels of free theophylline associated with bronchodilatation in patients ($2-5 \times 10^{-5}$ mol/l). Therapeutic plasma levels of theophylline cause only 10%–15% inhibition of phosphodiesterase in vitro.

2. Drugs such as dipyridamole and papaverine are more potent inhibitors of phosphodiesterase enzymes in vitro than theophylline but do not cause bronchodilatation in patients with asthma.

3. The action of β-agonists and theophylline should be synergistic in vivo as they are in vitro if theophylline is acting through PDI. Most studies in asthmatic patients have shown a less than additive increase in $FEV_1$ or PEF when both drugs are administered.

4. Studies in vitro have not shown the expected increase in intracellular cyclic AMP levels with theophylline-induced smooth muscle relaxation, nor in man has

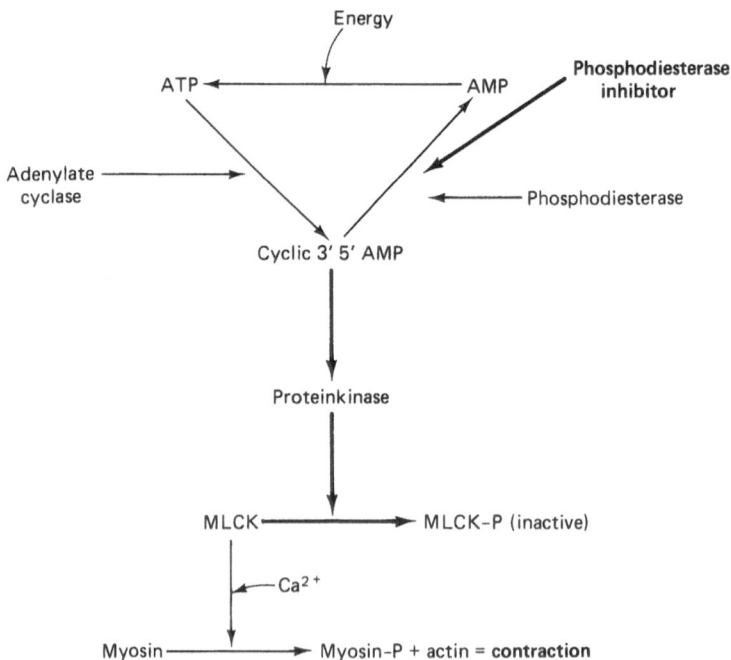

**Fig. 17.4.** Effect of phosphodiesterase inhibition by theophylline on cyclic 3,5-AMP activity.

oral theophylline been associated with the increased levels of plasma cyclic AMP levels seen with β-agonists.

These observations do not exclude the possibility that theophylline may be causing effective intracellular inhibition of phosphodiesterase through preferential uptake of theophylline into the cell or via a phosphodiesterase enzyme which is particularly sensitive to theophylline. There is, however no direct evidence for this, and several possible alternative actions are currently being investigated, including the following:

1. *Release of catecholamines.* Theophylline has been shown to release catecholamines from the adrenal medulla in animals and to produce a small increase in plasma and urinary catecholamines in man. Part of the bronchodilatation following intravenous aminophylline and oral theophylline in normal subjects is attenuated by propranolol, suggesting that it is mediated via β-adrenoreceptors. It is unlikely, however, that catecholamine release makes a large contribution to the actions of theophylline in patients since the increase in catecholamine levels is modest, the side-effects of theophyllines differ from those of catecholamines, and the increase in plasma cyclic 3,5-AMP levels after oral theophylline is small.

2. *Adenosine antagonism.* Adenosine is a naturally occurring purine nucleoside which, when inhaled, causes bronchoconstriction in asthmatic patients. Plasma adenosine levels are increased following antigen challenge in asthmatic patients, so endogenous adenosine release may be relevant to asthma. Theophylline competitively antagonises many actions of adenosine in vitro at concentrations which are lower than those needed to inhibit phosphodiesterase. Studies of inhaled adenosine in asthmatic patients have shown some inhibition of bronchoconstriction by theophylline, but the effect was less than would be expected if this were theophylline's main mechanism of action. Adenosine antagonism appears to make a greater contribution to some of the other actions of theophylline, including gastric acid secretion, central nervous system stimulation, natriuresis and release of free fatty acids. Enprofylline, a xanthine which is said to cause less adenosine antagonism, causes less tremor and gastric acid secretion than theophylline. It causes more nausea and headache however, which is surprising if these effects of theophylline are due to adenosine antagonism.

Changes in intracellular calcium distribution and prostaglandin metabolism have also been proposed as mechanisms whereby theophylline might induce bronchodilatation but supporting data are sparse. So far, none of the suggested mechanisms adequately explains the known actions of theophylline. Its effects may be due to more than one action.

# Pharmacokinetics

## Absorption

Predictability and rate of absorption are particularly important for theophylline because of its small therapeutic window. Following oral administration, serum theophylline levels depend on the proportion of drug absorbed and the rate of absorption. Anhydrous theophylline is completely and rapidly absorbed from liquids or uncoated tablets to produce peak plasma levels 2 h after ingestion on an empty stomach and a steady fall thereafter. With slow-release formulations, peak levels usually occur 6–12 h after administration. Most retain 100% bioavailability, though incomplete absorption has occurred with some of the new formulations, with some enteric-coated tablets, and with some methylxanthines other than theophylline. Absorption appears to be slower at night and is usually delayed if the tablet is taken after food or antacids. This delay is usually small but it has been as long as 24 h with high doses of some slow-release theophyllines.

Absorption from rectal suppositories is both greater and more rapid when they are presented in a hydrophyllic base (100% bioavailability; peak serum levels at 1.5 h) than in a fatty base (bioavailability around 40%; peak effect 3–8 h). Absorption from retention enemas is rapid, although incomplete, producing maximum serum levels at around 1 h.

## Distribution

Approximately 40% of theophylline in serum is protein bound, almost entirely to albumin, and this varies little between subjects. Measured serum concentrations normally include both bound and free theophylline. Theophylline concentrations in saliva are very close to serum levels of free or physiologically active theophylline; i.e. approximately 60% of total serum concentrations. The free fraction is increased in patients with an acidosis or low plasma proteins so serum concentrations should be kept in the low therapeutic range in these patients. It has been suggested that protein binding decreases as serum theophylline concentrations rise, but this is disputed. Any concentration-related protein binding effect around the therapeutic range is, at the most, small but disproportionate increases in serum levels may occur with higher doses.

Theophylline passes freely across the placenta, into breast milk and across the blood–brain barrier. Concentrations in the cerebrospinal fluid are about 90% of serum concentrations.

## Metabolism

Ten per cent of theophylline is excreted unchanged in urine; the remainder undergoes biotransformation in the liver by one of several cytochrome P-450 enzyme-dependent pathways to produce relatively inactive metabolites (Fig. 17.5). Some of the pathways appear to follow first order kinetics, i.e. at a rate proportional to theophylline concentration, whereas others follow saturable (zero order) kinetics. Single dose theophylline studies in adults have usually shown first order kinetics with serum levels in the therapeutic range. Saturable kinetics may occur in children or with higher doses in adults, leading to a disproportionate increase in serum concentrations and side-effects with further increases in dose. In neonates the proportion of theophylline metabolised to caffeine is increased, producing concentrations which increase respiratory drive.

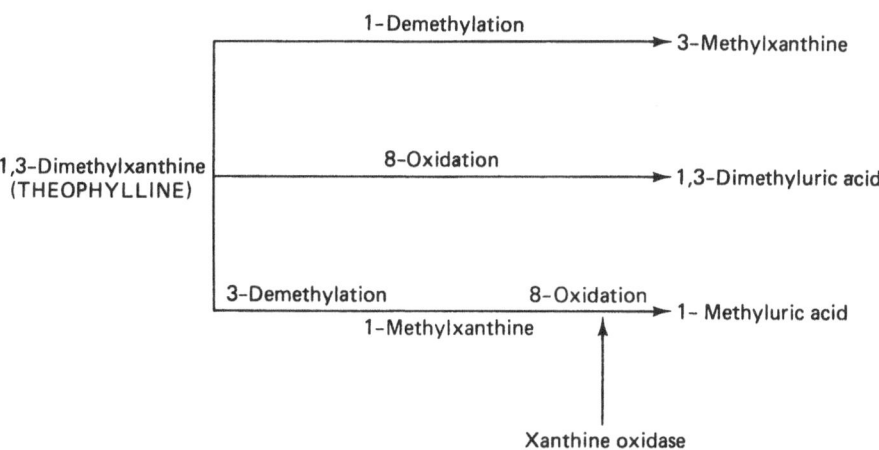

**Fig. 17.5.** Metabolism of theophylline.

The main problem with theophylline is that a given dose produces widely different plasma theophylline concentrations in different subjects, largely due to intersubject variation in hepatic drug metabolism. The wide range of theophylline half-life seen in different subjects (4–26 h) can, to some extent, be accounted for by factors known to alter hepatic enzymes (Table 17.1). Neonates and children differ markedly from adults. Heart failure and cirrhosis decrease theophylline clearance whereas cigarette smoking increases it, a heavy smoker on average requiring almost twice as much theophylline as a non-smoker to achieve serum concentrations in the therapeutic range. Even when allowance has been made for known factors such as cigarette smoking and liver function, there is an as yet unexplained residual three- to fourfold difference between adults.

A number of drugs have been shown to interact with theophylline by inhibiting or inducing cytochrome P-450 mixed function oxidase activity, and the list is slowly increasing (Table 17.2). A change in medication or a viral infection can convert a well controlled theophylline regimen into a toxic one.

**Table 17.1.** Effect of age on half-life of theophylline

|  |  | Half-life (h) | Average daily dose (mg/kg) |
| --- | --- | --- | --- |
| Neonates |  | 30 |  |
| Children | <1 year | 20 | 4 |
|  | 1–6 years | 3 |  |
|  | 6–17 years | 4 |  |
| Adult | Non-smoker | 8 | 9 |
|  | Smoker | 4–5 |  |
|  | Heart failure | 23 |  |
|  | Alcoholic cirrhosis | 26 |  |

**Table 17.2.** Factors known to affect theophylline half-life

| Factors increasing theophylline clearance | Factors decreasing theophylline clearance |
|---|---|
| *Diet and smoking* | |
| Smoking | |
| Low carbohydrate, high protein diet | |
| Methylxanthine-containing foods | |
| Alcohol | |
| *Disease* | |
| Cystic fibrosis | Heart failure |
| | Alcoholic cirrhosis |
| | Viral infection |
| | Pneumonia |
| | BCG |
| *Drugs* | |
| Phenytoin | Cimetidine |
| Carbemazepam | Allopurinol (600 mg/day) |
| Rifampicin | Propranolol |
| Barbiturates | Erythromycin |
| | Oral contraceptives |

Antacids, by altering pH, may increase diurnal swings in plasma theophylline concentrations from certain slow-release preparations, e.g. Nuelin.

# Pharmacological Actions

The main actions of theophylline are summarised in Table 17.3. Its bronchodilator action is considered to be largely due to a direct effect on bronchial smooth muscle and this is supported by the rapidity with which bronchodilatation occurs following intravenous administration. Other mechanisms, such as a reduction in the release of local mediators, change in mucus production or mucociliary clearance, may also contribute but this is difficult to confirm. Theophylline probably has at most a small effect on mucociliary clearance since conflicting results have occurred in subjects with airflow obstruction.

Theophylline has a direct central respiratory stimulant effect. This appears to be useful for apnoeic infants but it has not been shown to be of value to patients with respiratory failure. Intravenous aminophylline causes distressing air hunger when given too rapidly. Some studies suggest that theophylline may have a direct effect on the force of contraction of the fatigued diaphragm but this is disputed. Any such effect is likely to be small at most and more valuable to patients with respiratory failure than to those with asthma.

Theophylline has complex cardiovascular effects due to the combination of a direct chronotropic and inotropic effect on the heart, and a relaxant effect on both veins and arteries. The chronotropic effects cause tachycardia and arrhythmias which can be fatal. The peripheral actions cause large postural changes in blood pressure and heart rate: a mean fall in systolic blood pressure of 15 mmHg and

**Table 17.3.** Main actions of theophylline

| | |
|---|---|
| 1. Respiratory | Bronchodilatation |
| | Reduction in mediator release from mast cells |
| | Increased mucociliary clearance |
| | Respiratory stimulation |
| | Increased force of contraction of fatigued diaphragm (disputed) |
| 2. Cardiovascular | Direct chronotropic and inotropic effect |
| | Arrhythmias |
| | Systemic venodilatation ⟍ |
| | Systemic vasodilatation ⟋ ⟶ Postural hypotension |
| | Pulmonary vasodilatation |
| | Increased resistance of cerebral arterioles |
| | Stimulation of vagal and vasomotor centre |
| 3. Central nervous system | Stimulation — insomnia, vomiting, fits, confusion, agitation, lack of concentration |
| 4. Renal | Diuresis |
| 5. Skeletal muscle | Tremor |
| 6. Stomach | Increased gastric acid secretion |
| | Reduced oesophageal sphincter pressure |
| 7. Metabolic | Hypokalaemia |

increase in heart rate of 20 beats/min in normal subjects after therapeutic doses of both intravenous and oral theophylline. Theophylline has been shown to increase both right and left ventricular ejection fraction and heart rate in patients with chronic bronchitis.

# Theophylline Serum Concentrations, Effects and Side-effects

## Relationship Between Serum Theophylline Concentrations, Bronchodilatation and Side-effects

The bronchodilator effect of theophylline increases linearly with log serum theophylline concentration (Fig. 17.6). Bronchodilatation can be detected with serum concentrations as low as 5 μg/ml and increases progressively with increasing plasma concentrations up to 20 μg/ml. Higher doses have not been studied systematically for safety reasons.

Toxic effects are also related to plasma theophylline concentrations (Fig. 17.6). They are relatively unusual with serum concentrations below 20 μg/ml and become increasingly common with levels exceeding 25–30 μg/ml. Serum theophylline levels of 10–20 μg/ml are generally considered to be optimum since they combine a reasonable amount of bronchodilatation with a low incidence of side-effects. In Europe, where theophylline is used infrequently as sole therapy, a more cautious therapeutic range of 7.5–15 μg/ml is often preferred.

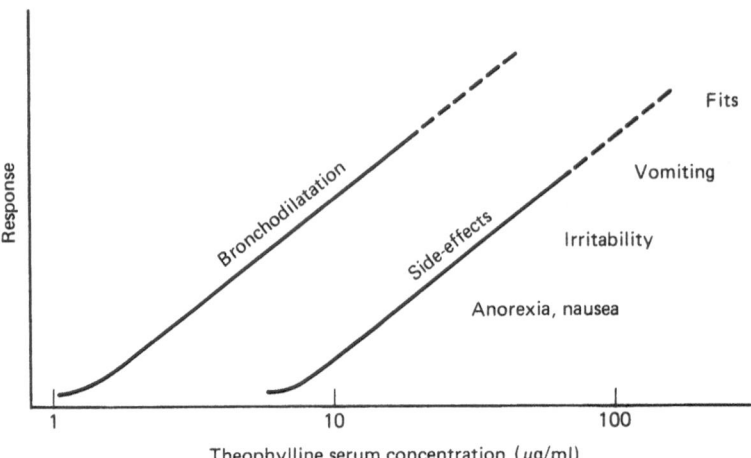

**Fig. 17.6.** Diagrammatic representation of the relationship between theophylline serum levels, bronchodilator response and side-effects.

There are large intersubject differences in the plasma theophylline concentration at which side-effects occur and in the nature of the presenting side-effect. At one extreme, 1% of children and 4% of adults are unable to tolerate plasma theophylline levels within the therapeutic range, whereas an occasional patient with serum concentrations in excess of 100 µg/ml has had no symptoms. Fits have occurred with serum levels as low as 25 µg/ml, though in a series of eight patients with grand mal fits, the mean theophylline plasma concentration was 53 µg/ml.

## Side-effects and Toxicity

Local effects of theophyllines include gastric irritation and oesophageal ulceration presumably due to the tablet sticking in the oesophagus. These are much less common than systemic effects. With higher doses of theophylline, nausea, vomiting and anorexia are common, followed by headache and insomnia. These occur with both parenteral and oral administration and are mainly related to plasma concentrations. Children may present with behaviour problems, lack of concentration, irritability or fits and elderly patients with confusion and disorientation.

Intravenous aminophylline can cause collapse and sudden death, particularly if the injection is given too rapidly. Death appears to be commoner in patients with pre-existing heart disease and is probably due to cardiac arrhythmias. Animal studies have shown arrhythmias to be commoner when theophylline is combined with high doses of β-agonist and this is likely to be true in man, though difficult to ascertain. Collapse may also occur from postural hypotension or fits. Patients on oral maintenance theophylline are particularly at risk and should not receive intravenous aminophylline until serum drug levels have been determined. Ethylenediamine is a common contact allergen and patients given aminophylline can develop urticaria, erythema and exfoliative dermatitis.

## Treatment of Toxicity and Overdosage

Theophylline toxicity is being seen with increasing frequency as a result of deliberate self-poisoning, after chronic inadvertent overdosage or when intravenous aminophylline is given to patients on regular oral therapy. The effects of acute and chronic poisoning are similar. With deliberate overdosage, however, there are likely to be a large number of tablets in the gastrointestinal tract, particularly if slow-release tablets have been taken, and serum concentrations may continue to rise for up to 24 h. The features of theophylline overdosage are varied and include hyperventilation, tremor, tachycardia, nausea, vomiting, abdominal pain, restlessness and confusion. More recently, rhabdomyolysis and hypocalcaemia have been described. Patients may have a respiratory alkalosis or a metabolic acidosis depending on whether hyperventilation or cardiac problems predominate. The main risk to life is from hypokalaemia, arrhythmias, hypotension and fits. The symptoms and signs do not correlate well with serum levels. Treatment should be guided by serial serum theophylline measurements.

Patients at risk should be looked after in an intensive care area with electrocardiographic monitoring. Gastric lavage or induced vomiting is worthwhile up to 12 h after ingestion of an overdose. Activated charcoal should then be given and repeated 2-hourly; it is safe, reduces absorption and, although not of proven value in theophylline overdosage, it is known to increase clearance of therapeutic doses of theophylline. General supportive measures include prompt correction of hypokalaemia, acidosis and dehydration. Sinus tachycardia may not require treatment, though β-adrenoceptor antagonists are recommended if the patient is not asthmatic. Arrhythmias will require a drug such as verapamil if the patient has asthma.

Benzodiazepines should be given to patients with convulsions and considered on a prophylactic basis for patients with serum concentrations above 40–60 µg/ml. Charcoal haemoperfusion and haemodialysis increase plasma theophylline clearance and may be helpful in intractable vomiting. Haemoperfusion has been recommended for patients with serum levels above 40–60 µg/ml but there is no evidence as yet that it improves outcome. Since it is associated with a small risk and supportive therapy gives very good results, more evidence of benefit is required. Peritoneal dialysis is relatively ineffective.

## Theophylline Assays

Serum theophylline levels should be measured in all patients suspected of having theophylline toxicity or of having taken an overdose of theophylline, and in patients on regular theophylline who develop severe asthma in whom intravenous aminophylline is considered necessary. Elective theophylline assays are necessary for optimal theophylline treatment to be given (see below).

Theophylline can be assayed in most biological fluids by radio- or enzyme immunoassay, gas chromatography or high performance liquid chromatography. Serum assays are invasive so alternative methods have been investigated. Theophylline concentrations in stimulated saliva collected at least 2 h after drug administration have correlated closely with free plasma theophylline concentrations, the two values usually being within 1 µg/ml. Total plasma theophylline concentrations can be calculated by assuming a free to total theophylline ratio of 0.6 and again will usually be within 1 µg/ml. This is close enough to allow saliva theophylline concentrations to replace plasma levels for most clinical purposes, though timing of the measurement is important.

Recently, theophylline has been assayed from a dried blood spot collected from a finger prick by the patient. The results correlated closely with venous plasma theophylline concentrations and raise the possibility of home measurements by patients in the future.

# Which Theophylline?

## Oral

When an oral theophylline is required, a slow-release preparation should be given (Table 17.4). These are absorbed more reliably, have a better time profile, cause less gastric irritation and provide better asthma control and compliance than plain anhydrous theophylline. Anhydrous theophylline needs to be administered frequently to maintain reasonable serum theophylline concentrations and compliance is poor, around 50%. Even 6-hourly administration causes large differences in peak and trough serum levels, so that patients run the dual risk of overdosage and undertreatment. Patients are unlikely to take theophylline at regular intervals throughout the day. In one investigation the mean intervals between doses prescribed three times daily were 5.5, 6 and 12.5 h.

The differences between the different slow-release preparations are small. On a twice-daily regimen, the difference between peak and trough levels will be relatively small in non-smokers (5–10 µg/ml) but greater in smokers, who may be better on an 8-hourly regimen. A once-daily regime will cause a greater peak-to-trough difference, usually of the order of 10–15 µg. The tablets should be taken after food if possible to reduce peak-to-trough differences and minimise gastric

**Table 17.4.** Slow-release theophylline preparations

| Drug | Slow-release preparation | Dose per tablet (mg) | Free theophylline equivalence (mg) |
|------|--------------------------|----------------------|------------------------------------|
| Aminophylline | Phyllocontin continus | 100, 225, 350 | 85, 200, 320 |
| Choline theophyllinate | Sabibal SR 90; 270 | 142, 424 | 90, 270 |
| Theophylline | Nuelin SA | 175, 250 | |
| | Slo-Phyllin | 65, 125, 250 | |
| | Theo-Dur | 200, 300 | |
| | Theograd | 350 | |
| | Uniphyllin Continus | 200, 400 | |

**NB** Aminophylline = ethylenediamine 15% + theophylline 85%.
  Choline theophyllinate = choline 36% + theophylline 64%.

intolerance. When taken without food, the tablet should be accompanied by a drink to prevent oesophageal ulceration, particularly when taken late in the evening.

Many compound bronchodilator tablets containing theophylline are still available. These are dangerous and have resulted in overdosage from the unwitting simultaneous administration of two theophylline preparations.

### Intravenous

Patients receiving regular oral theophylline therapy should only be given intravenous aminophylline if the serum theophylline concentration is below the therapeutic range. The dose of aminophylline needs to be adjusted in the light of the current and anticipated serum concentrations since with slow-release preparations peak plasma levels can be delayed for up to 24 h after administration. Aminophylline should be used unless ethylenediamine sensitivity is present.

# Dose

### Oral

If theophylline is to be effective and safe, measurement of drug concentrations in serum or saliva is necessary. This is less important if a single dose of theophylline is given at night for nocturnal symptoms, though optimal management requires an early morning serum level.

Side-effects are less likely to occur if patients are started on a small dose which is increased gradually. Weinberger and Hendeles (1983) have made recommendations for establishing therapy in ambulatory patients and these are distributed with FDA approved drugs in the United States. A small initial dose of theophylline based on body weight is followed by further increments after 3 and 6 days if tolerated and a serum theophylline assay 3 days later, 4 h after the last dose of theophylline. Further dose adjustments are made if necessary, to obtain serum levels in the therapeutic range. Serum levels should then be checked every 6–12 months, or more often if there are problems or in a growing child. Patients with low plasma proteins should have lower serum theophylline concentrations. This regimen produces a relatively low incidence of side-effects but the dose increments depend on calculations based on age and weight and the scheme is unlikely to be implemented widely.

Attempts have been made to predict the optimum oral maintenance dose for an individual patient from plasma levels following a single oral or intravenous dose of theophylline. These predictions give some guide to oral maintenance requirements, but the range of peak concentrations following the calculated dose is still wide and further serum assays are necessary once the patient is stable.

### Intravenous

In patients not receiving oral theophylline, the present recommendation is 6 mg/kg over 30 min followed by 0.5 mg/kg per hour maintenance (i.e. for a 70-kg person, 420 mg loading dose followed by 280 mg 8-hourly). The maintenance dose should be reduced in patients with hepatic disease or cardiac failure. This regimen will produce mean peak theophylline levels of 10 μg/ml, but the range is wide (95% confidence limits 4–22 μg/ml in one study), emphasising the need for serum theophylline monitoring for optimum use.

# Clinical Indications

### As Regular Treatment

There are large variations in the use of theophylline in different countries, ranging at one end of the spectrum from its use as the preferred initial treatment for asthma to the belief that the small risk of serious side-effects means that it is rarely justified. Countries with long experience with inhaled $\beta_2$-agonists and inhaled steroids, such as the United Kingdom, tend towards the latter view.

There are no long-term comparisons of inhaled $\beta_2$-agonists and oral theophylline. Short-term studies have shown $\beta_2$-agonists to be equally effective or slightly more effective than theophylline in terms of bronchodilatation when optimum serum theophylline levels were achieved. The comparative convenience, side-effects and risks of each treatment should determine the choice for initial treatment. In support of theophylline it is argued that many patients, particularly children, find a tablet less conspicuous and more convenient to take than an inhaled medication and that the incidence of side-effects has been low when theophylline plasma levels are monitored and the dosage titrated appropriately. Its effectiveness has been shown to be maintained over a year. However, many patients will not tolerate theophylline, it cannot be used on demand and the process of monitoring plasma levels is expensive, time consuming and invasive. In contrast, the use of long-term $\beta_2$-agonists by metered dose inhaler is associated with maintained effectiveness, measurement of plasma drug concentrations is unnecessary and patients can adjust their therapy within prescribed limits themselves. The incidence of minor side-effects with $\beta$-agonists given by metered dose inhaler is very low, and there is no evidence of severe toxicity.

The risk of serious side-effects from theophylline is difficult to establish with certainty but it is clearly related inversely to the time and trouble taken to control therapy. When serum levels are monitored and both the patient and the doctor appreciate the complexity of theophylline clearance, the risk with theophylline therapy is probably similar to that with oral $\beta_2$-agonists. However, this situation requires much effort and is seldom achieved. In practice the majority of patients in the United Kingdom have no serum levels measured after receiving theophylline. They are usually given a low dose in the knowledge that it is likely to have a less than optimal effect, but in the hope that the risk of adverse effects is low. Several surveys have shown that the majority of patients have subtherapeutic levels, a minority have serum levels in the therapeutic range and a small but important proportion have toxic levels. In one large retrospective study in London, 8% of patients had theophylline levels in the toxic range, of whom 3 had convulsions and 2 died. Several other studies support the view that theophylline, administered as it is in the United Kingdom, is causing appreciable morbidity and some deaths. Since theophylline has no clear-cut advantage over $\beta_2$-agonists and presents a greater potential hazard, it should not be the first choice treatment for patients with either asthma or chronic bronchitis. In patients not well controlled on inhaled bronchodilator and steroid therapy, a trial of theophylline is reasonable but it should only be continued if benefit is demonstrated.

## The Combination of Theophylline with a β-agonist

The majority of studies have found a less than additive increase in $FEV_1$ or PEF when theophylline and a β-agonist have been combined. When a large dose of inhaled $\beta_2$-agonist has been taken, the effect of additional theophylline has usually been very small, suggesting that a ceiling effect for response is being reached. It has been argued that taking a small dose of each drug would maximise bronchodilatation and minimise side-effects, but there is no good evidence to show that the side-effects with this combination are less than those with a larger dose of inhaled $\beta_2$-agonist alone.

## Nocturnal Asthma

Patients who continue to have nocturnal symptoms despite maximum treatment with inhaled β-agonists and steroids may benefit from a single nocturnal dose of a slow-release theophylline. There is limited information on how theophylline compares with other remedies, such as high doses of inhaled steroids or $\beta_2$-agonists, or slow-release oral $\beta_2$-agonists in patients with severe nocturnal asthma. There is evidence that theophylline impairs the quality of sleep as judged by the electroencephalogram and this could be a problem with long-term treatment.

## Acute Episodes of Asthma

Intravenous aminophylline is effective in the majority of episodes of acute asthma seen outside hospital where the attacks are short lived. It is probable that a nebulised $\beta_2$-agonist is as effective and safer, but clear evidence for this is lacking. Giving a drug over 15 min is difficult for the general practitioner or casualty officer and some of the problems reported with intravenous aminophylline are probably due to excessively rapid injection.

## Summary of Use of Theophylline

At present we believe that theophylline has a relatively small place in the treatment of airways obstruction. The main indications are:

1.  A single dose of theophylline may be given at night to patients whose nocturnal asthma is not controlled by other measures (see Chap. 4).
2.  Oral theophylline should not be used as first line treatment for asthma. It has a place as additional therapy in patients with asthma who are not controlled on maximum doses of inhaled β-agonists and inhaled steroids. It should only be prescribed if there is clear-cut benefit, if there are no significant side-effects, and when the patient does not have complicating problems which will cause variable changes in theophylline clearance.
3.  Intravenous aminophylline has a role in the management of acute severe asthma, though in the first instance nebulised $\beta_2$-agonists should be tried.

The value of theophylline in patients with chronic bronchitis is debatable. Inhaled $\beta_2$-agonists or antimuscarinic drugs are equally effective in causing bronchodilatation and should be tried in the first instance. Older patients run greater risks from regular theophylline treatment so it should only be prescribed if there is clear evidence of benefit.

### Contraindications

Theophylline should be avoided in patients with epilepsy or peptic ulcer and in those with fluctuating hepatic function or heart failure. Patients should be told to halve the dose when febrile and to question whether any new drugs they are given might interfere with theophylline metabolism.

## Useful References

Cushley M, Holgate ST (1984) Theophylline. In: Buckle DR, Smith H (eds) Development of anti-asthma drugs. Butterworths, London, pp 205–223

Dahlqvist R, Billing B, Ripe E (1984) Theophylline — clinical pharmacokinetics and therapeutic drug monitoring. Eur J Resp Dis 65 (Suppl. 136): 81–94

Ebden P, Leopold D, Buss D, Smith AP, Routledge PA (1985) Relationship between saliva and free and total plasma theophylline concentrations in patients with chronic airflow obstruction. Thorax 40: 526–529

Isles AF, MacLeod SM, Levison H (1982) Theophylline. New thoughts about an old drug. Chest 1: 49S–54S

Mountain RD, Neff TA (1984) Oral theophylline intoxication. A serious error of patient and physician understanding. Arch Intern Med 144: 724–727

Moxham J, Green M (1985) Aminophylline and the respiratory muscles. Bull Eur Physiopath Resp 21: 1–6

Persson CGA (1983) The profile of action of enprofylline, or why adenosine antagonism seems less desirable with xanthine antiasthmatics. In: Morley J, Rainsford KD (eds) Pharmacology of asthma, agents and actions, supplement 13. Birkhäuser Verlag, Basel

Rhind GB, Connaughton JJ, McFie J, Douglas NJ, Flenley DC (1985) Sustained release choline theophyllinate in nocturnal asthma. Br Med J 291: 1605–1607

Vaughan LM, Weinberger MM, Milavetz G, Tillson S, Ellis E, Jenne J, Szefler SJ, Wiener MB, Conboy K, Shaughnessy T, Carrico J (1986) Multicentre evaluation of disposable visual measuring device to assay theophylline from capillary blood sample. Lancet I: 184–185

Weinberger M, Hendeles L (1983) Slow release theophylline. Rationale and basis for product selection. N Engl J Med 308: 760–764

Woodcock AA, Johnson MA, Geddes DM (1983) Theophylline prescribing, serum concentrations, and toxicity. Lancet II: 610–612

# 18 Corticosteroids

Naturally occurring steroids consist of glucocorticoids affecting glucose metabolism and having associated anti-inflammatory activity, mineralocorticoids acting predominantly on renal handling of salt and water, and sex hormones.

Corticosteroid drugs have assumed a major role in the management of respiratory disorders since the first patient with asthma received ACTH in 1949. The beneficial actions are associated with glucocorticoid and anti-inflammatory activity. Attempts to separate beneficial from unwanted effects have led to the production of synthetic analogues largely lacking in mineralocorticoid or sex hormone activity, and to the development of steroids with high topical activity for use by inhalation. It has not been possible to separate glucocorticoid activity from anti-inflammatory activity.

## Chemistry

Molecular manipulation has made it possible to synthesise steroids with either mineralocorticoid or glucocorticoid activity. The features associated with glucocorticoid and anti-inflammatory activity are shown in Fig. 18.1.

Lipid-soluble steroids with marked topical activity have been produced for use by inhalation. Topical activity appears to be related to esterification of the 17 and 21 positions and formation of 16, 17-acetonide derivatives.

## Formulation

The drugs used most often in respiratory medicine, prednisolone, hydrocortisone and the topically active steroids, betamethasone valerate, beclomethasone dipropionate and budesonide, are discussed in most detail (Table 18.1). Triamcinolone

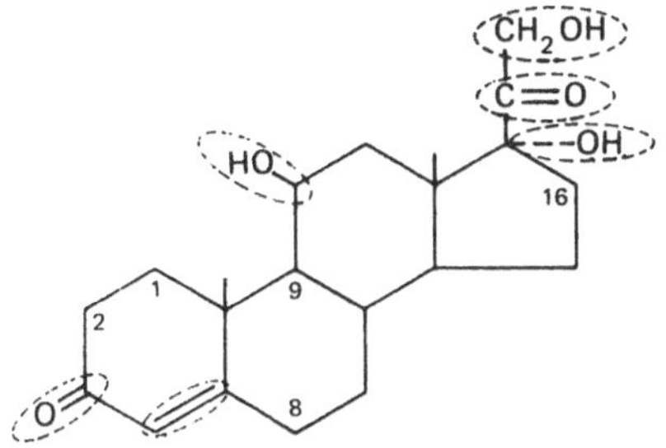

**Fig. 18.1.** Chemical features of cortisol associated with anti-inflammatory activity; the important features are ringed. (From Harding 1984, reproduced with permission.)

and methylprednisolone are mentioned briefly. For oral administration, prednisone and prednisolone are used most widely and since prednisone has to be converted into prednisolone it is sensible to use prednisolone in the first place. There is no evidence that any other oral corticosteroid offers any advantage. Enteric-coated preparations are available, though the value of enteric coating in preventing gastrointestinal problems is unproven.

The inhaled route confers bronchial selectivity for all steroids, but in addition the drugs available for inhalation have much higher topical activity than other steroids. Beclomethasone dipropionate was introduced for inhalation in 1972, since when two other steroids have become available for inhalation — betamethasone valerate and a non-halogenated steroid, budesonide — both of which appear to be of roughly similar potency to beclomethasone dipropionate.

All three drugs are available in a metered dose inhaler. Beclomethasone dipropionate is also available as a nebuliser solution and as a dry powder for use in a turbo inhaler (Table 18.2). The dry powder appears to be roughly equipotent to the formulation in the metered dose inhaler. Spacing devices increase lung absorption from the metered dose inhaler and reduce the incidence of candidiasis.

**Table 18.1.** Relative potencies and equivalent doses of corticosteroids

|  | Relative anti-inflammatory potency | Relative sodium-retaining potency | Duration of biological action | Approximate equivalent oral or i.v. dose (mg) |
|---|---|---|---|---|
| Cortisol (hydrocortisone) | 1 | 1 | S | 20 |
| Prednisone | 4 | 0.8 | I | 5 |
| Prednisolone | 4 | 0.8 | I | 5 |
| 6-Methylprednisolone | 5 | 0.5 | I | 4 |
| Cortisone | 0.8 | 0.8 | S | 25 |
| Triamcinolone | 5 | 0 | I | 4 |
| Triamcinolone acetonide | 50 | 0 | L | 0.3 (i.m.) |
| Dexamethasone | 25 | 0 | L | 0.75 |

S = short = 8–12 h half-life.
I = intermediate = 12–36 h half-life.
L = long = 36–72 h half-life.

**Table 18.2.** Formulations and available doses of inhaled steroids

|                              | Form               | Dose (µg)    |
| ---------------------------- | ------------------ | ------------ |
| Beclomethasone dipropionate  | MDI                | 50, 250      |
|                              | + volumatic spacer |              |
|                              | Rotahaler          | 100, 200     |
|                              | Nebuliser solution | 50 µg/ml     |
| Betamethasone valerate       | MDI                | 100          |
| Budesonide                   | MDI                | 200          |
|                              | + Nebuhaler        |              |
|                              | Paediatric MDI     | 50           |

MDI = metered dose inhaler.

Hydrocortisone and methylprednisolone are the preferred corticosteroids for intravenous administration. Why hydrocortisone is used for asthma and methylprednisolone for the adult respiratory distress syndrome is not clear; the different approaches appear to be based on custom rather than pharmacological rationale or evidence of benefit.

ACTH and its synthetic analogue tetracosactrin can be given by intramuscular injection but are rarely indicated for respiratory problems. Depot or slow-release steroid preparations are available for intramuscular injection. They produce a more variable response than oral steroids and should only be used for short periods when fine titration of dose is not important, to allow a patient with hay fever to take an examination, for example.

# Mode of Action

### At Intracellular Level

Many of the actions of corticosteroids are now known to be due to a specific effect on enzyme induction (Fig. 18.2). Corticosteroids diffuse rapidly across cell membranes and bind to cytoplasmic steroid receptors. After undergoing conformational change the steroid–receptor complex migrates to the nucleus where it becomes attached to specific acceptor sites on nuclear chromatin. This causes transcription of RNA and subsequent coding for the production of regulatory peptides and proteins such as the proteinkinases. These enzymes, which may have either stimulatory or inhibitory actions, appear to be responsible for most of the observed effects of steroids.

One of the recently documented actions of corticosteroids likely to be important in respiratory disease is inhibition of phospholipase $A_2$ by a specific protein, identified in 1980 and named macrocortin (UK), lipomodulin (USA) and, more

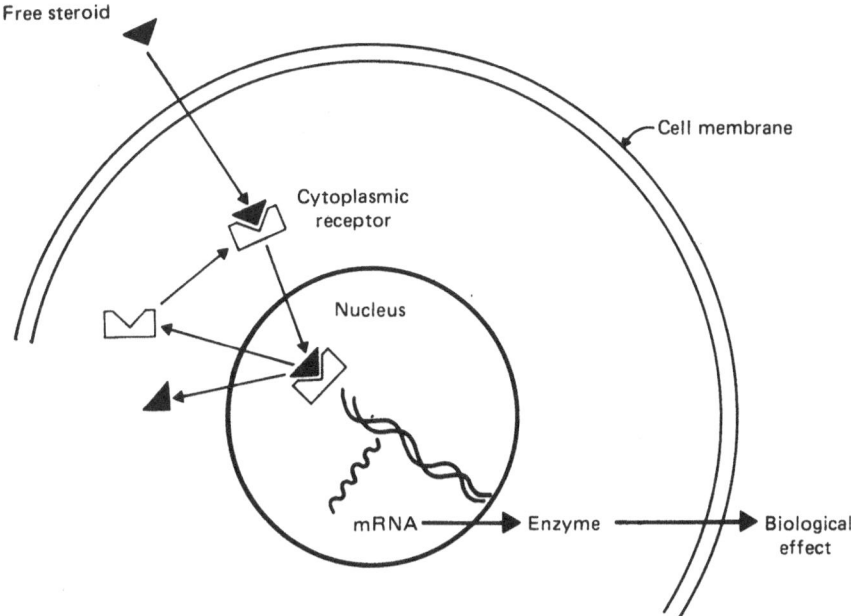

**Fig. 18.2.** Intracellular action of corticosteroids.

recently, lipocortin. By inhibiting phospholipase $A_2$ lipocortin prevents degradation of membrane phospholipids to arachidonic acid and so reduces synthesis of leukotrienes, prostaglandins and thromboxane (Fig. 18.3).

Some of the actions of corticosteroids, such as suppression of ACTH, occur much more rapidly and non-nuclear mechanisms appear to be involved, possibly in this case a direct effect of the steroid–receptor complex on cytoplasmic enzymes. Steroid effects mediated by proteins synthesised in the nucleus, such as lipocortin, differ from non-nuclear steroid actions in that they occur with very low drug concentrations and their peak pharmacological effect is delayed for several hours.

## At Tissue Level

Although many of the physiological effects of corticosteroids are well documented, relatively little is known about how they modify disease activity, and how the intracellular action of steroids described above relates to their effect on the inflammatory and immunological response in disease. It is likely that the action of lipocortin in preventing arachidonic acid metabolism and the release of inflammatory and bronchoconstrictor mediators is important (see Fig. 18.3), but its precise role in different disease processes has not been clarified.

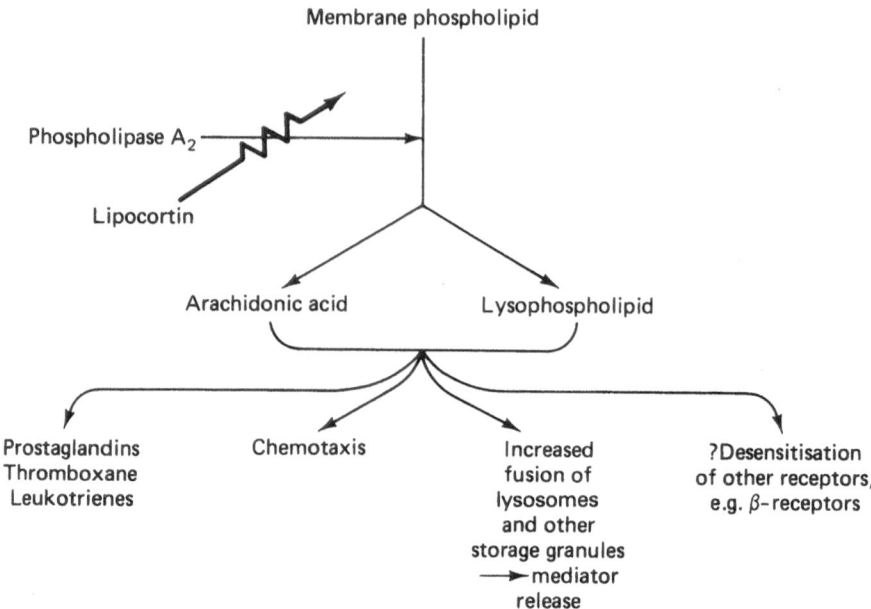

**Fig. 18.3.** Effect of the action of lipocortin on phospholipase A$_2$ activity.

The main tissue effects of steroids which may be important in respiratory disease are summarised. The evidence for some of their actions is indirect or based on animal studies.

1.  Changes in inflammatory cell numbers and reduced chemotaxis as a consequence of the reduced conversion of saturated fatty acids to unsaturated arachidonic acid (Table 18.3). When inflammation is present, inhibition of neutrophil–endothelial interaction may also play a role.

2.  Reduction in mucosal oedema. This is a specific glucocorticoid effect associated with vasoconstriction and a reduction in capillary permeability.

3.  Enhancement of effect of β-agonists. In-vitro work suggests that steroids should increase the response to β-agonists as a result of increased β-receptor expression, enhanced proteinkinase activity and blockade of post-synaptic uptake$_2$ mechanism for removing catecholamines. The evidence in man, however, is unconvincing. Patients with asthma who are responsive to β-agonists show only an additive response when steroids are given with β-agonists rather than the synergistic response which would be expected if receptor responsiveness were increased (Fig. 18.4).

### In Vivo

1. *Reduction of response to antigen challenge*. The late response to antigen challenge in asthmatic patients is inhibited by a single dose of steroids. The early

**Table 18.3.** Effect of corticosteroids on inflammatory cells

*Neutrophils*
Circulating neutrophils increased
Reduced migration to sites of inflammation
?Reduced endothelial adherence

*Lymphocytes*
Circulating lymphocytes usually reduced
Effect on lymphocyte function unclear

*Eosinophils*
Circulating eosinophils fall dramatically (probably due to sequestration)

*Macrophages*
Macrophage numbers reduced
Secretion of mediators responsible for migration and recruitment of inflammatory cells reduced
Release of fibronectin and alveolar macrophage derived growth factor (both implicated in the
    development of lung fibrosis) not reduced, at least in patients with fibrosing alveolitis

*Mast cells*
Mast cell function apparently unaffected by steroids
No change in serum antibody levels including IgE
Some of the consequences of antigen–antibody reactions suppressed

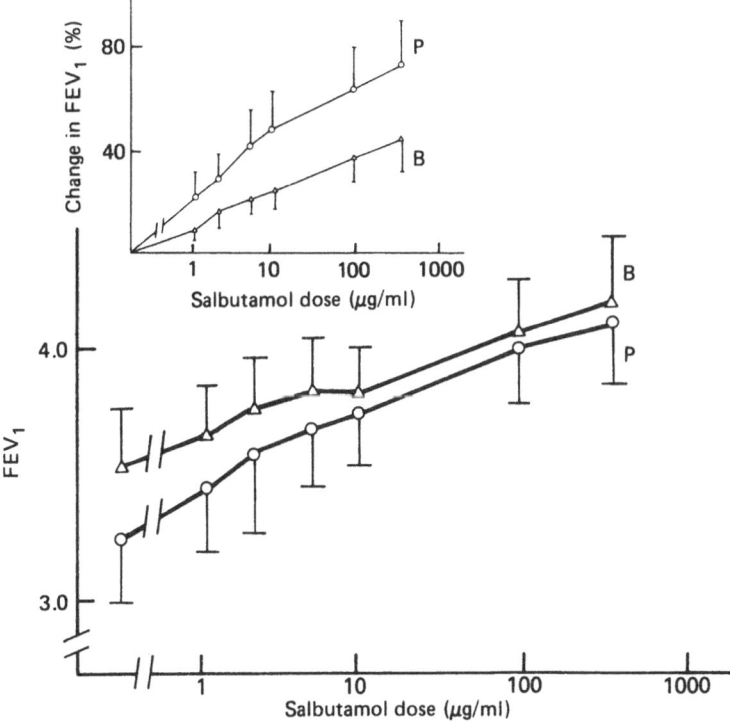

**Fig. 18.4.** Dose–response curve to inhaled salbutamol before and after 2 weeks inhaled beclo-methasone (B) and placebo (P) in 6 asthmatic subjects. (From Harrison, Richards and Tattersfield, unpublished.)

response is not inhibited by a single dose, but is reduced progressively after several days of steroid treatment. There is no immediate response to steroids in anaphylaxis.

2. *Enhancement of mucociliary clearance.* Clearance is increased after 4 weeks of oral steroids in asthmatic patients, but this may be a non-specific effect as a result of clinical improvement. Steroids have been shown to decrease mucus secretion in human airways in vitro.

### Inhaled Steroids

The steroids available for inhalation such as beclomethasone dipropionate and budesonide are very effective when given by this route. This is due to three factors: slightly greater potency (around tenfold) than hydrocortisone for glucocorticoid receptors, bronchial selectivity due to the inhaled route of administration, and pharmacokinetic factors. Once absorbed, the drugs are avidly extracted and metabolised by the liver and this allows higher doses to be inhaled without side-effects.

# Pharmacokinetics

### Absorption

Prednisone and prednisolone are rapidly and consistently absorbed after oral administration, with peak plasma levels at 1–2 h. Different formulations show some variation in the rate of absorption but they almost always show 100% bioavailability. Absorption is unaffected by gastric pH, antacids or $H_2$-receptor antagonists. It may be delayed by meals and enteric coating, but total absorption is normally unchanged.

The topically active steroids available for inhalation are absorbed rapidly from the lung and more slowly from the gastrointestinal tract. ACTH is readily absorbed after intramuscular injection. Following intravenous administration, it has a half-life of only 15 min.

### Protein Binding

Secretion of cortisol and corticosterone by the adrenal cortex follows the diurnal rhythm of ACTH secretion, most of the daily output in normal subjects being released between 0400 h and 1600 h, with peak levels around 0600 h and trough levels around midnight. Corticosteroids cannot be stored and continuous synthesis is required to maintain secretion. Ninety per cent of endogenous cortisol is reversibly bound to protein, mainly to a specific $\alpha_1$-glycoprotein, transcortin, but also to albumin. Only the free unbound cortisol is biologically active. Transcortin binding shows high affinity but low total binding capacity; albumin binding in contrast has low affinity but high total capacity. Under basal physiological conditions, most cortisol is bound to transcortin. When cortisol concentrations are increased both the albumin-bound and free cortisol fractions increase.

Change in protein binding has little effect on endogenous cortisol production, since ACTH secretion is determined by free cortisol levels. It is important with exogenous steroids such as prednisolone. Patients with low serum albumin levels show higher free steroid levels and an increased incidence of side-effects for a given steroid dose.

With low doses of prednisolone, the normal diurnal rhythm of cortisol secretion is not fully suppressed. Competition for binding sites between endogenous cortisol and prednisolone results in reduced prednisolone binding and increased free prednisolone levels, particularly in the morning when cortisol levels are highest. Diurnal changes in cortisol secretion are suppressed by high doses of prednisolone.

Protein binding of prednisolone is non-linear so prednisolone shows dose-dependent pharmacokinetics, the volume of distribution and plasma clearance increasing with increasing dose. This means that the increase in pharmacological effect is proportionally less than the increase in dose.

Cortisol appears to penetrate well into the lung, though whether this is true for all corticosteroids and for all respiratory disorders is not known.

## Metabolism and Excretion

Prednisone, which is biologically inactive, is rapidly and virtually completely converted by the liver to its active form, prednisolone, so the effects of the two drugs are normally identical (Fig. 18.5). Conversion is occasionally delayed in patients with hepatic disease. The first pass metabolism of both prednisone and prednisolone is about 20%, so that 80% of the oral dose is bioavailable.

The plasma half-life of different steroids varies considerably: 80 min for cortisol, 2–3 h for prednisolone, and 5 h for dexamethasone (see Table 18.1). There is some variation between subjects, but plasma half-life is not affected by age or smoking. Prednisolone half-life is unchanged in patients with asthma but may be increased in those with ventilatory failure.

Both endogenous and synthetic corticosteroids are mainly deactivated in the liver by reduction or side chain removal followed by conjugation to form water-soluble glucuronides or sulphate esters (Fig. 18.5). About 75% of the conjugated forms appears in the urine, the remainder in the faeces. Hepatic enzyme inducers such as rifampicin, phenytoin and barbiturates may reduce the half-life of prednisolone by up to 50% and can cause clinically adverse changes in steroid-controlled diseases such as asthma. In one study the administration of rifampicin to steroid-dependent asthmatic patients caused a fall in peak flow rate of 50 l/min despite an increase in steroid dose. Oral contraceptives decrease prednisolone clearance, but their net effect on steroid pharmacokinetics is complex since they also increase transcortin levels.

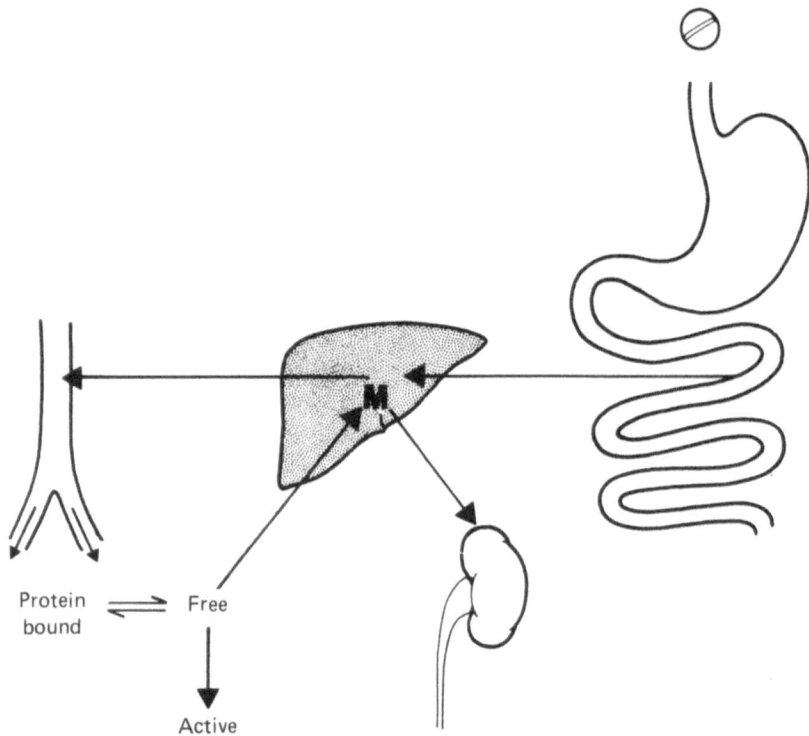

**Fig. 18.5.** Absorption and metabolism (M) of oral prednisolone.

Hepatic metabolism of the lipid-soluble corticosteroids given by inhalation is far more rapid than that of prednisolone. Following absorption from the lung or gut, about 80%–90% of the drug is removed by first pass metabolism. They also have a larger apparent volume of distribution and greater clearance.

## Pharmacological Actions

The pharmacological effects of corticosteroids in the lung are difficult to define. They appear to suppress disease activity in a wide range of disorders of both airways and alveoli. They are described as a prophylactic treatment for asthma though bronchodilatation and relief of symptoms are sometimes seen within hours.

The peak time course of action for many steroid effects is much longer than the relatively short plasma half-life (Fig. 18.6). The delay is due to the time taken for enzyme induction to occur (6–12 h), and because the anti-inflammatory and

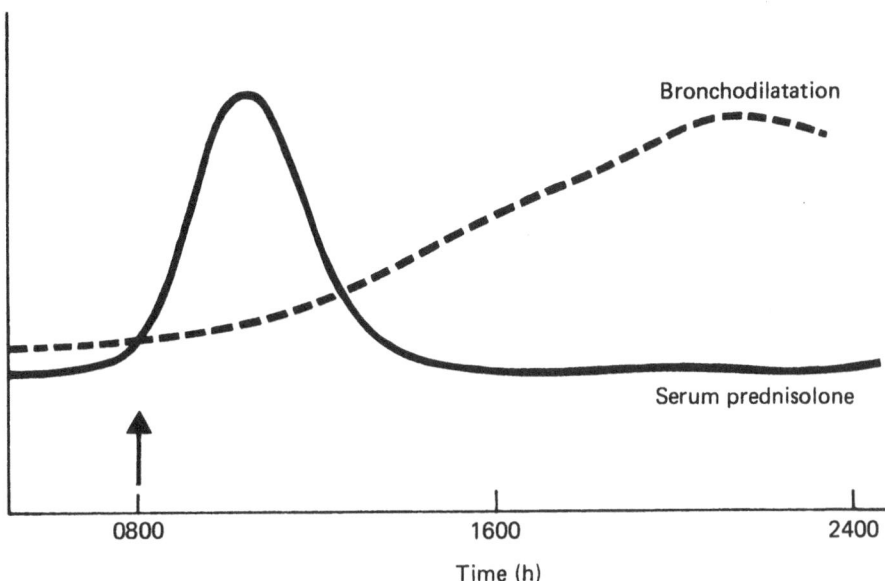

**Fig. 18.6.** Diagrammatic representation of time course of serum prednisolone and bronchodilatation following oral prednisolone at 0800 h in a patient with mild asthma.

immunological actions take time to be effective. In the few time course studies in patients with mild asthma, the response to inhaled, oral or intravenous steroids peaked between 6 h and 12 h, and returned to baseline by 24–48 h. However, in patients with more severe asthma, maximum benefit may not be seen for several days, and in other diseases such as sarcoid and fibrosing alveolitis it may be several weeks before the maximum response is seen.

The time course of action may vary for different steroid effects. It has been suggested that the actions causing adverse effects are of shorter duration than those causing benefit. If this is true, a relatively infrequent dosage regimen such as alternate day steroids would then be beneficial, permitting the desired action and minimising side-effects. One advantage of giving prednisolone as a single dose in the morning is that the drug is cleared in a few hours, allowing endogenous free cortisol levels to fall in time for ACTH to be stimulated.

## Side-effects

The side-effects of corticosteroids are well known (Table 18.4). The following are of particular relevance in the treatment of respiratory disease.

**Table 18.4.** Side-effects of oral corticosteroids

| | |
|---|---|
| Skin and general appearance | Moon face |
| | Central fat distribution |
| | Striae |
| | Atrophic skin |
| | Excessive bruising and purpura |
| | Increased weight |
| | Hirsutism, acne |
| | Poor wound healing |
| Metabolic | Glucose intolerance |
| | Hypokalaemia |
| | Protein catabolism |
| Fluid balance | Oedema |
| | Hypertension |
| Gastrointestinal | Indigestion |
| | Complications from peptic ulceration |
| Musculoskeletal | Myopathy |
| | Osteoporosis with crush fractures |
| | Aseptic necrosis |
| Immunity | Increased predisposition to infection, particularly candidiasis |
| Eyes | Posterior subcapsular cataracts |
| | Glaucoma |
| Psychiatric | Variable euphoria/depression |
| Endocrine | Growth retardation |
| | Suppression of hypophyseal–pituitary–adrenal axis |
| | Menstrual irregularities |
| General | Masking signs of acute illness such as perforated ulcer, severe infection |

## Oral Steroids

1. Weight gain.
2. Dyspepsia. Reflux symptoms are common. The risk of peptic ulceration or gastrointestinal haemorrhage is approximately doubled in patients taking a short course of oral steroids.
3. Impairment of glucose tolerance. This is common with higher doses and may require temporary treatment with insulin.
4. Osteoporosis. Not uncommon with long-term high dose oral steroids.
5. Increased skin fragility. Especially in women on long-term oral therapy.
6. Fluid, electrolytes and blood pressure. Fluid retention and hypertension are not common. Hypokalaemia is usually seen in patients who are also taking diuretics and β-agonists.
7. Adrenal suppression. Some degree of adrenal suppression is universal with oral therapy and it will be complete with high doses. It should always be assumed to be present. Steroid doses must be increased appropriately to cover stress such as acute intercurrent illness and surgery.

All patients on oral steroids should be given careful instructions about dosage and drug side-effects. They should always be given a steroid card and should in addition be told about:

The dangers of running out of tablets

The indications for changing the dose

The need to inform other doctors and dentists about their treatment.

## Inhaled Steroids

Side-effects from inhaled steroids (Table 18.5) are relatively uncommon. Candidiasis is due to the local immune suppressant effect of high concentrations of steroids in the oropharynx. It is seen most frequently when steroids are given by metered dose inhaler since this causes considerable impaction with high local concentrations. Candidiasis is clinically apparent in between 5% and 10% of patients in reported studies, though cultures are positive more often. The incidence of candidiasis is related more to frequency of dose than to absolute dose, and it has not been more common with the high dose inhalers. Its occurrence is reduced if the drug is given twice daily and by drinking water after inhalation. The use of a spacing device with a metered dose inhaler to reduce impaction has been very effective — reducing the incidence of candidiasis by 90% in one study. Amphotericin or nystatin lozenges can be used to treat candidiasis which fails to respond to these measures.

Dysphonia is an infrequent complication of inhaled steroids, due to an adductor deformity of the vocal cords. It has been attributed to a local steroid myopathy, although it can occur surprisingly quickly after the start of treatment. When it occurs, inhaled steroids should be reduced or discontinued. Response to steroid withdrawal can be slow.

Change in hypophyseal–pituitary–adrenal (HPA) function is very rare on doses of beclomethasone dipropionate up to 1500 μg/day. Patients on 2000 μg/day show slightly impaired adrenal function, although it is usually still within the normal range. Growth of children is not retarded by inhaled steroids. In patients on high doses of inhaled steroids (>1500 μg/day) major events such as surgery or severe infection should be covered with parenteral or oral steroids, and patients should carry a steroid card.

HPA function normally improves gradually following the change from oral to inhaled steroids. There may be clinical evidence of hypoadrenalism or an acute arthralgia during the change-over period.

**Table 18.5.** Side-effects of inhaled corticosteroids

*Direct*
Candidiasis
Dysphonia — rare
Bronchoconstriction — recorded but *very* rare
Minimal suppression of HPA axis with very high doses

*Indirect*
Addisonian problems and arthralgia during change
   from oral to inhaled steroids, particularly if change is
   too rapid

## Parenteral Steroids

There is virtually no indication for the use of ACTH or tetracosactrin in respiratory disease. The main problem is that the cortisol response varies considerably between patients so the therapeutic response is unpredictable. It was suggested that ACTH might have advantages over oral corticosteroids in children since it would interfere less with adrenal function and growth hormone secretion, but the evidence for clinical benefit has been inconsistent. It can produce hypersensitivity reactions and involves the discomfort of an injection.

Hydrocortisone sodium succinate given intravenously in doses up to 1200 mg/day rarely produces significant side-effects in the short term other than some hypokalaemia. With prolonged treatment, problems with hypokalaemia are common and an acute steroid myopathy can occur. It has occasionally caused bronchoconstriction, usually in patients with aspirin-sensitive asthma. High dose methylprednisolone may cause transient weakness, flushing and a bitter taste, and temporary hypotension has been noted. There is some concern that it may cause avascular necrosis of bone.

Triamcinolone has no sodium-retaining properties and the main side-effects differ to some extent from those of prednisolone, with easy bruising, menstrual disturbance, weight loss, hirsutism and myopathy being the most frequent. The injectable preparation, triamcinolone acetonide, is ten times more potent than oral triamcinolone and prednisolone, and this has caused confusion and excessive prescribing to some patients.

# Clinical Indications (Table 18.6)

### Asthma

Most patients with asthma respond well to corticosteroids. The indications for their use are as follows.

### *Acute Asthma*

All patients with acute severe asthma should be given parenteral or high dose oral steroids. They are safe when given for short periods and may be life saving. Several prospective placebo-controlled trials have shown clear benefit in the steroid-treated group.

The recommended doses are empirical. Hydrocortisone 200 mg 4-hourly intravenously is widely used followed by oral prednisolone 40 mg/day when the patient is obviously improving. Higher intravenous doses have been tried but they conferred no advantage and were associated with a higher incidence of side-effects. However, the intravenous route may not be necessary for most patients. In a recent study, oral prednisolone 45 mg was found to be as effective as intravenous

**Table 18.6.** Respiratory indications for oral or
parenteral corticosteroids

*Good evidence of benefit*
Acute severe asthma
Chronic severe asthma
Acute allergic aspergillosis
Fibrosing alveolitis (only a minority will respond)
Pulmonary eosinophilia
Vasculitis

*Evidence of efficacy lacking*
Adult respiratory distress syndrome

*Occasional use*
Sarcoidosis
Severe tuberculosis
Allergic alveolitis
Terminal lung cancer

hydrocortisone. The effect of oral prednisolone will lag 1–2 h behind that of an intravenous drug, and this delay is only likely to be important in patients with very severe asthma. Adverse reactions to intravenous hydrocortisone have been reported more often than reactions to oral prednisolone, though they are still extremely rare.

## Chronic Asthma

Most patients with chronic asthma inadequately controlled on full bronchodilator therapy respond well to inhaled steroids. The early studies of the equivalence of inhaled and oral steroids suggested that 400 µg of beclomethasone dipropionate was as effective as 7 mg prednisolone. These studies were carried out on patients previously maintained on oral steroids and many were able to stop them completely or markedly reduce the dose. Subsequent studies with higher doses of inhaled beclomethasone dipropionate, up to 2000 µg/day, showed that an even greater reduction in prednisolone dose is possible. We usually start patients on 100 µg beclomethasone dipropionate b.d. and either 50 µg or 200 µg budesonide b.d., depending on severity, and then adjust the dose in the light of the patient's response. Twice daily dosage for inhaled steroids is as effective as more frequent dosing and more convenient. The maximum recommended doses of beclomethasone dipropionate and budesonide at present are 2000 µg/day and 1200 µg/day respectively, though we occasionally give higher doses.

## Deteriorating Asthma

Many patients with relatively mild and easily controlled asthma will have episodes of deterioration when they require a short course of oral steroids. The length of the course depends on the severity and duration of the deterioration (see Chap. 4). Many patients keep a supply of oral steroids at home and administer a short reducing course themselves.

## More Severe Chronic Asthma

If adequate control of symptoms is not obtained by maximum doses of bronchodilators and inhaled steroids, oral steroids may be required. A formal steroid trial should be carried out as described below. Giving a high dose enables the reversibility of airflow obstruction to be assessed and establishes a target optimum value for lung function for the future. When good control of symptoms and function has been obtained, a further determined attempt should be made to withdraw oral steroids under cover of high doses of inhaled steroids before accepting the necessity for long-term oral steroid therapy. Alternate day steroids may be feasible in some patients, but control of asthma often deteriorates towards the end of the 48 h. The evidence that alternate day steroids benefit growth in children is conflicting. The objectives of treatment have to be more modest in patients with more severe asthma and need to balance symptomatic benefit against the side-effects of steroids.

A minority of patients with chronic severe asthma are not controlled satisfactorily by the combination of oral steroids and maximum doses of inhaled steroids and they continue to have disabling breathlessness or unacceptable side-effects, usually weight gain. Intramuscular depot triamcinolone acetonide has been reported to be helpful in this situation, but this was mainly because a much higher dose equivalent was given, with a consequent increase in side-effects. There is no good evidence that a patient not responding to one steroid can obtain a better balance of benefit and side-effects from a second.

However, the studies necessary to determine this are difficult to carry out because of problems in determining equipotent doses and because side-effects take a long time to become apparent and are difficult to quantify. Since the side-effects with triamcinolone acetonide differ from those of prednisolone — with weight loss, hirsutism and myopathy being more common — it may be worth trying in patients with excessive side-effects and weight gain due to prednisolone, assuming that the side-effects of triamcinolone are tolerable and care is taken to avoid doses causing myopathy.

## Steroid "Resistance"

A few patients with asthma, possibly around 5%, do not respond to steroids despite having a good response to β-agonists, and these patients have been labelled as being "corticosteroid resistant". It is not clear whether they are a distinct subgroup or one end of a spectrum of responsiveness. Corticosteroid-resistant patients have abnormal monocyte responses to steroids in vitro.

## Allergic Aspergillosis

Episodes of allergic bronchopulmonary aspergillosis with lung shadowing on the chest X-ray should be treated with a course of oral steroids, starting with 30 mg or 40 mg daily for 2–3 weeks and then reducing gradually. Some patients require intermittent courses of oral steroids but continuous oral therapy is necessary for those showing progressive deterioration in pulmonary function or frequent acute episodes of pulmonary infiltration. Asthma should be treated conventionally with inhaled β-agonists and steroids but inhaled drugs do not appear to prevent acute episodes of aspergillosis.

### Restrictive Lung Disease

The indications for steroids in restrictive disorders such as sarcoid and fibrosing alveolitis depend on the primary diagnosis (see Chaps. 9 and 10). When patients are being considered for long-term treatment, a formal trial should be undertaken, though in a few patients who are deteriorating rapidly steroids have to be given empirically.

### Adult Respiratory Distress Syndrome

Patients with ARDS, or those at high risk of developing it, are often given high dose pulsed methylprednisolone (30 mg/kg as an infusion in 30 min, repeated three times at 12-h intervals). Steroids could have a beneficial action by inhibiting mediator release and reducing capillary permeability, but clinical benefit still requires confirmation from adequate prospective studies. Such evidence as is available suggests that the earlier steroids are given, the more likely they are to be effective.

## Occasional Indications for Steroids

### Tuberculosis

Patients with severe tuberculosis and acute systemic illness may improve if oral steroids are added to their antituberculous chemotherapy. This effect seems to be non-specific (see Chap. 8). Steroids are also given to try to prevent some of the late fibrotic complications of tuberculosis when it involves serous surfaces such as the pleura, pericardium, meninges and peritoneum, though benefit is not proven. However, steroids are generally safe as long as effective antituberculous chemotherapy is given, though there is a risk that complications such as bowel perforation may be masked.

### Lung Cancer

Patients with terminal cancer are sometimes helped by oral steroids, presumably through their non-specific euphoriant effects. Short-term symptomatic benefit may be produced in patients with superior vena caval or upper airways obstruction while the effects of radiotherapy or chemotherapy are awaited. High dose dexamethasone (12 mg/day) usually provides worthwhile temporary relief of symptoms in patients with brain metastases.

# Steroid Trial

Steroids should only be taken long term by patients who have demonstrated unequivocal evidence of a response. Assessment may be difficult when response is delayed. Subjective response to steroids is common so a formal trial must include an objective assessment of lung function whether the problem is airways obstruction or a restrictive disorder such as fibrosing alveolitis. Steroids should be discontinued in those who are not responsive.

## Airways Obstruction

The indications for a trial of oral steroids are:

1.  Asthmatic patients who are poorly controlled on maximum doses of inhaled β-agonists and inhaled steroids
2.  Patients with severe airways obstruction. Asthma masquerades as irreversible airways obstruction with sufficient frequency to justify a steroid trial in all patients.

Patients with airways obstruction should be clinically stable and have stable spirometric values before the trial and should be on maximal treatment with β-agonists. Prednisolone 30–40 mg/day should be given for 2 weeks and the patient reassessed. If there is a 15% improvement or more in $FEV_1$ or PEF, then inhaled steroids should be added in full dose, and the oral steroid reduced to the minimum dose required to maintain satisfactory control. Complete discontinuation of oral steroids should be the objective provided that symptom control is reasonable and function remains satisfactory. The figure of 15% is an arbitrary one and, in patients with a low $FEV_1$, needs to be interpreted with caution. Fortunately most patients with moderate or severe asthma show a larger change and most of those with chronic bronchitis considerably less than 15%. In patients with an equivocal result, the effect of reducing or stopping steroids should be carefully monitored.

## Restrictive Disorders

Criteria for assessment of response should include an improvement in symptoms, pulmonary function, particularly vital capacity, and clearing of the chest X-ray. High doses of prednisolone (30–40 mg) should be given following stable baseline measurements and the response observed after 3–4 weeks. In general, high doses should be continued until maximum improvement is attained and this may take several months. The dose should then be reduced gradually to the minimum levels which maintain the improvement. Reducing the dose too rapidly tends to result in relapse or suboptimal control of the disease. The required duration of treatment clearly depends on the underlying disorder, but is usually prolonged. If there is no response at 3–4 weeks, it is unlikely that a longer trial of treatment will produce a response.

A few patients feel that they have benefited from corticosteroids but the objective evidence is indeterminate. In this situation more detailed monitoring during withdrawal is helpful. Long-term therapy is probably justified if there is significant deterioration on withdrawal.

# Useful References

Blackwell GJ, Carnuccio R, Di Rosa M, Flower RJ, Parente L, Persico P (1980) Macrocortin: a polypeptide causing the anti-phospholipase effect of glucocorticoids. Nature 287: 147–149

British Thoracic and Tuberculosis Association (1976) A controlled trial of inhaled corticosteroids in patients receiving prednisone tablets for asthma. Br J Dis Chest 70: 95–102

Chang KC, Miklich DR, Barwise G, Chai H, Miles-Lawrence P (1982) Linear growth of chronic asthmatic children: the effects of the disease and various forms of steroid therapy. Clin Allergy 12: 369–378

Clark TJH, McAllister WAC (1983) Corticosteroids. In: Clark TJH, Godfrey S (eds) Asthma. Chapman and Hall, London, pp 372–392

Fanta CH, Rossing TH, McFadden ER (1983) Glucocorticoids in acute asthma. Am J Med 74: 845–851

Gambertoglio JG, Amend WJC, Benet LZ (1979) Pharmacokinetics and bioavailability of prednisone and prednisolone in healthy volunteers and patients: a review. J Pharmacokinet Biopharm 8: 1–52

Harding SM (1984) Corticosteroids. In: Buckle DR, Smith H (eds) Development of anti-asthma drugs. Butterworths, London, pp 297–313

Liddle GW (1961) Clinical pharmacology of the anti-inflammatory steroids. Clin Pharmacol Ther 2: 615–635

Messer J, Reitman D, Sacks HS, Smith H, Chalmers TC (1983) Association of adrenocorticosteroid therapy and peptic-ulcer disease. N Engl J Med 309: 21–24

Smith MJ, Hodson ME (1983) Effects of long term inhaled high dose beclomethasone dipropionate on adrenal function. Thorax 38: 676–681

# 19 Sodium Cromoglycate and Related Drugs

Altounyan, a research scientist with asthma, made the somewhat surprising observation 20 years ago that a khellin derivative with no bronchodilator properties
reduced his response to inhaled antigen. Its effects were too shortlived to be useful, but it led to the investigation of several hundred derivatives of khellin, from
which sodium cromoglycate emerged for clinical evaluation in 1965.

Sodium cromoglycate inhibits the bronchoconstrictor response to exercise and
inhaled antigen in patients with asthma. It is usually referred to as a prophylactic
drug since it does not cause immediate bronchodilatation. It is worth stressing,
however, that any prophylactic drug should cause bronchodilatation in the full-
ness of time if it is preventing bronchoconstriction.

## Chemistry

Sodium cromoglycate is a bis-chromone, i.e. two chromone molecules (ben-
zopyrone rings) linked together (Fig. 19.1). It is highly acidic, almost completely
ionised and poorly lipid soluble.

## Formulation

Sodium cromoglycate is available in several formulations. It has usually been
administered for asthma from a capsule containing 20 mg of finely powdered drug
mixed with lactose to prevent clumping. The capsule is placed in a turbo inhaler
(Spinhaler R) which the patient rotates to break the capsule before inhaling the
dry powder. Children over the age of 4 or 5 years can usually inhale the drug once
the capsule is in place. Those up to the age of 7 or 8 years and patients with arthritis
may have difficulty in putting the capsule into the inhaler. Recently, metered dose

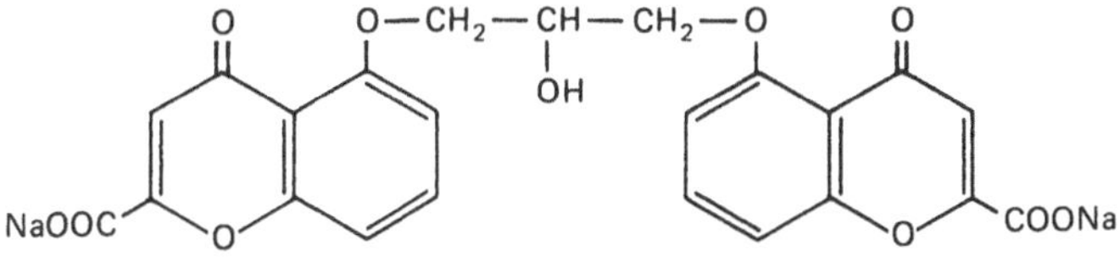

Fig. 19.1. Sodium cromoglycate.

inhalers containing 1 mg and 5 mg per metered dose have been marketed and a nebuliser solution is available for children unable to use a Spinhaler or metered dose inhaler.

Sodium cromoglycate is available as eye-drops for allergic conjunctivitis and as a dry powder, drops or spray for intranasal use for hay fever and allergic rhinitis. An oral preparation has been used for gastrointestinal disorders.

# Mode of Action

Much of the early investigation on mechanism of action was carried out in the rat where sodium cromoglycate is a potent inhibitor of both IgE and chemically induced mast cell degranulation. Sodium cromoglycate reduces the intracellular accumulation of calcium following mast cell stimulation by a mechanism which has not been fully clarified. Mast cell stabilisation was assumed to be the mechanism underlying the effects of sodium cromoglycate in asthma, but it now appears that the rat is a poor model of the findings in man. When dispersed human mast cells have been studied, the effect of sodium cromoglycate on degranulation has been more variable and considerably less than that seen with therapeutic concentrations of β-agonists. The mast cell stabilisation hypothesis also fails to explain how sodium cromoglycate inhibits the bronchoconstrictor response to stimuli where mast cell mediator release appears not to be involved, such as cold air, sulphur dioxide and adenosine. Finally, several drugs which cause greater inhibition of human mast cell degranulation in vitro than sodium cromoglycate have not been effective when given clinically.

The early view that sodium cromoglycate achieves its effect in asthma by mast cell stabilisation is therefore being reconsidered and other possible modes of action are under investigation. These include inhibition of local axon reflexes within the lung, blockade of potential mediators such as PAF-acether, and inhibition of vagal activity, either by reducing sensory irritant fibre discharge or by modulating transmission through parasympathetic ganglia. Very high doses of drug inhibit mast cell phosphodiesterase activity but this is unlikely to be relevant with the drug concentrations achieved in man. Sodium cromoglycate has no effect on human basophils.

# Pharmacokinetics

Because sodium cromoglycate is not lipid soluble it must be applied locally to the bronchial, nasal or conjunctival mucosa. Following inhalation, 5%–10% of the total dose is absorbed. The half-life of sodium cromoglycate in blood is 1–1.5 h. It is not metabolised and is excreted unchanged in urine and bile in roughly equal amounts. Only 1%–2% is absorbed after oral administration.

# Pharmacological Actions

The main use of sodium cromoglycate is as a prophylactic drug in asthma. It is effective if taken immediately before exercise or allergen challenge but requires regular administration for days or weeks to be useful in chronic asthma. Much of the controversy about the role of sodium cromoglycate in the treatment of asthma is due to a failure to appreciate that studies in vitro and in induced asthma may not be relevant to "everyday" asthma. There is also a paucity of good dose–response and time course data in patients with asthma.

Sodium cromoglycate has been of modest benefit to patients with hay fever, allergic rhinitis and allergic conjunctivitis and some success has been claimed for its use in eczema, though this has not been widely studied. Oral sodium cromoglycate has helped some patients with food allergy. It has not been helpful in other conditions such as ulcerative colitis.

### Induced Asthma

Sodium cromoglycate inhibits bronchoconstriction induced by antigen, exercise and aspirin. A single 20 mg dose will usually inhibit most of the early response to antigen (see Chap. 4) when given up to 1 h prior to challenge, but it is progressively less effective when given after challenge. It reduces the severity of the late reaction in most subjects, but not all. The bronchoconstrictor response to exercise is also largely inhibited by sodium cromoglycate 20 mg by Spinhaler or 2 mg by metered dose inhaler, if given at any time from a few minutes to 3 h before exercise. Some studies have found a progressive inhibition of exercise-induced asthma with increasing doses of sodium cromoglycate, whereas others have been unable to relate the response to the dose administered. When sodium cromoglycate 20 mg was compared with salbutamol 200 µg in patients undergoing antigen and exercise challenge, the β-agonist was more effective in inhibiting both histamine release and bronchoconstriction (Holgate et al. 1984).

Sodium cromoglycate has had a negligible effect on the bronchoconstrictor response to histamine and cholinergic agents in acute studies. A small effect has sometimes been present with long-term treatment.

### Clinical Asthma

The majority of long-term studies of sodium cromoglycate in patients with asthma have shown it to give some benefit, though this has often been more apparent in terms of patient assessment or reduction in the use of bronchodilator inhalers than in objective measures such as improvement in $FEV_1$. It has been difficult therefore to determine the time course of action of sodium cromoglycate. Several studies suggest that it takes a few weeks for its maximum effect to be apparent, and that, once the drug is discontinued, there may be a carry-over effect for a few weeks. The relationship between dose and response has also not been clarified and there are insufficient data to know whether tolerance is a problem.

## Side-effects

Sodium cromoglycate is one of the safest drugs available and serious side-effects, mainly hypersensitivity reactions, are extremely rare. The powder is hygroscopic and may clump in humid countries. The exit port of the metered dose inhaler can become blocked by drug and should be washed every 2–3 weeks. The powder can also be irritant and may cause dryness of the mouth and throat, or transient cough. Wheezing and bronchoconstriction occur very infrequently, presumably due to the irritant effect of the powder in patients with hyperreactive airways since they usually occur with the inactive powder also.

## Clinical Indications

Several studies have shown sodium cromoglycate to be better than placebo but the important clinical question is how it compares with the alternative drugs available. There are few good comparisons, but sodium cromoglycate in general has been less effective in both children and adults than the alternative prophylactic treatment, inhaled steroids. Most clinicians find sodium cromoglycate to be useful in a relatively small number of adult patients and overall to be considerably less effective than inhaled steroids. The main indications for its use are as follows.

1. In mild asthma. A β-agonist is normally the drug of first choice for both children and adults with asthma. When symptoms are not controlled on a β-agonist alone, a prophylactic drug is usually added — the choice lying between sodium cromoglycate and an inhaled steroid. Both have a very good safety profile. Sodium cromoglycate is in general more effective in children than adults and is a reasonable second drug to try in children or young adults, particularly if atopic. In adults, preference has moved from sodium cromoglycate to an inhaled steroid.

2. Although sodium cromoglycate is an effective prophylactic for exercise-induced asthma if taken a few minutes before exercise, most patients find an inhaled β-agonist more convenient and equally or more effective.

# Nedocromil Sodium

Nedocromil sodium is a new prophylactic drug for use by inhalation, currently undergoing clinical evaluation.

# Oral Antiallergic Drugs

At a time when respiratory physicians are pressing the advantages of the inhaled route of administration for delivery of drugs to asthmatic patients, the pharmaceutical industry has been looking for an effective oral antiallergic drug. The advantage of the oral route is that it would allow patients with asthma, hay fever and rhinitis to be treated by a single drug; the disadvantage is that much larger doses need to be given and side-effects are more likely. In-vitro tests appear to be poor predictors of clinical efficacy and none of the 30 or so drugs investigated over the last decade is now on the market, due to lack of clinical effectiveness or the occurrence of side-effects. Ketotifen, sometimes described as an oral antiallergic drug, has pharmacological actions which suggest it is better described as an antihistamine.

# Useful References

Altounyan REC (1975) Developments in the treatment of asthma with disodium cromoglycate (lomudal). Acta Allergol 30 (Suppl. 12): 65–86

Buckle DR (1984) Disodium cromoglycate and compounds with similar activities. In: Buckle DR, Smith H (eds) Development of anti-asthma drugs. Butterworths, London, pp 261–297

Church MK (1985) The biochemical basis of pulmonary and antiallergic drugs. In: Devlin JP (ed) Pulmonary and antiallergic drugs. Wiley, New York, pp 43–121

Godfrey S (1983) Anti-allergic agents. In: Clark TJH, Godfrey S (eds) Chapman and Hall, London, pp 359–371

Holgate ST, Church MK, Cushley MJ, Robinson C, Mann JS, Howarth PH (1984) Pharmacological modulation of airway calibre and mediator release in human models of bronchial asthma. In: Kay AB, Austen KF, Lichtenstein LM (eds) Asthma — physiology, immunopharmacology and treatment. Academic Press, London, pp 391–415

Howarth PH, Durham SR, Lee TH, Kay AB, Church MK, Holgate ST (1985) Influence of albuterol, cromolyn sodium and ipratropium bromide on the airway and circulating mediator responses to allergen bronchial provocation in asthma. Am Rev Resp Dis 132: 986–992

Northern General Hospital, Brompton Hospital and Medical Research Council Collaborative Trial (1976) Sodium cromoglycate in chronic asthma. Br Med J 1: 361–364

# 20 Respiratory Stimulants

An effective respiratory stimulant should be helpful for patients with acute ventilatory failure following an exacerbation of chronic bronchitis, and for the longer-term management of patients with chronic ventilatory failure where increased ventilation and oxygenation would be expected to produce useful symptomatic improvement. The drugs available at present have a relatively small stimulant effect and a fairly high incidence of side-effects, so their role in both circumstances is limited. A carbonic anhydrase inhibitor, acetazolamide, is used prophylactically for acute mountain sickness and the place of respiratory stimulants in the treatment of the sleep apnoea syndrome is currently being explored.

Respiratory stimulants have no role in the management of patients with hypoxaemia associated with a normal or low arterial $PCO_2$ since ventilation is clearly adequate, nor in the management of patients with ventilatory failure due to neuromuscular or chest wall problems. In general, they have no place in the treatment of central respiratory depression due to drugs, apart from the very occasional use of doxapram to counter the delayed effect of anaesthetic drugs. Naloxone, an opioid antagonist, is used to reverse opioid-induced respiratory depression.

Respiratory stimulants comprise a heterogeneous group of drugs with different mechanisms and sites of action. Drugs such as nikethamide, although used as respiratory stimulants, cause general stimulation of the central nervous system. Side-effects are common and they are rarely used today. Drugs which act by stimulating peripheral chemoreceptors appear to have fewer side-effects. In this section the drugs used most often for ventilatory failure, acute mountain sickness, sleep apnoea and opioid overdosage are discussed — namely, doxapram, carbonic anhydrase inhibitors, protriptyline and naloxone — and a new drug, almitrine, currently under investigation for chronic ventilatory failure.

## Doxapram

Doxapram is the only respiratory stimulant used with any frequency for acute ventilatory failure. It acts as a stimulant of the respiratory centre both directly and indirectly through stimulation of peripheral chemoreceptors.

## Formulation

Doxapram is available for intravenous administration. Since it has a short duration of action, of 10–15 min only, it is usually given as a continuous intravenous infusion though it can be given as a bolus injection. The infusion rate is determined by the patient's condition, side-effects and arterial blood gas measurements.

## Indications

Doxapram is used for some patients with acute ventilatory failure due to exacerbations of chronic bronchitis. The first priority in this situation is to keep the patient alert and able to cough effectively so that bronchial secretions are removed. If the patient fails to make progress on conservative treatment (vigorous physiotherapy, nebulised $\beta_2$-agonists, antibiotics, diuretics if indicated and 24% oxygen — see Chap. 6), a decision has to be made as to whether mechanical ventilation is indicated, and if not, whether doxapram should be tried. The decision depends on several factors including experience and local facilities, the cause of the recent deterioration and other medical considerations. Doxapram provides a small additional drive to ventilation only, and patients with problems unlikely to resolve in a few hours are usually better managed by mechanical ventilation. Doxapram can limit the increased respiratory depression which follows oxygen therapy and may be used either as a short-term measure in an attempt to avoid mechanical ventilation, or in patients for whom mechanical ventilation would not be appropriate. Because of its side-effects it should normally be reserved for patients who are drowsy or in whom the $PaCO_2$ has risen to above 10 kPa (75 mmHg).

Excessive sedation following intravenous diazepam for endoscopy or after general anaesthesia has occasionally been helped by doxapram.

### Side-effects

Doxapram appears to cause fewer side-effects than drugs such as nikethamide which only act centrally. It does, however, cause some generalised stimulation of the central nervous system including the vasomotor centre. Side-effects include a metallic taste, tachycardia, mild hypertension, agitation, tremor and a generalised feeling of warmth. More serious symptoms include vomiting and hallucinations. It should be avoided in patients with epilepsy, severe hypertension, coronary artery disease and those on a monoamine oxidase inhibitor. It has caused bronchoconstriction in asthmatic subjects.

# Almitrine

There is at present no satisfactory oral respiratory stimulant for long-term use in patients with chronic ventilatory failure. There is considerable interest in the piperazine derivative, almitrine bismesylate, since it is taken up and concentrated in the carotid body and appears to act entirely on peripheral chemoreceptors — hence it causes a greater increase in ventilation in hypoxaemic patients. It also increases pulmonary vascular resistance in patients with chronic airflow obstruction. Ventilation–perfusion matching in the lung improves following almitrine, but this appears to be secondary to improved ventilation since the drug has no effect in patients with bilateral carotid body resection.

### Formulation and Pharmacokinetics

At present almitrine is only available on a named patient basis. It is absorbed rapidly following oral administration and is highly protein-bound. It has a half-life of around 2 days and is excreted in bile, partly unchanged and partly as inactive metabolites.

### Efficacy and Side-effects

Information on efficacy and side-effects is still limited. In short-term studies in patients with chronic airways obstruction almitrine has increased $PaO_2$ by 1–2 kPa (7–15 mmHg), reduced $PaCO_2$ by 1 kPa (7 mmHg) or slightly less and reduced nocturnal hypoxaemia. Improvements have been maintained for up to 6 months. The drug was apparently acceptable, although with higher doses the increase in ventilation was uncomfortable. The long-term effects of increased pulmonary vascular resistance are uncertain. Peripheral neuropathy has been described, though its relationship to the use of almitrine has been disputed.

# Carbonic Anhydrase Inhibitors

Carbonic anhydrase (CA) catalyses the reaction

$$H_2O + CO_2 \overset{CA}{\underset{}{\rightleftharpoons}} H_2CO_3 \rightleftharpoons HCO_3^- + H^+$$

Inhibitors of carbonic anhydrase such as acetazolamide and dichlorphenamide slow the uptake of carbon dioxide by red cells, thus increasing carbon dioxide tension in tissues, including the brain, and reducing its elimination. In the kidney, carbonic anhydrase inhibition causes reduced $H^+$ secretion by the renal tubule, with increased bicarbonate loss in the urine, and a resulting metabolic acidosis. Ventilation is increased as a result of the acidosis and possibly by the local increase in carbon dioxide tension in the brain. Carbonic anhydrase inhibitors should not be used in acidotic patients and hence are contraindicated in acute ventilatory failure.

## Formulation

Acetazolamide and dichlorphenamide are available as tablets.

## Indications

Both acetazolamide and dichlorphenamide have too many side-effects to be widely accepted for the treatment of chronic ventilatory failure. They are occasionally helpful in patients in whom ventilatory failure appears to be disproportionate to the degree of airways obstruction.

If taken prior to ascent to altitude, acetazolamide will help to prevent acute mountain sickness, increase exercise performance and help to prevent the reduction in muscle mass which normally occurs at altitude. The metabolic acidosis from acetazolamide helps to counter the respiratory alkalosis seen at altitude, causing a further rise in ventilation and an increase in arterial $PO_2$, both awake and asleep. The reduction in nocturnal hypoxaemia may be particularly important since sleep apnoea is common at altitude and the hypoxaemia can be very severe. The diuretic effect of acetazolamide is also helpful.

## Side-effects

Acetazolamide can cause paraesthesia and hyperchloraemia, though when taken for acute mountain sickness it is well tolerated. Dichlorphenamide causes less chloride retention, but it produces headache and gastrointestinal symptoms in many patients.

# Naloxone

Naloxone is a competitive opioid antagonist rather than a respiratory stimulant, but is discussed here for convenience. It reverses respiratory depression due to opioid drugs. It has some agonist activity at very high concentrations but this is not important clinically. It is ineffective in other forms of ventilatory failure.

## Formulation

The peak pharmacological effect of naloxone lasts for only 10 min after an intravenous bolus so it is normally given by infusion. When used as a diagnostic test, an initial dose of 0.8–2.0 mg should be given as an intravenous bolus and repeated every 2–3 min up to a maximum dose of 10 mg. If the patient clearly responds, the drug can continue to be given as an infusion in a dose of up to 5 mg/h.

### Indications

Naloxone should be given to all patients with respiratory depression due to opioids and as a diagnostic test in coma of unknown origin where opioid overdose is possible. It may need to be continued for several days in patients who have taken an overdose of long-acting opioids such as methadone and in this situation mechanical ventilation is an alternative form of treatment to be considered. When respiratory depression is present in opioid addicts, naloxone may be used but caution is needed since it may precipitate withdrawal symptoms. Respiratory depression due to non-opioid drugs will not respond to naloxone.

## Protriptyline

Protriptyline is used for sleep apnoea only. The mechanism of action is unclear but a reduction in rapid eye movement sleep or an increase in motor nerve discharge to upper airways may be responsible. Its place in relation to other forms of treatment is discussed in Chapter 6.

## Other Drugs

Theophyllines are sometimes used to stimulate respiration in the newborn. They have not been shown to be useful in older patients with acute or chronic ventilatory failure.

Nocturnal oxygen therapy may also be helpful in the sleep apnoea syndrome, presumably by reversing the central depressant effect of hypoxia which tends to propagate the apnoeic episodes. Other drugs, including medroxyprogesterone, almitrine and methylxanthines, have been tried but await formal assessment.

## Useful References

Henry J, Volans G (1984) Analgesics: opioids. Br Med J 289: 990–993

Howard P (1984) Almitrine bismesylate (Vectarion). Clin Resp Physiol 20: 99–103

Meredith T, Caisley J, Volans G (1984) ABC of poisoning. Emergency drugs: agents used in the treatment of poisoning. Br Med J 289: 742–748

Milledge JS (1983) Acute mountain sickness. Thorax 38: 641–645

# 21 Antituberculous Chemotherapy

The principles of antituberculous chemotherapy were considered in Chapter 8. This chapter is concerned with the antituberculous drugs in current use and with the commoner problems arising during treatment.

## Isoniazid

Isoniazid was discovered in 1912 but was not recognised to have antituberculous activity until 1952. A number of related compounds have some antituberculous activity but only isoniazid is clinically useful.

### Mode of Action

Isoniazid acts only against *Mycobacterium tuberculosis*. It penetrates cells freely and is active against both intracellular and extracellular organisms. It is taken up by growing mycobacteria, and inhibits mycolic acid synthesis. In consequence, cell wall permeability increases and the organisms lose acid-fastness. Within a few hours the action becomes irreversible, but growth continues for at least one generation. It has good sterilising activity, but its delayed action makes it less effective than rifampicin against slowly dividing or intermittently active organisms, and disappearance of organisms is slower than with rifampicin. There is no cross-resistance with other antituberculous drugs, including ethionamide which also inhibits mycolic acid synthesis.

Isoniazid is a good resistance preventer, though if it is given with a poorly chosen accompanying drug, isoniazid resistance is readily acquired. Primary resistance is not uncommon, ranging from just over 1% in the United Kingdom to 20% in some Far Eastern countries.

## Absorption, Distribution, Metabolism and Excretion

Isoniazid is readily absorbed from the gastrointestinal tract, peak serum concentrations being attained within 2 h of oral administration. There is no significant binding to plasma proteins. The high tissue concentrations attained (1–2 µg/ml) are 20–50 times greater than the in vitro minimum inhibitory concentration (mic) for *M. tuberculosis*. Isoniazid is widely distributed, penetrating most tissues, including the cerebrospinal fluid, in effective concentrations. It is metabolised mainly in the liver, initially by acetylation to acetyl-isoniazid, with subsequent hydrolysis and conjugation. The metabolites are excreted in the urine, together with some unchanged isoniazid. None of the metabolites has antituberculous activity.

The serum half-life of isoniazid is mainly a function of the rate of acetylation, which is genetically determined. There is an approximately threefold difference in rate between rapid and slow acetylators, with a half-life of 1.1–1.5 h for rapid acetylators and 3–4 h for slow acetylators. There are racial differences in the proportion of rapid and slow acetylators, some ethnic groups such as the Chinese and Japanese being predominantly rapid acetylators while others such as the Caucasians have an approximately equal distribution of rapid and slow acetylators. There is no evidence that acetylator status has therapeutic significance with standard doses of isoniazid, although toxic effects may be more common in slow acetylators when high dose regimens are used. In practice it is not necessary to determine acetylator status. Half-life does not change with age, but may be prolonged in severe renal failure.

## Interactions

Isoniazid interacts with pyridoxine to produce an inactive compound which is rapidly excreted and this can result in pyridoxine deficiency. Much less commonly, isoniazid inhibits the synthesis of nicotinamide. In slow acetylators it may interact with anticonvulsants.

## Toxic Effects

Minor gastrointestinal intolerance does occur, but is not common. Exacerbation of pre-existing acne may be troublesome. Hypersensitivity with rash and fever occurs in up to 5% of patients.

The main toxic effects are hepatic and neurological. Hepatotoxicity occurs in a relatively small proportion of patients (1%–2%), but, unlike the toxicity from rifampicin, it tends to be more serious, with perhaps a 10% mortality for patients with "hepatitis" (jaundice with elevated enzyme levels). Hepatic toxicity is commoner in older patients and in those with pre-existing liver disease. Peripheral neuropathy due to pyridoxine deficiency can be prevented by routine administration of pyridoxine supplements. Once present it does respond, although less satisfactorily, to treatment with pyridoxine. Nicotinamide deficiency is rare and supplementation is not required. Other neurological toxic effects such as optic neuritis, psychotic reactions and convulsions occur very rarely, although convulsions are a prominent feature in patients taking an overdose of isoniazid.

Blood disorders have occasionally been reported, as have a wide variety of other side-effects.

Isoniazid appears to be effective and safe in pregnancy. Although it penetrates the fetus, there is no evidence that it has a significant toxic or teratogenic effect.

## Dose

(For oral dose and preparations, see Tables 21.1 and 21.2.)

An intravenous preparation (ampoule 50 mg in 2 ml) is given in the same dose as for oral administration. It is compatible with other drugs in intravenous solutions.

Intrathecal therapy is not required in tuberculous meningitis. Isoniazid penetrates well into the CNS and should be given orally in high dose (8–12 mg/kg). Pyridoxine supplements are essential.

**Table 21.1.** Normal doses of antituberculous drugs

| Intermittent | Adult | Children Dose (mg/kg per day) | Twice-weekly dose |
|---|---|---|---|
| Isoniazid | 300 mg/day | 5–10 | 15 mg/kg |
| Rifampicin | <50 kg — 450 mg/day<br>>50 kg — 600 mg/day | 10–20 | 600–900 mg |
| Pyrazinamide | <50 kg — 1.5 g/day<br>>50 kg — 2.0 g/day | 40 | <50 kg — 3 g<br>>50 kg — 3.5 g |
| Streptomycin | <50 kg or >40 years<br>—0.75 g/day<br>>50 kg and <40 years<br>—1.0 g/day | 20 | No dose increase,<br>i.e. 0.75 g or 1.0 g |
| Ethambutol | Low — 15 mg/kg per day<br>High — 25 mg/kg per day | As for adults | 45 mg/kg |
| Thiacetazone | 150 mg/day | 2–4 | — |
| Prothionamide | <50 kg — 750 mg/day<br>>50 kg — 1 g/day | — | — |
| Cycloserine | 500 mg/day | — | — |

See text for dose in renal failure and tuberculous meningitis.

# Rifampicin

Rifampicin was discovered in 1963. It is a rifamycin produced by *Streptomyces mediterranei*.

**Table 21.2.** Combined preparations of antituberculous drugs

Isoniazid and rifampicin ("Rifinah" or "Rimactizid")
Two-tablet strengths:
    "150" — isoniazid 100 mg, rifampicin 150 mg
      Dose 3 tablets/day
    "300" — isoniazid 150 mg, rifampicin 300 mg
      Dose 2 tablets/day
Isoniazid, rifampicin and pyrazinamide ("Rifater")
  Isoniazid 50 mg, rifampicin 120 mg, pyrazinamide 300 mg
    Dose 3–6 tablets/day depending on weight
Isonazid and ethambutol ("Mynah")
  Four-tablet strength:
    All contain 100 mg isoniazid
      "200" — 200 mg ethambutol
      "250" — 250 mg ethambutol
      "300" — 300 mg ethambutol
      "365" — 365 mg ethambutol
    Dose 3 tablets/day

## Mode of Action

Rifampicin inhibits protein synthesis in susceptible bacteria by blocking transcription and synthesis of messenger RNA. It is active against a wide variety of organisms including some strains of mycobacteria. *M. tuberculosis* is normally fully sensitive. Other mycobacteria show wide variation in susceptibility to rifampicin, and some, such as *M. fortuitum*, *M. intracellulare* and *M. avium*, are highly resistant.

Rifampicin has very high sterilising activity, presumably because of its rapid action and effect on intermittently dividing organisms. There is no cross-resistance between rifampicin and other antituberculous drugs. Natural resistance is rare, but resistant mutants occur at a rate between $1 \times 10^{-8}$ and $1 \times 10^{-10}$. Primary resistance is still rare in the United Kingdom (<1%), but is not uncommon where rifampicin has been widely and carelessly used (up to 25%). Rifampicin is a good resistance preventer. When it is given in combination with isoniazid, emergence of resistance during treatment is very unusual. Patients who relapse after treatment with rifampicin-isoniazid usually have organisms which are still sensitive on laboratory testing, and the drugs can be used in retreatment with good hope of success. The emergence of resistant strains in patients treated with two good resistance preventers like rifampicin and isoniazid reflects particularly poor antituberculous chemotherapy.

## Absorption, Distribution and Excretion

Rifampicin is rapidly absorbed from the upper gastrointestinal tract, with peak serum concentrations 2–4 h after an oral dose. Absorption is more rapid in the fasting state, the peak being delayed and the peak level lower if the drug is taken after food. The peak concentrations attained with therapeutic doses (10 µg/ml) are of the order of 100 times greater than the mic for sensitive strains of *M. tuberculosis*. The drug is widely distributed, with good tissue penetration and high tissue levels in almost all normal tissues including bone and serous exudates. Rifampicin does not penetrate the normal blood–brain barrier, but penetrates well in the presence of inflammation.

Approximately 90% of the drug is excreted in the bile, either unchanged or following acetylation to desacetyl-rifampicin. Rifampicin itself is reabsorbed and undergoes significant enterohepatic circulation producing very high concentrations in bile. Desacetyl-rifampicin is not reabsorbed and most of the drug is excreted in this form in the faeces. The remainder is excreted in the urine, in which very high peak concentrations (over 200 µg/ml) are attained, producing a strong orange coloration. Rifampicin induces hepatic enzymes, including those concerned with its own metabolism, so the mean serum half-life of the drug tends to fall in the first few days of treatment.

There are variations in the extent to which protein binding occurs, but these are not clinically significant.

### Interactions

Enzyme induction by rifampicin affects the handling of many drugs and physiologically active compounds, usually by promoting their metabolism and impairing their effect. These include anticoagulants, oral contraceptives, antidiabetic drugs, steroids, digoxin, anticonvulsants and vitamin D. For most drugs this effect can be countered by change in dose, but it is difficult to restore the full effect of some drugs (vitamin D and steroids), while for others the effect of increasing the dose is unpredictable (the contraceptive pill).

### Toxic Effects

Minor degrees of gastrointestinal intolerance are not uncommon and can usually be reduced by taking the drug after food. Severe intolerance is not common. Rifampicin penetrates all secretions, including tears, and may cause staining of soft contact lenses. Hypersensitivity reactions are common, but major reactions are rare. Minor transient thrombocytopenia, leucopenia and eosinophilia occur but are usually mild and do not justify routine monitoring. With intermittent therapy, immune reactions associated with antibodies to rifampicin are more frequent and can be serious. They range from febrile reactions, the "flu" syndrome, to thrombocytopenic purpura and renal damage. The occurrence of any immune reaction greater than a febrile reaction should be regarded as an absolute contraindication to further treatment with rifampicin.

The major side-effects of rifampicin are hepatic, either direct toxic effects or as a consequence of enzyme induction. A transient minor rise in bilirubin, SGOT and SGPT is very common in the early stages of treatment. These changes normally disappear with continued therapy, and are usually of no significance. Routine monitoring of liver function should be undertaken only if there is known to be pre-existing hepatic dysfunction. Changes in liver function usually reverse quickly following discontinuation of therapy, and it is generally safe to monitor liver function clinically by watching for the development of jaundice.

Teratogenic effects have been observed in rats and mice on high doses of rifampicin, but not in the rabbit. There is no evidence of teratogenicity in the human, but rifampicin should be avoided in the first 3 months of pregnancy unless the patient has an acute life-threatening illness. Rifampicin is safe in the later months of pregnancy. In patients with active tuberculosis it is generally desirable to avoid pregnancy, and this is particularly important if rifampicin is being used in treatment. In view of its unpredictable effect on the efficacy of the contraceptive pill, other measures should be recommended during treatment.

### Dose

(For oral dose and preparations see Tables 21.1 and 21.2.)

For parenteral therapy, an intravenous preparation is available from the manufacturers on a named user basis. The same dose is given as for the oral preparation.

# Pyrazinamide

It was known that nicotinamide had weak antituberculous activity, and a search of related compounds for a more active drug led to the introduction of pyrazinamide in 1954.

Pyrazinamide is active only at acid pH, and hence is effective only against organisms within the cell. Pyrazinamide has high sterilising activity against intracellular organisms which are normally actively dividing. It has no effect against extracellular or dormant organisms. Pyrazinamide is useful only in the first 2–3 months of chemotherapy, during which time there are still viable intracellular organisms. Thereafter all intracellular organisms have normally been killed, and pyrazinamide loses its effect. Its mechanism of action is unknown. Cross-resistance with other antituberculous drugs does not occur. Pyrazinamide is a relatively weak resistance preventer.

### Absorption, Distribution, Metabolism and Excretion

Pyrazinamide is readily absorbed from the gastrointestinal tract, with peak concentrations of approximately 60 µg/ml occurring within 2 h of an oral dose. The plasma half-life is about 10 h. It diffuses into most tissues, including the cerebrospinal fluid. Pyrazinamide is metabolised in the liver and the metabolites, mainly pyrazinoic acid, are excreted in the urine.

## Interactions

Pyrazinoic acid blocks uric acid excretion in the kidney and may cause hyperuricaemia. It also interferes with urine testing by "Acetest" and "Ketostix".

## Toxic Effects

Minor gastrointestinal intolerance has been reported. Gout may be precipitated as a result of interference with uric acid metabolism. Sensitivity reactions including fever, arthralgia and skin rashes have been reported. Sideroblastic anaemia has been produced.

The main site of toxicity is the liver, with a range of reactions from a mild hepatitis-like illness to severe hepatic failure. Severe reactions were at first thought to be common, and this belief was in large part responsible for virtually the entire discontinuation of its use in most regimens in the early 1970s. As now used, in rather lower dosage in the initial phase of chemotherapy, hepatotoxicity does not appear to be greater than that of rifampicin or isoniazid.

## Dose

Pyrazinamide can only be given orally (see Table 21.1 for dosage).

# Streptomycin

Streptomycin, an aminoglycoside antibiotic, was one of the first drugs recognised to have activity against *M. tuberculosis* and was in use by the late 1940s. Aminoglycosides are effective only against metabolically active organisms, in which they interfere with protein synthesis. There are wide variations in the antibacterial activity of the aminoglycosides, largely determined by their uptake and penetration into the bacterial cell. Of the group, only streptomycin, dihydrostreptomycin and hydroxystreptomycin have major antituberculous activity. Viomycin and capreomycin have weak activity. Gentamycin, kanamycin, neomycin and the other aminoglycosides are not effective. Partial cross-resistance occurs between aminoglycosides, with complete cross-resistance between capreomycin and viomycin.

Streptomycin has a rapid sterilising action against extracellular organisms, but is ineffective against intracellular organisms. Uptake of streptomycin by bacteria is pH dependent and is inhibited at acid intracellular pH. It is a moderately good resistance preventer.

## Absorption, Distribution, Metabolism and Excretion

Streptomycin is not absorbed from the gastrointestinal tract and is given by intramuscular injection. It is widely distributed and penetrates well into most tissues except the normal CSF. It is not metabolised and is mainly excreted unchanged by the kidney. Its excretion is dependent on glomerular filtration. Small amounts are also excreted in the bile. Serum half-life, normally about 3 h, is prolonged in the neonate and the elderly, and markedly prolonged in renal failure.

## Interactions

There are no interactions of note, but the effect of age and renal function on toxicity must be remembered.

## Toxic Effects

Sensitisation is common, both in patients receiving the drug and in those who give it. Dermatitis in nursing staff is a problem requiring scrupulous care with technique. In the patient, febrile reactions and skin rashes are common. Streptomycin is ototoxic, producing damage to both auditory and vestibular neurons. The changes are only partially reversible and the damage is cumulative with increasing exposure to the drug. In adults the vestibular division is most affected. The incidence of ototoxicity increases with increasing age, and it is much more common in patients with renal failure. Recovery is at best slow and often incomplete. For anything other than transient minor giddiness or hearing impairment at the time of injection, streptomycin should be discontinued. Although streptomycin is not teratogenic, it is contraindicated in pregnancy. Fetal ototoxicity is liable to cause permanent deafness.

Other toxic effects are much rarer and are probably due to hypersensitivity reactions. They include renal damage and blood dyscrasias.

## Dose

Streptomycin can only be given by intramuscular injection. Its use is normally contraindicated in renal failure. If it has to be given, peak and trough blood levels should be measured and dosage appropriately adjusted. As ototoxicity is cumulative, the total dose given should not exceed 100 g and the duration of its use should not exceed 120 days. (For details of dose see Table 21.1.)

# Ethambutol

Ethambutol was introduced in 1961. It has weak sterilising activity, but is a moderately good resistance preventer. It has supplanted PAS as a companion drug for isoniazid in 18-month regimens, and is currently used in the intensive phase of short course chemotherapy in the United Kingdom, although it is not clear how much it contributes to this regimen. Most studies have failed to show an additional effect from ethambutol in regimens based on isoniazid and rifampicin. The mode of action of ethambutol is unknown, but probably differs from that of the other antituberculous drugs as cross-resistance does not occur.

## Absorption, Distribution, Metabolism and Excretion

Ethambutol is readily absorbed after oral administration, effective plasma concentrations being achieved within 2–4 h of an oral dose. Most of the drug is excreted unchanged in the urine, although a small proportion also appears in the urine as inactive metabolites. In patients with renal failure the dose must be reduced.

Ethambutol appears to diffuse widely into body tissues. It penetrates into the CSF in patients with meningitis, but not in normal subjects.

## Toxic Effects

The major toxic effect is retrobulbar neuritis with loss of visual acuity. Although the lesion is normally reversible, with recovery taking up to 1 year, permanent blindness may be produced if ethambutol is not promptly discontinued. Ocular toxicity is dose dependent, being uncommon at a dose of 15 mg/kg, and occurring in about 20% of patients with doses greater than 30 mg/kg. The incidence of toxicity is increased by renal failure. Regardless of the dose used, all patients to whom ethambutol is given should be warned about the possible effects on vision and advised to discontinue treatment promptly if they notice any deterioration in eyesight. Routine testing of visual acuity and fundal examination should be carried out before ethambutol is given. Reduction in visual acuity or significant ophthalmological abnormality should be regarded as a contraindication to treatment with ethambutol as they render the detection of toxicity more difficult. Particular care is required in children in whom detection of early signs of ocular toxicity is difficult. High doses of ethambutol should not be given. Routine testing of visual acuity during treatment is not helpful in detecting early toxicity. Impairment of colour vision is a late sign of toxicity, and routine testing of colour vision is not useful.

Gastrointestinal disturbances and allergic reactions have been reported, as have a wide variety of other side-effects, including renal failure, but these are infrequent. Although there is some evidence that the drug is teratogenic in animals, there are no reports of adverse effects in pregnancy or of fetal abnormality.

No major drug interactions have been reported.

## Dose

Efficacy is a function of dosage. Two dose levels are used, 15 mg/kg, which can be expected to produce a serum level of about 4 µg/ml, and 25 mg/kg, which produces a serum level around 8 µg/ml. The mic for *M. tuberculosis* ranges between 0.5 µg/ml and 8 µg/ml. The lower dose is likely to be effective against most but not all sensitive strains. High dose ethambutol is effective against most sensitive strains but, in view of the greater risk of ocular toxicity, its use should be confined to the initial phase of treatment and the management of patients with resistant organisms. The lower dose should be used in continuation chemotherapy. Because of the increased incidence of ocular toxicity with the higher dose, many physicians use only the lower dose.

Ethambutol is available as tablets or a syrup. It is generally used in a combined tablet with isoniazid. (For details of dosage see Table 21.1, p. 251.)

# Thiacetazone

Thiacetazone is a thiosemicarbazone, one of a group of drugs with antibacterial, antiviral and antitumour activity. Its mode of action against *M. tuberculosis* is unknown. There is some cross-resistance with ethionamide, which suggests an action on the mycolic acid pathway, but this has not been confirmed.

Thiacetazone has little sterilising activity but is a moderate preventer of drug resistance.

### Absorption, Distribution and Excretion

Thiacetazone is well absorbed from the gut, with peak plasma concentrations at about 4 h and a half-life of about 12 h. It is metabolised mainly in the liver and excreted in the urine.

### Toxic Effects

There is considerable variation in the severity of the side-effects which appears to be geographical and may also be partly based on race. Gastrointestinal upset, skin rashes and vertigo occur frequently. Skin reactions include exfoliative dermatitis and toxic epidermal necrolysis, and have been fatal. Various other side-effects, including liver damage, are reported.

In view of the very considerable variation in toxicity, local susceptibility to toxic effects should be carefully assessed before thiacetazone is introduced into any wide-scale treatment programme.

## Interactions

Thiacetazone may displace streptomycin from its sites of protein binding and increase ototoxicity.

## Dose

Thiacetazone is given orally, usually combined with isoniazid. Its main attraction is its low cost. (For details of dosage see Table 21.1, p. 251.)

# Para-amino Salicylic Acid

Para-amino salicylic acid (PAS) was one of the early drugs used to treat tuberculosis. Salicylic acid stimulates the respiration of *M. tuberculosis* and PAS was introduced as a compound which would interfere with salicylic acid utilisation. More recent evidence suggests that it does not act in this way, but that it interferes with either folic acid synthesis or with iron uptake. PAS has no action on other bacteria and cross-resistance with other antituberculous drugs does not occur.

PAS has relatively little sterilising activity but is a moderate resistance preventer. It was almost invariably given in combination with isoniazid in continuation chemotherapy. Although reasonably effective, it is unpleasant to take, and has been almost entirely superseded.

As its sodium salt, PAS is readily absorbed orally, producing effective peak concentrations within 1–2 h. It is excreted rapidly in the urine, approximately equally as unchanged PAS and in an acetylated form. It is widely distributed in effective concentration in most tissues, but only penetrates the CSF in the presence of meningitis. It is unpalatable and large doses must be taken. Gastrointestinal side-effects are common despite a wide variety of different formulations and presentations designed to overcome them. Hypersensitivity reactions are frequent, usually in the first month of treatment. They commonly include skin rashes and fever, but a wide variety of other allergic reactions may be found. Toxicity to liver and bone marrow may occur. Any toxic or hypersensitivity reaction produced by salicylate or the p-amino side chain will also be produced by PAS.

Drug interactions are similar to those of salicylates, and range from interference with simple quantitative urine testing for sugar to impairment of iodine uptake by the thyroid gland, which in prolonged treatment may lead to goitre and hypothyroidism.

PAS is unstable in aqueous solution. In the crystalline form it is hygroscopic and tablets and cachets deteriorate if conditions of storage are poor.

## Dose

Because of the gastrointestinal side-effects, PAS is normally given twice daily shortly after meals. (For details of dosage see Table 21.1, p. 251.)

# Prothionamide

Prothionamide acts in a way similar to isoniazid by inhibiting mycolic acid synthesis. However, there is a lack of cross-resistance to isoniazid, indicating a different action on mycolic acid synthesis, although the source of the difference has not been identified. There is cross-resistance between prothionamide and the thiosemicarbazones, suggesting some common feature of bacterial uptake, metabolism or action.

Prothionamide has little sterilising activity. Its action appears to be mainly as a resistance preventer. Its place in therapy has been limited by side-effects.

### Absorption, Distribution, Metabolism and Excretion

Although relatively insoluble, it is readily absorbed from the gut and widely distributed throughout the body, including the nervous system. Peak concentrations in blood are attained within 2 h, and the biological half-life is between 2 and 4 h. It is metabolised in the liver and subsequently excreted in the urine, almost entirely as inactive metabolites. Excretion is impaired in renal failure, when the dose should be reduced.

### Interactions

There are no important interactions.

### Toxic Effects

Gastrointestinal side-effects are common and often severe. They include excessive salivation with an unpleasant taste in the mouth, nausea and vomiting and diarrhoea. A wide variety of other toxic actions and hypersensitivity effects have been reported including hypoglycaemia. There appear to be some racial differences in tolerance.

### Dose

It is suitable for oral administration only. (For details of dosage see Table 21.1, p. 251.)

# Cycloserine

Cycloserine is active against a wide range of bacteria, including the mycobacteria. Chemically it resembles alanine and it inhibits the utilisation of alanine in the synthesis of cell wall peptidoglycan. It appears to be able to penetrate mycobacteria which lose acid-fastness. In culture the organisms disintegrate, but clinically it has only weak sterilising and resistance-preventing activity.

### Absorption, Distribution and Excretion

Cycloserine is rapidly absorbed after oral administration. It is widely distributed to all tissues, and is relatively slowly excreted, mainly in the urine. In patients with renal failure, toxic levels are readily produced.

### Toxic Effects

Cycloserine is toxic to the nervous system, producing psychotic reactions, convulsions, and a wide variety of other neurological side-effects. These side-effects greatly limit the use of what is not a particularly effective drug.

### Dose

The dose for adults is 250 mg twice daily.

# Drug Resistance and Antituberculous Chemotherapy

Patients have to be treated when the sensitivity of the infecting organisms is unknown. Even when culture and sensitivity testing can be carried out, the results are not available for 2–3 months and treatment must be started before then. In Third World countries where tuberculosis is common, culture and sensitivity testing are usually not available. The choice of regimen must be based on background information about the general pattern of drug sensitivity, and the particular circumstances of the individual patient, including a detailed history of previous antituberculous chemotherapy and the patient's response to it. Initial triple therapy with isoniazid, rifampicin and pyrazinamide is adequate to deal with the small possibility of primary resistance in patients in the United Kingdom. If resistance is thought likely, at least one further drug should be added, in the first instance ethambutol, streptomycin or ethionamide. The continuation regimen should be reviewed in the light of clinical progress and culture results. Many patients respond clinically, even when laboratory testing suggests that their organisms are resistant. If the patient is responding, treatment should be continued regardless of the laboratory result. If response is poor, laboratory sensitivity testing should be used as a guide for selection of a different drug regimen. A second-choice regimen which does not include rifampicin or isoniazid is likely to be much less effective. If drugs with weaker sterilising activity are used, continuation therapy should be with three drugs rather than two, and careful supervision is essential. Patients known to be unco-operative and to have resistant organisms should have supervised chemotherapy.

If it is thought likely that the patient has multiply resistant organisms, treatment should if possible be deferred until results of sensitivity testing are available. If the organisms are still sensitive to either isoniazid or rifampicin, an effective regimen can be given, although treatment will have to be more protracted. If they are resistant to both drugs, it will be necessary to use second line drugs of limited efficacy. It is then desirable to give at least three drugs to which the organism is sensitive and to treat for 18 months. In ill patients for whom it is not possible to wait for sensitivity results a clinical assessment of likely sensitivity should be made, paying particular attention to previous chemotherapy, and the results of previous sensitivity tests if any. A minimum of three drugs should be given.

Occasionally with multiply resistant organisms, surgical treatment to control the disease may have to be considered. Resection of infected tissue and measures leading to cavity closure reduce the total bacterial burden and favour healing.

# Hypersensitivity Reactions

Hypersensitivity reactions to antituberculous drugs are not uncommon. They tend to occur in the first few weeks of treatment and are usually characterised by itching and erythematous skin rashes. If the reaction is severe, there may by pyrexia and general malaise, the skin lesions may progress to exfoliative dermatitis, and occasionally there is hepatic or renal involvement. For any reaction worse than trivial skin itching, the drugs should be discontinued until the reaction settles. Patients with tuberculosis are rarely so ill that temporary discontinuation of therapy is impossible. For the very sick an empirical judgement must be made and drugs not thought likely to have caused the reaction should be continued. The offending drug should be identified by giving test doses of each drug, starting with a small dose (25–50 mg isoniazid or 50–100 mg rifampicin). If there is no reaction to these two drugs, consideration should be given to the use of a two-drug regimen using rifampicin and isoniazid which can often be used without major problems. Hyposensitisation is rarely necessary and should only be undertaken if the sensitising drug is essential for the continuation of treatment. The dose of the drug is slowly increased over 2–3 weeks until the full dose is tolerated. Steroid therapy is sometimes required for severe reactions and may occasionally be necessary to permit hyposensitisation. The occurrence of severe exfoliative dermatitis or of major hepatic or renal reaction should be regarded as an absolute contraindication to continued use of the sensitising drug.

# Antituberculous Chemotherapy and Liver Disease

Patients requiring antituberculous chemotherapy may have pre-existing liver disease due to tuberculosis itself or to other causes such as cirrhosis or alcohol abuse, or they may develop liver damage as a result of treatment, either as part of a severe generalised hypersensitivity reaction or as a direct toxic effect of the antituberculous drugs. It can be difficult to determine the cause of abnormalities in liver function, and when they are due to drugs it may be difficult to identify the causative drug with any certainty as drugs are always given in combination and most are potentially hepatotoxic. The three major antituberculous drugs — isoniazid, rifampicin and pyrazinamide — are all potentially hepatotoxic, with a similar incidence of significant reactions — about 1%. With all the drugs severe toxic reactions usually show a picture of hepatocellular damage with elevation of bilirubin as well as of liver enzymes. With lesser reactions enzyme abnormalities alone are found. The abnormalities usually disappear when treatment is discontinued.

Liver damage with isoniazid is more common in older subjects, and in those with underlying liver disease. There is no evidence that hepatic toxicity is related to acetylator status. Unlike the liver damage associated with rifampicin, there is a significant mortality from isoniazid liver damage — about 10% of cases, most of whom have pre-existing liver disease or other major systemic illness. Evidence of significant hepatic dysfunction in patients on isoniazid should always be treated seriously.

During the first few weeks of treatment with rifampicin minor evidence of liver dysfunction with transient elevation of alanine or aspartate transaminase is common and the abnormalities disappear despite continued treatment. Routine monitoring of liver function is not required. More severe reactions occur in about 1% of patients, but unlike liver damage due to isoniazid, the prognosis is relatively favourable.

It was initially thought that pyrazinamide was particularly hepatotoxic, producing major problems in 5% of patients undergoing treatment, but the doses then used were high. Subsequent experience with the current conventional doses suggests that the incidence of liver damage is no greater than with isoniazid or rifampicin, and that the prognosis is good.

In all patients with liver disease a baseline measurement of liver function should be made at the start of treatment, and liver function should be routinely monitored for the first 3 months, the period of greatest risk of adverse reaction. If after 3 months there is both clinical improvement and improvement in liver function, it is very unlikely that serious problems will be encountered subsequently. Despite the possibility that problems may be encountered, there is no evidence that the use of any of the three main drugs is contraindicated. There is no method of predicting serious adverse reactions, save that there is some evidence that hepatotoxicity may be dose related. Care should be taken that recommended doses are not exceeded. With that proviso, full conventional therapy can be given and the response to treatment monitored by observing liver function tests.

When hepatotoxicity occurs, treatment should be discontinued until the liver function tests return to normal. Each drug should then be re-introduced singly to exclude hypersensitivity reactions. If that is the problem, the drug involved should be withdrawn. In most patients it is possible to achieve a satisfactory alternative treatment regimen. Rifampicin and ethambutol are usually safe and effective when there has been major toxicity from isoniazid.

Concern about hepatotoxicity is particularly great for prophylactic chemotherapy. Risks that may be acceptable in the treatment of active disease are not acceptable in prophylaxis. In a major trial of isoniazid prophylaxis the overall incidence of isoniazid-related hepatic damage was 5.2/1000, with a clear increase with increasing age from 2.8/1000 for those aged less than 35 years to 7.7/1000 for those aged more than 55 years. A stronger indication for isoniazid chemo-prophylaxis is required in older patients.

## Antituberculous Chemotherapy in Renal Failure

The metabolism of isoniazid, rifampicin, pyrazinamide and ethionamide is not affected by renal failure, and they can be given in normal dose. They are the pre-ferred drugs for patients in renal failure for they are both safe and effective.

Streptomycin and ethambutol are dependent on renal excretion and should if possible be avoided in renal failure. When they have to be given, dose reduction is required to prevent toxic effects. For streptomycin, blood levels should be deter-mined and the dose adjusted so that the trough concentration is below toxic levels (4 µg/ml). The dose of ethambutol should be reduced to 8–10 mg/kg per day. If the patient is being dialysed, the drugs should be given 4–6 h before dialysis; they will then be removed before they can produce toxic effects.

## Treatment of Tuberculosis in Pregnancy

Most antituberculous drugs are widely distributed in the body and penetrate the placenta and fetus. Those which are potentially toxic to the fetus or are potentially teratogenic must be avoided during pregnancy. Streptomycin is ototoxic and should not be given. Isoniazid, ethambutol and PAS are not toxic and not known to be teratogenic and may safely be given during pregnancy. Rifampicin has not yet been shown to be definitely non-teratogenic and its use should be avoided if possible in the first 3 months of pregnancy. During this time isoniazid plus etham-butol is the preferred regimen. Thereafter, isoniazid plus rifampicin should be used. If the patient is acutely ill, full chemotherapy with rifampicin, isoniazid and pyrazinamide should be given since the small potential risk of fetal damage is out-weighed by the greater efficacy of the regimen.

## Pregnancy in Patients on Antituberculous Chemotherapy

Pregnancy is generally best avoided when any medication is being taken. There are particular problems with rifampicin which may be teratogenic, and women of childbearing age taking this drug should take particular care with contraception. Rifampicin increases the metabolism of the hormones in the contraceptive pill and makes its effect uncertain, and therefore other contraceptive methods should be used. If a patient does become pregnant while taking rifampicin, it is probably reasonable to offer termination of the pregnancy, although there is thus far no strong evidence of a significant teratogenic effect and there have been many reports of normal pregnancies, occurring in women taking the drug.

# Useful References

American Thoracic Society (1983) Treatment of tuberculosis and other mycobacterial diseases. Am Rev Respir Dis 127: 790–796

British Thoracic Society (1984) A controlled trial of six months' chemotherapy in pulmonary tuberculosis: final report. Br J Dis Chest 78: 330–336

British Thoracic Society (1985) Short course chemotherapy for tuberculosis of lymph nodes: a controlled trial. Br Med J 290: 1106–1108

Dutt AK, Moers D, Stead WW (1984) Short course chemotherapy for tuberculosis with mainly twice weekly isoniazid and rifampin. Am J Med 77: 233–242

Girling DJ (1984) Hepatic toxicity of antituberculosis regimens. Tubercle 65: 1–4

IUAT Committee on Prophylaxis (1982) Efficacy of various durations of isoniazid preventive therapy for tuberculosis: five years of follow-up. Bull IUAT 60: 555–564

Leader (1983) Isoniazid prevention of tuberculosis. Lancet I: 395–396

McAllister WAC, Thomson PJ, Al-Habet SM, Rogers HJ (1983) Rifampicin reduces effectiveness and bioavailability of prednisolone. Br Med J 286: 923–925

Medical Research Council Tuberculosis and Chest Diseases Unit (1985) Treatment of pulmonary tuberculosis in patients notified in England and Wales 1978–9: chemotherapy and hospital admission. Thorax 40: 113–120

Medical Research Council Working Party on Tuberculosis of the Spine (1985) A 10-year assessment of controlled trials of in-patient and out-patient treatment and of plaster-of-Paris jackets for tuberculosis of the spine in children on standard chemotherapy. J Bone Jt Surg 67B: 103–110

Mitchison DA (1985) The action of antituberculous drugs in short course chemotherapy. Tubercle 66: 219–225

Ross JD, Horne NW (1983) Modern drug treatment in tuberculosis, 6th edn. The Chest, Heart and Stroke Association, London

Snider DE, Farer LS (1984) Preventive therapy for tuberculosis: an intervention in need of improvement. Am Rev Respir Dis 130: 355–356

Steen JSM, Stainton-Ellis DM (1977) Rifampicin in pregnancy. Lancet II: 604–605

# 22 Drugs Affecting Cough and Sputum

Cough and hypersecretion are part of the protective response of the airways to irritation, and expectoration serves a useful purpose in draining secretions. When faced with a patient with cough and sputum production, it is important to identify and deal with the underlying cause; this has a much better chance of success than purely symptomatic treatment such as the use of mucolytic agents and cough suppressants. Irritant environmental factors such as cigarette smoke should be removed if possible, pulmonary infection treated with antibiotics, and dehydration, which may cause sputum to be tenacious, should be corrected. In patients with cough due to lung cancer or mediastinal nodes, local radiotherapy should be considered. The natural history of the condition being treated should also be taken into account. Patients may be prepared to tolerate a symptom when they realise it will be shortlived and less prepared to do so when they know it is likely to persist.

Self-limiting upper or lower respiratory tract infections do not normally require cough medicines. A demulcent such as linctus simplex may help to relieve a sore throat, as do traditional remedies such as sweetened drinks. The majority of patients with hypersecretion due to chronic bronchitis or bronchiectasis have no difficulty in expectoration and require neither expectorants nor cough suppressants. Some patients with thick tenacious sputum may need help, as for example in cystic fibrosis, bronchiectasis or severe asthma. Drainage and removal of secretions are the mainstay of treatment and drugs play little part. In patients with reversible airways obstruction bronchodilators may help to remove secretions.

## Cough Medicines

Despite the paucity of evidence showing benefit from "cough medicines", they constitute one of the most commonly prescribed groups of drugs, with 75 million prescriptions each year in the United Kingdom. The British National Formulary listed 67 preparations under the heading of "Expectorants, demulcents and compound preparations" in 1985, prior to the introduction of the limited list. The drugs under this heading are a diverse collection — irritants, sedatives, antihistamines, bronchodilators and cough suppressants, singly and in combination. Many traditional remedies such as ipecacuanha, ammonium chloride and iodine-containing compounds would not find a place in a rational pharmacopoeia and cannot be recommended, nor would compound decongestants, some of which have been associated with hallucinations in children and hypertensive crises in patients on monoamine oxidase inhibitors. Only the mucolytic agents justify consideration.

# Mucolytic Agents

## Formulation

Acetylcysteine, carbocisteine, bromhexine and methylcysteine are available for oral use and bromhexine for intravenous and intramuscular use also. Tyloxapol can be given by inhalation though care is needed since the drug can attack rubber equipment and are degraded by certain metals.

## Modes of Action

Mucolytic agents were so named when it was recognised that these drugs liquefied sputum in vitro. This effect is due to disruption of disulphide cross-linkage within and between mucous glycoproteins. Their action in vivo, however, may be related to other properties which are not strictly "mucolytic", including reduced mucus synthesis, protection against oxidant lung damage from irritants such as tobacco smoke, and replenishing glutathione so that covalent binding of reactive metabolites to cell proteins is reduced. The precise way in which each drug exerts its effect is unclear. It may well vary between drugs so the results from one cannot be extrapolated to another.

A decrease in sputum viscosity should be helpful when sputum is too viscid, though too great a reduction would make cilia and coughing ineffective. Since neither the optimum viscoelastic properties of sputum nor the precise mode of action of these drugs in vivo are known, the drugs must be judged by their clinical effects.

## Clinical Studies

Inhalation of mucolytic agents has shown little evidence of clinical benefit, possibly because excessive mucus secretion prevents drug access where it is most needed. The drugs can cause bronchoconstriction in patients with asthma. There is no indication for their use by this route.

Oral mucolytic agents have usually caused a reduction in sputum viscosity, but in most instances no convincing change in mucociliary clearance. There has been inconsistent evidence of clinical benefit in patients with chronic bronchitis.

Acetylcysteine, which has been studied most, is rapidly absorbed and slowly excreted. Three recent large placebo controlled trials of oral acetylcysteine 200 mg b.d. in patients with chronic bronchitis have shown a small reduction in exacerbations of bronchitis — 0.5 to just over 1 exacerbation in 6 months. There were no clear-cut changes in pulmonary function though one trial showed some decrease in the severity of cough, difficulty in expectoration and sputum volume. Bromhexine and S-carboxymethylcysteine have been tried on smaller numbers of patients and usually for shorter periods. Results have been conflicting, but there may be slight benefit in less ill patients. The results in both acute and chronic asthma have been unimpressive. The oral drugs are normally well tolerated, with occasional epigastric discomfort, nausea and an increase in serum aspartate transaminase levels, though oral acetylcysteine has recently been suspected of having caused allergic reactions, including asthma and anaphylaxis.

### Clinical Indications

The potential benefit of reducing exacerbations of bronchitis by between one-half and one episode each winter would not appear to justify the regular oral administration of acetylcysteine to patients with chronic bronchitis. In the occasional patient with particular difficulty in coughing up sticky sputum, a trial of oral acetylcysteine is reasonable.

# Antitussive Agents

In patients with chronic cough the cause should be identified (Table 22.1) and treated if possible. Patients with persistent cough should stop smoking and avoid dusty or irritant environments. Persistent cough without obvious cause is usually due to asthma or to a continuing irritant response after a respiratory tract infection. If there is any doubt about the diagnosis of asthma, a therapeutic trial of bronchodilators and inhaled steroids should be undertaken.

Cough suppression is clearly inappropriate when cough is producing sputum, as in bronchiectasis. Occasionally, however, in conditions such as lung cancer, cough can be distressing whilst serving no useful purpose and an effort should then be made to suppress it. Attempts at cough suppression may be worthwhile in whooping cough.

The most effective cough suppressants are the opioids, which appear to reduce not only the frequency and intensity of cough, but also the subjective reactions to it. In general the dose required for effective cough suppression is rather less than the analgesic dose. Codeine, widely used for cough, undergoes less first-pass metabolism than other opioids so its effect is more predictable after oral administration. It is largely metabolised to inactive compounds though some is demethylated to morphine. Codeine has low affinity for opioid receptors and its antitussive action is probably due to binding to other receptors. Pholcodine 10 mg appears to

**Table 22.1.** Causes of cough

| | | |
|---|---|---|
| Infections | Upper respiratory tract infection | |
| | Whooping cough | |
| | Acute bronchitis | |
| | Pneumonia | |
| Neoplasia | Lung cancer particularly | |
| | Mediastinal glands | |
| Allergies | Dry irritating cough in patients with allergic rhinitis | |
| Chronic airways obstruction | Asthma | |
| | Chronic bronchitis | |
| Aspiration | Gastric contents | |
| | Foreign body | |
| | Postnasal drip | |
| Inhalation | Fumes and irritants including cigarette smoke | |
| Other lung disorders | Fibrosing alveolitis | |
| | Pulmonary congestion and oedema | Relatively rare |
| | Sarcoid | |

be as effective as codeine 15 mg but with no analgesic activity; methadone is more potent. All opioids cause constipation and are potentially dangerous in patients with impaired control of ventilation, as in chronic bronchitis and asthma where they may precipitate respiratory depression. Morphine and diamorphine are the most potent antitussive agents and extremely useful for the treatment of cough associated with advanced lung carcinoma. Opioids should be given when other treatment, such as antibiotics for intercurrent infections or palliative radiotherapy, is unable to help. Addiction is not a problem in these patients, though it severely limits the use of opioids in other conditions. Drowsiness tends to disappear with continued use. Constipation is always a problem with opioids and should be anticipated, by starting patients on a high-fibre diet for example.

Drugs related to the opioids but without the potential for addiction include dextromethorphan and noscapine. There is relatively little information on their effectiveness, and clinical experience in the United Kingdom is limited.

# Useful References

Boman G, Backer U, Larsson S, Melander B, Wahlander L (1983) Oral acetylcysteine reduces exacerbation rate in chronic bronchitis: report of a trial organised by the Swedish Society for Pulmonary Diseases. Eur J Resp Dis 64: 405–415

British Thoracic Society Research Committee (1985) Oral N-acetylcysteine and exacerbation rates in patients with chronic bronchitis and severe airways obstruction. Thorax 40: 832–835

Hughes DTD (1978) Diseases of the respiratory system: cough suppressants, expectorants, and mucolytic agents. Br Med J I: 1202–1203

Lopez-Vidriero MT (1984) Lung secretions. In: Clarke SW, Pavia D (ed), Aerosols and the lung. Butterworths, London, pp 19–48

# 23 Oxygen Therapy

## Indications

Oxygen therapy is a symptomatic form of treatment. It is usually given for a relatively short period to relieve "dangerous" hypoxaemia in the course of an acute illness such as pneumonia, exacerbations of bronchitis and left heart failure. The hypoxaemia is almost always the result of impaired gas exchange, and is at least partially relieved by the increase in alveolar oxygen concentration produced by increasing inspired oxygen concentrations. Long-term oxygen therapy has a limited place in the management of chronic respiratory disease.

Decisions about oxygen therapy are usually made on the basis of arterial blood gas measurements, and assumptions about a "safe" arterial $PO_2$. In most acute illnesses a $PaO_2$ >8 kPa (60 mmHg) can generally be regarded as safe, provided that cardiac output and haemoglobin concentration are normal. The arterial oxygen saturation will be above 90% with a near-normal oxygen content, and the patient will be on the "flat" part of the dissociation curve where minor variations in arterial $PO_2$ do not cause much variation in oxygen saturation. A higher $PaO_2$ is occasionally required in order to ensure adequate oxygen delivery to tissues particularly dependent on oxygen, notably the brain. Following head injury and after neurosurgery, a higher $PaO_2$ should be maintained — at least 9 kPa (70 mmHg) and preferably >11 kPa (80 mmHg). In patients known or thought likely to have chronic hypoxaemia and underventilation, a lower value for a "safe" $PaO_2$ is appropriate. These patients have adapted to a lower $PaO_2$, and they are also likely to have reduced carbon dioxide sensitivity with dependence on the hypoxic drive for respiration. Pursuit of higher oxygen levels is liable to lead to progressive underventilation. When there is evidence of chronic elevation of $PCO_2$, it is reasonable to accept an arterial $PO_2$ >7 kPa (50 mmHg), if cardiac output and haemoglobin levels are normal.

## Sources of Oxygen Supply

Most oxygen is prepared by fractional evaporation of liquid air. It is completely dry and of high purity. It is distributed either in cylinders or as liquid oxygen for use in evaporators to supply pipeline systems. Pipeline and cylinder pressures are high, and must be lowered by the use of a reducing valve before delivery to the patient. Needle valves and flow meters are used to regulate the gas flow. More recently, two new sources of oxygen supply have become available, the oxygen concentrator, which uses a molecular sieve to retain nitrogen, and a membrane oxygen enricher using a semipermeable membrane which permits the passage of oxygen and water vapour to produce both high oxygen levels and high humidity. The majority of oxygen concentrators can produce oxygen concentrations of 80+% at flow rates up to 4 l/min. The main application of these machines is in domiciliary oxygen therapy.

# Methods

Oxygen, like water, is readily available and is essential for life, but in the sick patient oxygen, like water, may also be dangerous. It should be regarded as a drug, and used in the minimum concentration necessary to achieve the desired therapeutic effect. If oxygen is to be given with care, precision in dose is essential, and this is a function of the means of delivery. For most purposes oxygen masks are used. They are apparently simple devices, but they must:

1.  Be capable of reasonable precision in the concentration they deliver. For low concentration oxygen therapy, masks capable of delivering 24%, 28% and occasionally 32% oxygen are used. The concentration should be independent of oxygen flow rate and of the patient's ventilation.
2.  Provide an adequate volume flow so that the patient breathes in only the desired gas. Even on quiet tidal breathing, inspiratory flow rates are high (>30 l/min), and the normal tidal volume (500 ml) exceeds the dead space of most masks (70–100 ml). Unless there is a high gas flow through the mask as in the lower concentration venturi masks (60+ l/min), or a tightly fitting mask with a reservoir or demand valve, ambient air will also be inspired, reducing the effective oxygen concentration.
3.  Not permit rebreathing of expired air with the consequent risk of rise in $PCO_2$.
4.  Be comfortable, quiet and easily tolerated.

It is difficult to design the ideal oxygen mask, and a wide variety of devices is available. The problems are greatest with devices for delivering low oxygen concentrations (24%–32%) when the need for precision is greatest. At the moment venturi masks most nearly approach the ideal for providing low oxygen concentrations (Fig. 23.1). A jet of oxygen blown into the base of the venturi tube creates a partial vacuum and entrains ambient air through a series of apertures surrounding the jet. Once a critical driving gas flow rate has been achieved, the entrainment ratio is constant over a wide range of driving gas flow and is determined by the size of the entrainment apertures and their relationships to the driving jet of oxygen.

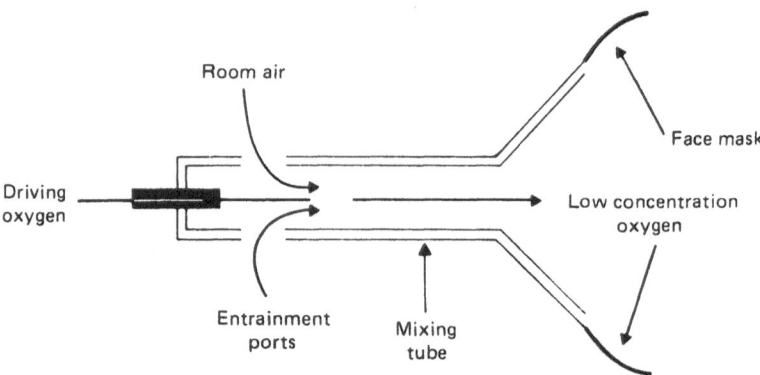

**Fig. 23.1.** Diagram of venturi mask showing how the jet of oxygen entrains room air to provide a low concentration of oxygen.

The driving oxygen and entrained air mix during their passage down the tube and are then delivered, usually by a loosely fitting plastic face mask. Venturi masks deliver a high gas flow which is adequate to match inspiratory flow rates and to wash out expired carbon dioxide, so ensuring that the patient breathes only the desired gas without rebreathing carbon dioxide. They are simple to use and work reliably so long as an adequate driving oxygen flow rate is used and the air entrainment holes are not blocked. They are usually well tolerated, although they are relatively noisy. The entrainment ratios and concentrations attained are shown in Table 23.1.

Other masks are much less satisfactory for low concentration oxygen therapy; they do not deliver an accurate oxygen concentration, and the concentration they give is inversely dependent on the patient's ventilation. Nasal prongs or catheters, while subject to these reservations, have major advantages in patient tolerance. At flow rates of 1–2 l/min they achieve effective inspired oxygen concentrations of 24%–28%, and permit coughing, talking, eating and drinking without hindrance. The flow rates are sufficiently low that local drying of the nasal mucosa is not a problem.

In the 32%–50% range, simple plastic face masks with a low dead space are most useful. In these masks the inspired volume exceeds the mask dead space and the inspirate is diluted with ambient air. The inspired oxygen concentration is a

**Table 23.1.** Venturi masks

| Concentration (%) | PIO$_2$ | | Entrainment ratio | Mask gas flow at driving O$_2$ flow | |
|---|---|---|---|---|---|
| | kPa | mmHg | | 4 l/min | 8 l/min |
| 24 | 23 | 170 | 21:1 | 88 | 176 |
| 28 | 27 | 200 | 10:1 | 44 | 88 |
| 32 | 31 | 230 | 6:1 | 28 | 56 |

function of both oxygen flow rate and the patient's ventilation and cannot be regulated with much precision. However, these oxygen concentrations are generally used in conditions when precision is less important and the masks are generally satisfactory. The low dead space minimises rebreathing, and the masks are usually comfortable.

Inspired concentrations above 50% are difficult to achieve with a conventional mask. A tight-fitting mask with a reservoir or a high flow demand valve is required. They are poorly tolerated by the sick patient. If the patient is ill enough to require oxygen concentrations above 50% to maintain a safe arterial $PO_2$, serious consideration should be given to intubation and mechanical ventilation.

# Monitoring

In patients with abnormal lungs, equilibration following change in inspired oxygen concentration is not immediate. The "final" value of arterial $PO_2$ is usually not reached for at least 15 min and will take longer if there is underventilation as a result of oxygen therapy. The rise in $PCO_2$ is usually a relatively slow process, taking several hours. As a general rule, arterial blood gases should be checked about 1 h after the start of treatment to ensure that the desired $PaO_2$ has been attained and that there has not been a large rise in $PCO_2$. If the desired $PaO_2$ has not been achieved, the appropriate changes should be made in inspired oxygen concentration. In patients in whom underventilation is thought likely, arterial blood gases should be checked again 3–4 h later, and once more on the following morning. Blood gases should always be checked if the patient becomes drowsy or if there is any reason to suspect that there might have been a rise in $PCO_2$.

If oxygen is indicated, it should be given continuously until the underlying condition improves. When an effective oxygen concentration has been determined, the blood gases need not be measured more than once daily unless the patient is acutely ill or in an unstable condition.

# Problems

### Progressive Underventilation

This is almost entirely an acute problem in patients with chronic respiratory disease and chronic underventilation. Loss of sensitivity to carbon dioxide makes the hypoxic drive more important in the control of ventilation. Abolition or significant diminution of hypoxaemia may lead to progressive respiratory depression with a rise in $PCO_2$ (see Chap. 6). This problem is commonly seen in patients recognised as having severe chronic respiratory disease, but it can also occur in those with less severe and sometimes undiagnosed chronic chest disease when treatment with high oxygen concentrations may depress respiration. If low oxygen concentrations are given, the possible rise in $PCO_2$ is limited, even if the patient underventilates to the extent that the initial $PaO_2$ is restored. In patients with chronic chest disease and an arterial $PCO_2$ >6 kPa (45 mmHg) or significant elevation of plasma bicarbonate, the starting oxygen concentration should always be 24%. Concentrations above 28% should virtually never be used.

## Drying of the Respiratory Tract

The drying effect of oxygen is only a problem when the upper respiratory tract is bypassed. The normal upper respiratory tract is capable of achieving full humidification of inspired air, even when admixed with up to 50% oxygen. Although oxygen from both cylinder and pipeline is completely dry, tracheal gas sampling shows 100% saturation with water vapour at 37°C in patients breathing through a normal upper respiratory tract. Humidification is only required if the upper respiratory tract is bypassed, by whatever means — tracheostomy, endotracheal tube or even an oral airway — and it is then required whether the patient is breathing air or air enriched with oxygen. In the absence of humidification, drying secretions tend to pile up against the end of the airway or tube where they form a viscid plug which can obstruct the airway completely. Drying of lower respiratory tract can also cause problems making secretions difficult to cough out or aspirate. If a humidifier is used, it must be capable of producing full saturation with water vapour at body temperature. This requires either a heated water humidifier or an ultrasonic humidifier. Heated water devices warm the inspired air to just above body temperature and saturate it with water vapour. Ultrasonic humidifiers supersaturate the air at ambient temperature so that full saturation is achieved at 37°C.

Humidification is not required with venturi masks or other low concentration oxygen devices. Attempts to provide it are usually unsatisfactory and are liable to impair the efficiency of the mask.

## Oxygen Lung Toxicity

High concentration inspired oxygen predisposes to absorption atelectasis. Oxygen also has a direct toxic effect on the lung which can be clearly demonstrated in the experimental animal. High alveolar oxygen concentrations produce free oxygen radicals and cause cell death. Type 1 pneumocytes and pulmonary endothelial cells appear to be particularly vulnerable, with reduced surfactant production and pulmonary oedema, producing a picture resembling that of the early stages of ARDS. Continued exposure to high concentrations produces fibroblastic proliferation and fibrosis. The important determinant of lung damage is alveolar oxygen tension, not inspired oxygen concentration. Normal subjects given "100%" oxygen for 24 h show transient abnormalities with evidence of alveolar capillary leak and increased albumin and transferrin in bronchoalveolar lavage fluid. Patients with severe lung abnormalities such as ARDS often require high inspired oxygen concentrations to maintain even a low arterial $PO_2$. After several days of treatment with oxygen concentrations above 50%, changes similar to those seen in animals are usually present. It is difficult to determine to what extent these are the result of the primary condition or of high concentration oxygen therapy. As oxygen therapy may be a contributory factor, an attempt should always be made to keep inspired oxygen below 50% using other measures such as PEEP or modification of ventilator patterns to maintain alveolar patency and improve $PO_2$.

Oxygen concentrations below 50% appear to be safe. As it is difficult to attain concentrations above 50% with a mask, oxygen toxicity is essentially a problem of ventilated patients, or those treated in hyperbaric chambers.

### Fire and Explosion

Whenever oxygen is used there is a fire and explosion hazard. Appropriate care should be taken to minimise this risk.

### Retrolental Fibroplasia

In the premature neonate requiring oxygen, the concentration must be carefully controlled so that the arterial $PO_2$ does not rise above 9 kPa (70 mmHg). Higher levels of arterial $PO_2$ produce retinal vascular damage with new vessel formation causing permanent blindness.

## Domiciliary Oxygen Therapy

Domiciliary oxygen may be used for the relief of symptoms in patients with severe respiratory disease. It is usually taken for relatively short periods of time, and oxygen cylinders are the most convenient form of supply. An assessment of the patient's response (e.g. improvement in walking distance) should be attempted before starting this form of treatment.

Long-term oxygen therapy has also been used in an attempt to improve the prognosis of patients with severe hypoxaemia from chronic chest disease (see Chap. 5). Oxygen for this treatment can be provided from cylinders but the number of cylinders required is large (at least 12 a week for 15 h treatment each day). This is expensive and cumbersome. The concentrator, despite the initial capital expense, is more convenient and cheaper to run, and is to be preferred once patients require more than 8 cylinders a week.

# Other Methods of Oxygen Therapy

## Oxygen Tents

Oxygen tents are occasionally used, especially for small children who have problems in tolerating masks or other oxygen therapy devices, but they are not particularly satisfactory. It is difficult to achieve and maintain the desired oxygen concentration in a tent. Gas flows have to be relatively high to remove carbon dioxide and prevent heat build-up. Patients in tents are relatively inaccessible and opening the tent for nursing or medical procedures tends to produce a protracted drop in oxygen concentration. Despite the difficulties in using masks for small children, most paediatric units find them more satisfactory.

## Incubators

Unlike oxygen tents, incubators have a relatively small volume and it is possible to control oxygen concentration in them with considerable accuracy. They are also less susceptible to the problems of carbon dioxide accumulation and fall in oxygen concentration with manipulation.

## "Portable Oxygen"

Portable oxygen devices are either small cylinders which can be refilled from a larger static cylinder in the patient's home or evaporators running from liquid oxygen. They are capable of providing oxygen at a flow rate of 4 l/min for up to 30 min. Their use may be justified in a few patients in whom a clinically worthwhile improvement in exercise tolerance can be demonstrated. The margins of benefit are small and the effort required to carry the device may offset the improvement produced by the oxygen.

## Hyperbaric Oxygen

Oxygen concentrations in hyperbaric chambers can be readily modified so that very high inspired oxygen tensions and consequently high arterial oxygen tension can be produced. The benefits are unclear, except in carbon monoxide poisoning, where oxygen supply can be maintained by dissolved oxygen and the dissociation of carbon monoxide from haemoglobin expedited. The half-life for elimination of carbon monoxide is 250 min when breathing air, 50 min when breathing 100% oxygen, and 22 min when breathing oxygen at 2.5 atmospheres. The inaccessibility of hyperbaric chambers greatly limits even this potential benefit. The fire hazards are great, and the risk of oxygen toxicity in the lung limits the time it can be used. Other clinical indications for hyperbaric oxygen therapy are not clear.

# Useful References

Bone RC, Pierce AK, Johnson RL (1978) Controlled oxygen administration in acute respiratory failure in chronic obstructive pulmonary disease: a reappraisal. Am J Med 65: 896–902

Editorial (1985) Long term domiciliary oxygen therapy. Lancet II: 365–367

Jackson RM (1985) Pulmonary oxygen toxicity. Chest 88: 900–905

Johns DP, Rochford PD, Streeton JA (1985) Evaluation of six oxygen concentrators. Thorax 40: 806–810

Jones HA, Turner SL, Hughes JMB (1984) Performance of the large-reservoir oxygen mask (Venti-mask) Lancet I: 1427–1431

Petty TL (1983) Selection criteria for long term oxygen therapy. Am Rev Resp Dis 127: 397–398

Stretton TB (1985) Provision of long-term oxygen therapy. Thorax 40: 801–805

Williams BT, Nichol JP (1985) Prevalence of hypoxaemic chronic obstructive lung disease with reference to long term oxygen therapy. Lancet II: 369–372

# Subject Index